Prostate Ultrasound

Christopher R. Porter • Erika M. Wolff

Editors

Prostate Ultrasound

Current Practice and Future Directions

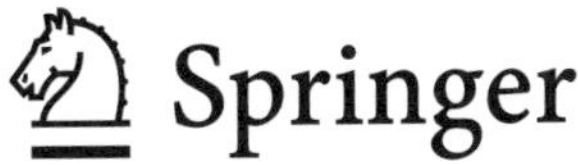
Springer

Editors
Christopher R. Porter, M.D., F.A.C.S.
Medical Director of Clinical Research
Co-Director Urologic Oncology
Section of Urology and Renal
  Transplantation
Virginia Mason
Seattle, WA, USA

Erika M. Wolff, Ph.D.
Section of Urology and Renal
  Transplantation
Virginia Mason
Seattle, WA, USA

ISBN 978-1-4939-5451-3   ISBN 978-1-4939-1948-2 (eBook)
DOI 10.1007/978-1-4939-1948-2
Springer New York Heidelberg Dordrecht London

Acknowledgments

The purpose of this book was to explore the science and theory of prostate ultrasound in a readable way. I am very fortunate to know and be associated with a fantastic group of authors who represent the pinnacle of ultrasound imaging and research in their respective fields. I am deeply indebted to them for all their hard work.

I am extremely grateful to the Assistant Editor, Erika M. Wolff, Ph.D., who has been present for the entire project, tirelessly editing the manuscripts and presenting fresh insight into the book.

I would like to especially acknowledge Dr. Ernie Feleppa, who has been a scientific mentor to me for nearly 15 years. His knowledge and friendship with Dr. William Fair set the foundation for my interest in ultrasound research.

I would also like to extend a special thanks to Dr. Pat Fulgham, perhaps the best teacher of ultrasound theory and practice that I have ever met.

It has been my privilege to work with this dedicated group of scientists, physicians, mentors, and teachers on this project and their collected wisdom will provide valuable insights into the theory and applications of Prostate Ultrasound for years to come.

Christopher R. Porter

Contents

Section C   The Future of Prostate Ultrasound

List of Contributors

Adnan Ali Department of Urology, Icahn School of Medicine, Mount Sinai Hospital, New York, NY, USA

Thenu Chandrasekar Department of Urology, University of California Davis Medical School, Sacramento, CA, USA

Anthony J. Costello Department of Urology, Royal Melbourne Hospital, Parkville, VIC, Australia

Wouter Everaerts Department of Urology, The Royal Melbourne Hospital, Parkville, VIC, Australia

Ernest J. Feleppa Biomedical Engineering Laboratory, Lizzi Center for Biomedical Engineering, Riverside Research, New York, NY, USA

Pat Fulgham Department of Urology, Texas Health Presbyterian Dallas, Dallas, TX, USA

Frederick A. Gulmi Department of Urology, Brookdale University Hospital and Medical Center, Brooklyn, NY, USA

Richard B. Johnston St. Joseph Medical Center, Tacoma, WA, USA

Anna M. Lawrence Department of Urology, Auckland Hospital, Auckland, New Zealand

Zachary Miller Department of Biomedical Engineering, Duke University, Durham, NC, USA

Kathryn Nightingale Department of Biomedical Engineering, Duke University, Durham, NC, USA

Khanh N. Pham Section of Urology and Renal Transplantation, Virginia Mason, Seattle, WA, USA

Miguel Pineda Department of Urology, Brookdale University Hospital and Medical Center, Brooklyn, NY, USA

Thomas Polascik Department of Urology, Duke Cancer Institute, Duke University Medical Center, Durham, NC, USA

Christopher R. Porter Section of Urology and Renal Transplantation, Virginia Mason, Seattle, WA, USA

Stephen Rosenzweig Department of Biomedical Engineering, Duke University, Durham, NC, USA

Kasra Saeb-Parsy Department of Urology, Addenbrookes Hospital, Cambridge University Hospitals NHS Trust, Cambridge, UK

Katsuto Shinohara Department of Urology and Helen Diller Family Comprehensive Cancer Center, University of California San Francisco, San Francisco, CA, USA

Bachir Taouli Department of Radiology, Icahn School of Medicine, Mount Sinai Hospital, New York, NY, USA

Ashutosh K. Tewari Department of Urology, Icahn School of Medicine, Mount Sinai Hospital, New York, NY, USA

Nikesh Thiruchelvam Department of Urology, Addenbrookes Hospital, Cambridge University Hospitals NHS Trust, Cambridge, UK

Section A

Basic Ultrasound Theory

Introduction

Christopher R. Porter

The human prostate, located at the center of the male pelvic floor, is much like the crossroads for the male genitourinary system as it can impact both fertility and urinary function. Indeed, the prostate holds significant health implications for a host of benign and malignant conditions. It is implicated in the pathophysiology of a range of conditions, from incontinence to cancer, that are estimated to cost the US health care system tens of millions of dollars each year.

This book has been written for the ultrasonographer, radiologist, and urologist. The book is divided into a basic theory section, an advanced imaging section, and a future of prostate ultrasound section. All three sections are germane to the practice of urology and the treatment of prostatic conditions. The scope of the book encompasses the physics of ultrasound, the technical aspects on the use of ultrasound, the actual present-day state of the art use of ultrasound in the treatment and diagnosis of men with prostatic issues, and its potential future applications.

While there are many texts on ultrasound and many more on prostatic conditions, unfortunately progress in ultrasound imaging of the prostate has effectively stalled. Although our images are sharper, the information conveyed remains a constant. We are only able to effectively visualize and measure the gland, we are not able to detect prostate cancer and we are only starting to be able to leverage ultrasound techniques to evaluate the dynamic role of the prostate in malignant and benign disease entities.

This book addresses the most up-to-date imaging techniques that incorporate ultrasound in the evaluation of prostate cancer. One of the most important aspects of the book is the focus on the applied physics of ultrasound and future techniques that promise to soon be routinely available as we continue to improve our ability to evaluate this optically illusive disease.

The prostate holds a particularly important place in benign conditions that in terms of real health care expenses are significantly larger than prostate cancer. Situated at the base of bladder just above the pelvic floor, with functional sphincters on either side, the prostate is implicated and often treated in men with significant urinary symptoms related to benign growth and infectious and inflammatory conditions. This book evaluates the imaging of the prostate for the diagnosis and treatment of these benign conditions and capitalizes on the skills of researchers in field to evaluate the future of pelvic floor ultrasound in the male.

It is my hope that this book will provide a framework for moving forward in our thoughts and endeavors to accurately image prostate cancer and to capture the dynamic role of the prostate in benign conditions. The exploration of the science of prostate ultrasound will ultimately facilitate improvements in the care available to our patients.

C.R. Porter, M.D., F.A.C.S.(✉)
Section of Urology and Renal Transplantation,
Virginia Mason, 1100 9th Ave,
Mailstop C7-URO, Seattle, WA 98101, USA
e-mail: Christopher.Porter@virginiamason.org

C.R. Porter and E.M. Wolff (eds.), *Prostate Ultrasound: Current Practice and Future Directions*,
DOI 10.1007/978-1-4939-1948-2_1, © Springer Science+Business Media New York 2015

History of Prostate Ultrasound

Richard B. Johnston and Christopher R. Porter

Sound

The range of the human ear in detecting and utilizing sound as a source of information is rather narrow. Under ideal laboratory conditions, humans can hear a sound as low as 12 Hz, but can comfortably detect sound in the range of 20 Hz to 20 kHz [1]. At sound frequencies below 20 Hz (termed infrasound) there are few, if any, useful medical applications. Sounds with frequencies above 20 kHz are referred to as ultrasound [1]. Many animals use sound at higher frequency for communication, locating prey, and navigating in the dark or underwater [2]. For example, Amazon River dolphins produce the highest frequency sound observed in mammals at above 110 kHz [2].

Ultrasound

Until the eighteenth century the science and understanding of sound was framed in terms of hearing. Consequently, there was no precise sci-entific concept of the infra or ultrasound range. Lorenzo Spallazani, an eighteenth century Italian biologist and physiologist, was the first to publish robust experimental proof that non-audible sound exists. In an elegant set of experiments he was able to demonstrate that blindfolded bats were able to fly and kill their prey unimpaired, yet bats with their mouths covered could not successfully fly or hunt. Later utilizing equipment that he and others developed, Spallazani was able to show that bats use a frequency of 100 kHz for their echolocation [3].

While scientists were able to demonstrate the existence of high frequency sound and its utilization by animals in the eighteenth century, it was not until the end of the nineteenth century and beginning of the twentieth century that advances in electrical research allowed investigators to develop sources of energy that could be regulated to produce ultrasound. Pierre and Jacques Curie discovered that voltage applied to certain crystals in alternating cycles produces expansion and compression—the so-called piezoelectric effect [4]. The Curies' combined their knowledge of pyroelectricity with their understanding of the underlying crystal structures in order to predict crystal behavior. However, decades of research were required to define the crystal structures that exhibited piezoelectricity. This resulted in the 1887 publication of Woldemar Voigt's "Üeber das Doppler'sche Princip (On the Principle of Doppler)," which first described the

R.B. Johnston, M.D., Ph.D.
St. Joseph Medical Center, Tacoma, WA, USA
e-mail: richard.b.johnston@gmail.com

C.R. Porter, M.D., F.A.C.S. (✉)
Section of Urology and Renal Transplantation,
Virginia Mason, 1100 9th Ave, Mailstop C7-URO,
Seattle, WA 98101, USA
e-mail: Christopher.Porter@virginiamason.org

C.R. Porter and E.M. Wolff (eds.), *Prostate Ultrasound: Current Practice and Future Directions,*
DOI 10.1007/978-1-4939-1948-2_2, © Springer Science+Business Media New York 2015

use of Doppler waves and their use as applied to ultrasonics [5].

Ironically it took an international disaster, the sinking of the Titanic, to open the gates on the research of ultrasound, currently one of the safest imaging modalities in medicine. The sinking of the "un-sinkable" vessel led to an intense interest in the remote detection of icebergs and the development of early sonar technology. The ensuing research over the early part of the twentieth century relied heavily on the piezoelectric effect and its ability to produce ultrasonic waves. The first real world application for piezoelectric devices was the hydrophone, first developed and used during World War I by the French as an ultrasonic submarine detector [6]. The detector consisted of a transducer, made of thin quartz crystals glued between two steel plates, and a hydrophone to detect the returned echo. This device emitted a single high frequency output and detected the returning wave after it had "bounced" off of an object. The duration of time it took for the wave to return was recorded, allowing for the calculation of the distance between objects, with up to a 50 mile radius.

Medical Application of Ultrasound

Military and commercial use of ultrasound continued at an increasing pace during the 1920s and 1930s. During this time ultrasound as an entity was being utilized more as a therapeutic tool and not as diagnostic imaging tool. It was not until 1936 that German scientist Raimar Pohlman described conversion of ultrasound return waves into a visual "real time" entity. He went on to describe the first therapeutic use of ultrasound in humans using high-intensity focused ultrasound (HIFU) [7]. This was quickly followed in 1942 by William Fry and Russell Meyers in their work on destruction of the basal ganglia to treat patients with Parkinson's disease [8]. Similarly, Peter Lindstrom reported ablation of frontal lobe tissue in moribund patients to alleviate their pain from metastatic cancer lesions utilizing high frequency ultrasound [9].

Between the First and Second World Wars, ultrasound was tried as a therapeutic tool for countless complaints and conditions, such as arthritic pains, gastric ulcers, eczema, asthma, thyrotoxicosis, hemorrhoids, urinary incontinence, elephantiasis, and even angina pectoris. Therapy was the principal objective of the American Institute of Ultrasound in Medicine (AIUM) from the early 1950s until the mid 1960s. Concerns over the harmful tissue damaging effects of ultrasound began mounting; unfocussed and uncontrolled ultrasound can depart much energy into tissue. Consequently, the development of ultrasound as an imaging modality was hampered [10].

Methods for real-time visualization of returning sound waves signals, a necessity for the development of an imaging modality, were immature compared to therapeutic applications for ultrasound. Early pioneer work in diagnostic ultrasound was performed by Douglass Howry, a radiologist at the Veteran's Administration Hospital in Denver, Colorado. Howry concentrated on the development of equipment to detect returning sound waves and he was able to demonstrate the existence of an ultrasonic echo interface between different tissues. Working with Howry, the nephrologist Joseph Homles, who was then the acting director of the hospital's Medical Research Laboratories, produced the "Somascope," a compound circumferential scanner, in 1954 [11]. The transducer of the somascope was mounted around the rim of a large metal immersion tank filled with water. The machine was able to make compound scans of an intra-abdominal organ from different angles to produce a "readable" picture. The sonographic images were referred to as "somagrams." The discovery and apparatus were published in the Medicine section of the LIFE Magazine® in 1954 (Fig. 1). The Somagram, although capable of producing 2-D, accurate, and reproducible images of body organs, required the patient to be immersed in water and remain motionless for long periods of time, which limited its widespread application.

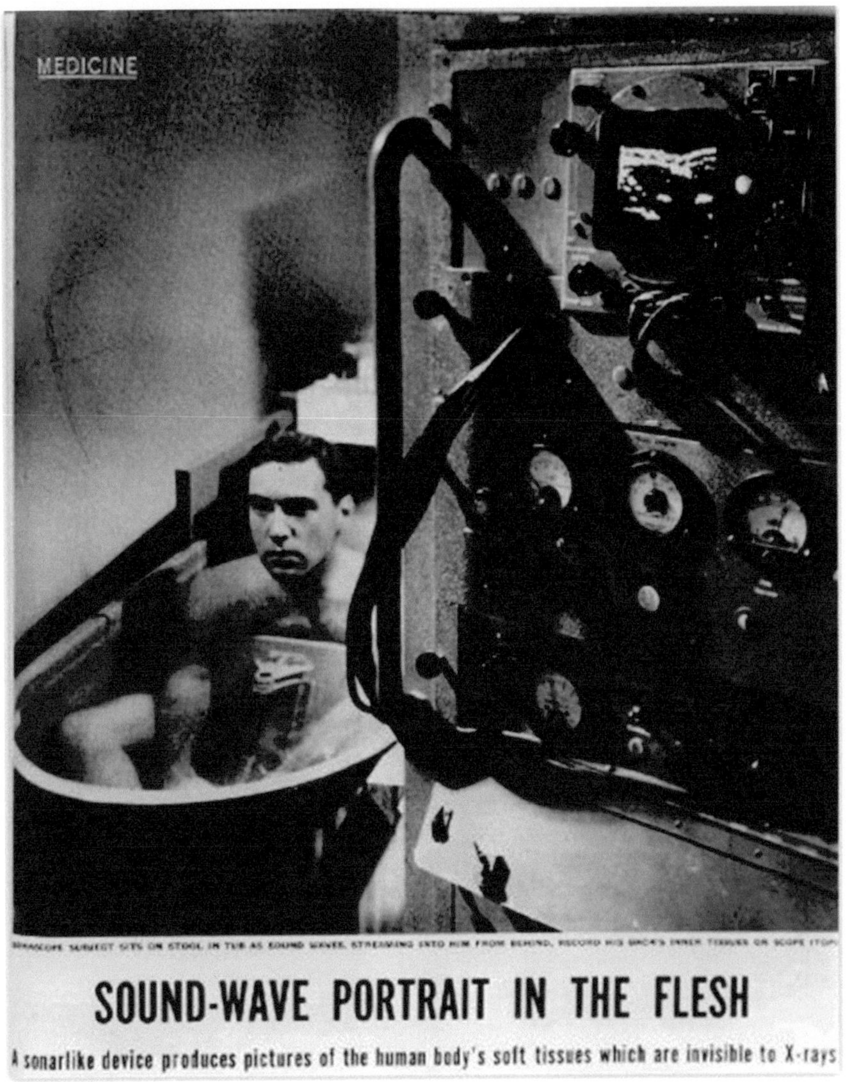

Fig. 1 Somagram device

Prostate Ultrasound

Over the next decade the use of ultrasound as a safe diagnostic imaging method began to gain acceptance and advances in ultrasound equipment development resulted in reduced size and increased reliability, readability, and usability. In 1963, the first trans-perineal ultrasonic examination of the prostate was published by two Japanese urologists, Takahashi and Ouchi.

However, the ultrasound images created with this array were of such poor quality that they had little medical utility [12] (Fig. 2).

The first clinically applicable images of the prostate obtained with trans-rectal ultrasound (TRUS) were described in 1967 by Watanabe et al. [13]. Watanabe used a 3.5 MHz transducer, which at that time was a significant improvement upon any previous probe and allowed clinicians to obtain clinically interpretable, real-time images. As ultrasound technology became more

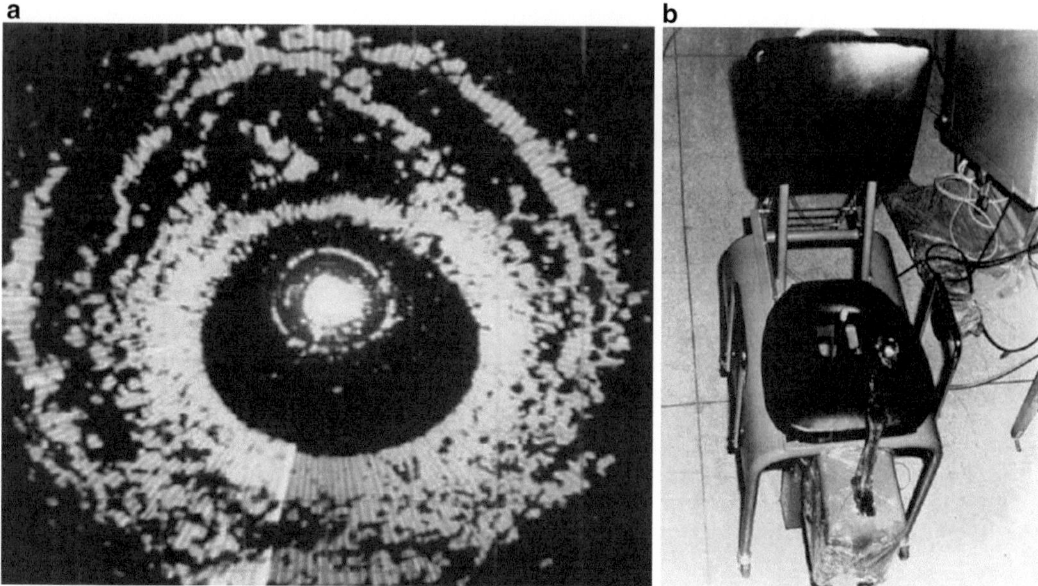

Fig. 2 (**a** and **b**) Early TRUS device and image (used with permission)

developed, the use of TRUS in the evaluation of prostatic disease increased. By the mid 1980s, the 7 MHz ultrasound probe, which more clearly delineated the architecture of the prostate, had become a standard diagnostic instrument of the urologist. Despite adequate visualization of the prostate by TRUS techniques, ultrasound guided biopsies were still performed via the transperineal route. In fact, it was not until 1987 that the first literature appeared describing the use of TRUS with trans-rectal biopsy. Since then, as ultrasound technology has become more refined, this technique has been described as a superior method of performing biopsy of the prostate [14].

Since the initial reports of TRUS of the prostate, substantial technologic advances have improved the diagnostic capabilities of this modality. The current TRUS probe that most urologists consider standard is a 5–8 MHz hand-held, high-resolution probe with multiaxial planar imaging capabilities, allowing for both transverse and sagittal imaging of the prostate in real time. These probes can be fitted with an adapter that accepts the needle of a spring-loaded biopsy gun, thus allowing multiple cores of tissue to be easily obtained. The visualization provided by the new higher resolution transducers, coupled with the ability to direct the biopsy needle into various regions of interest and provide uniform spatial separation of the areas to be sampled, has helped to make TRUS-guided prostate biopsy a standard technique in the diagnosis of prostate cancer.

References

1. Katz J. Handbook of clinical audiology. 5th ed. Philadelphia: Lippincott Williams & Wilkins; 2002. ISBN 9780683307658.
2. Heffner HE. Auditory awareness. Appl Anim Behav Sci. 1998;57(3–4):259–68.
3. "Spallanzani - Uomo e scienziato" (in Italian). Il museo di Lazzaro Spallanzani. Retrieved 07.01.2013; (google translate used Italian into English).
4. Curie JP, Curie. Développement par pression de l'é'lectricite polaire dans les cristaux hémièdres à faces inclinées. C R Acad Sci (Paris). 1880;91.
5. Voigt W. Ueber das Doppler'sche Princip (on the principle of Doppler). Göttinger Nachrichten. 1887;7:41–51. Reprinted with additional comments by Voigt in Physikalische Zeitschrift XVI, 381–6 (1915).
6. Chilowsky C.M. Langévin. M.P. (1916) Procídés et appareil pour production de signaux sous-marins dirigés et pour la localsation à distances d'obstacles sons-marins. French patent no. 502913.

7. Meyers R, Fry WJ, Fry FJ, Dreyer LL, Schultz DF, Noyes RF. Early experiences with ultrasonic irradiation of the pallidofugal and nigral complexes in hyperkinetic and hypertonic disorders. J Neurosurg. 1959;16:32–54.

8. Fry WJ, Barnard JW, Fry EJ, Krumins RF, Brennan JF. Ultrasonic lesions in the mammalian central nervous system. Science. 1955;122:517–8.

9. Ludwig GD, Ballantine HT. Ultrasonic irradiation of nervous tissue. Surgical Forum, Clinical Congress of the American College of Surgeons P. 400; 1950.

10. http://www.aium.org/aboutUs/history/articles/jum19.pdf. Accessed 21 Jun 2013.

11. Holmes JH, Howry DH, Posakony GJ, Cushman CR. The ultrasonic visualization of soft tissue structures in the human body. Trans Am Clin Climatol Assoc. 1954;66:208–23.

12. Takahashi H, Ouchi T. The ultrasonic diagnosis in the field of urology. Proc Jpn Soc Ultrasonics Med. 1963;3.

13. Langer JE. The current role of transrectal ultrasonography in the evaluation of prostate carcinoma. Semin Roentgenol. 1999;34:284–94.

14. Astraldi A. Diagnosis of cancer of the prostate: biopsy by rectal route. Urol Cutaneous Rev. 1937;41:421.

Applied Anatomy of the Male Pelvis

Wouter Everaerts and Anthony J. Costello

Abbreviations

APA	Accessory pudendal artery
DA	Detrusor apron
DVC	Dorsal vascular complex
EUS	External urethral sphincter
FTAP	Fascial tendinous arch of the pelvis
IPA	Internal pudendal artery
IUS	Internal urethral sphincter
LAF	Levator ani fascia
NVB	Neurovascular bundle
PF	Prostatic fascia
PPF	Peri-prostatic fascia
PPL	Puboprostatic ligaments
PVL	Pubovesical ligaments
SV	Seminal vesicles
TURP	Transurethral resection of the prostate

W. Everaerts, M.D., Ph.D. (✉)
Department of Urology, The Royal
Melbourne Hospital, Grattan Street,
Parkville, VIC 3050, Australia
e-mail: wouter.everaerts@med.kuleuven.be

A.J. Costello, M.D., F.R.A.C.S.
Department of Urology, The Royal
Melbourne Hospital, Grattan Street,
Parkville, VIC 3050, Australia

Epworth Healthcare Richmond,
32 Erin Street, Richmond, VIC 3121, Australia
e-mail: tony@tonycostello.com.au

Introduction

Although the ancient Egyptians started studying the anatomy of the human body as early as 1600 BC, the complex organisation of the male pelvis has long been poorly understood and is still a matter of debate today.

The description of the anatomical prostatectomy by Dr. P. Walsh, enabling to remove the prostate while preserving potency and continence and the increasing ability to detect prostate cancer in an early, organ-confined state, strongly increased the popularity of radical prostatectomy and the interest in prostate anatomy [1].

Moreover, since the introduction robotic-assisted surgery, with a tenfold magnification of the operative field, 3D view for better depth perception and integrated fluorescence imaging (Firefly™ Fluorescence), our visualisation of the peri-prostatic fasciae, nerves, and vessels is better than ever.

The improved visualisation of anatomical structures during surgery, combined with a revival of anatomical studies on cadavers as well as radical prostatectomy specimens have increased our knowledge about the anatomy of the male pelvis. In this book chapter we combine our own experience in the operation theatre and dissection lab, with recent literature to give an up-to-date overview of the functional anatomy of the male pelvis.

C.R. Porter and E.M. Wolff (eds.), *Prostate Ultrasound: Current Practice and Future Directions*,
DOI 10.1007/978-1-4939-1948-2_3, © Springer Science+Business Media New York 2015

Anatomy of the Prostate and Seminal Vesicles

Prostate

The prostate is a pyramidal-shaped, fibromuscular and glandular organ. It has a broad base adjacent to the bladder neck and a narrow apex contiguous to the urethral sphincter (Fig. 1). The normal prostate weighs about 20 g and is transversed by the prostatic urethra. Posteriorly, the prostate is perforated by the ejaculatory ducts, which pass obliquely to empty through the verumontanum on the floor of the prostatic urethra just proximal to the striated external urinary sphincter.

The prostate is composed of tuboalveolar glands surrounded by fibromuscular stroma. This stroma is composed of collagen and smooth muscle fibres that contract during ejaculation to express prostatic secretions into the urethra [2].

Prostatic Capsule

The so-called prostatic capsule is a condensed layer of fibromuscular tissue that encloses most of the external surface and determines the outer limits of the prostate. This structure is an important landmark in the pathological staging of prostate cancer, determining if the disease is still organ-confined. The capsule cannot be distinguished on the anterior aspect of the prostate, where the anterior fibromuscular stroma and detrusor apron are found. Moreover the capsule is absent at the apex and the base of the gland, where the prostate stroma blends with the muscle fibres of the urinary sphincter and detrusor muscle respectively [3–5].

Several authors have questioned the term "prostatic capsule" since the fibromuscular band is not a real anatomic capsule in the true sense of the word: first because it is incomplete at the apex and base, second because the fibromuscular band shows great homogeneity with the muscle content and muscle density of the prostatic stroma. Therefore is considered an extension of the parenchyma itself, rather than a distinct structure (Fig. 2) [3, 4, 6].

Zonal Anatomy of the Prostate

In 1968 McNeal introduced the concept that the glandular elements of the prostate can be divided into discrete regions or zones, each of which arises from a different part of the prostatic urethra

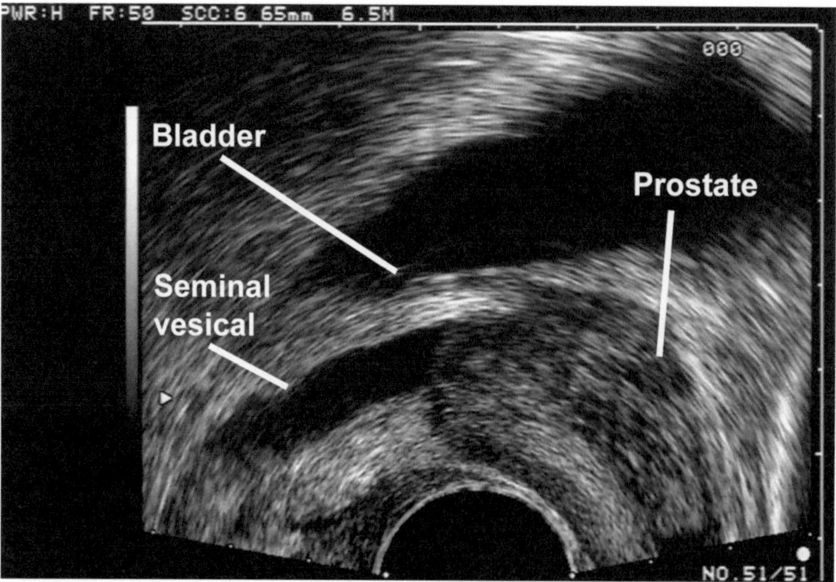

Fig. 1 Zonal anatomy of the prostate Reprinted from (2) with permission

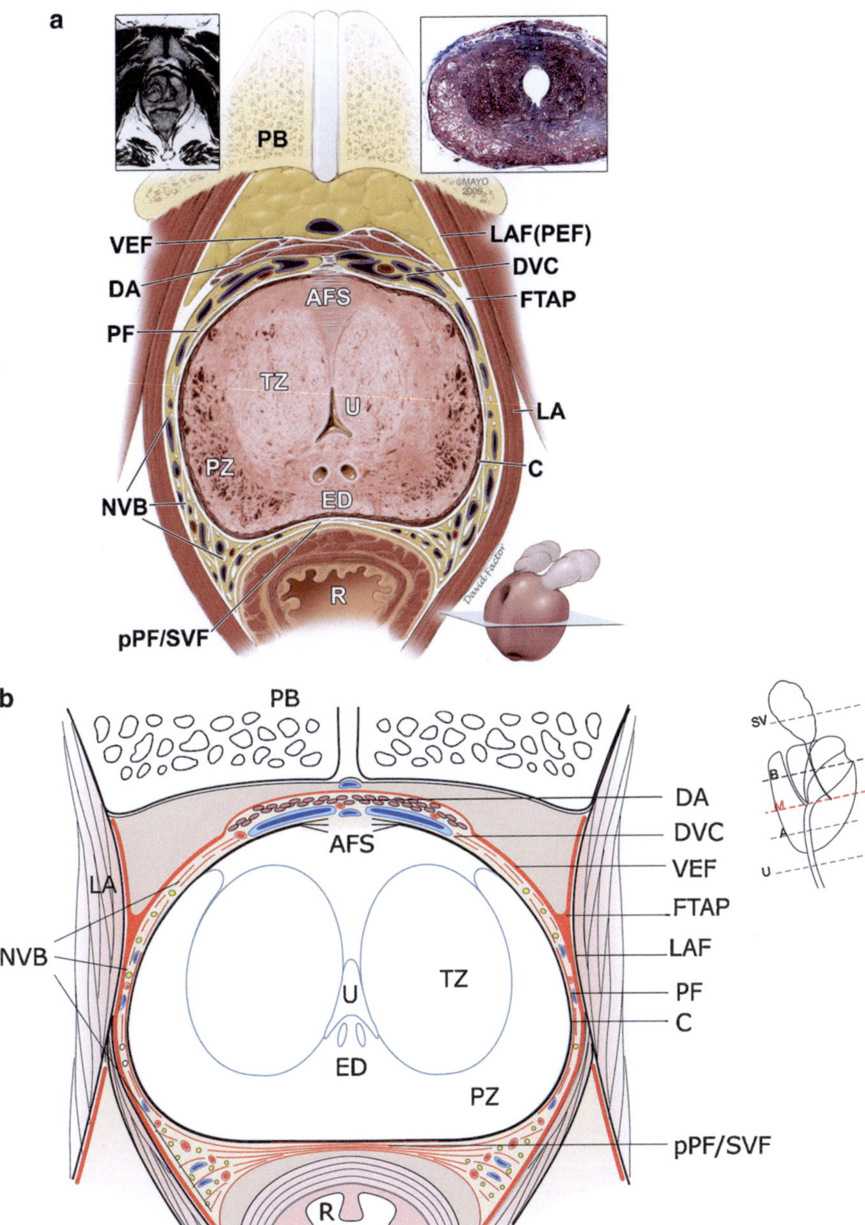

Fig. 2 Periprostatic fasciae. Axial section of prostate and periprostatic fascias at midprostate: (**a**) anatomic (reproduced with permission from the Mayo Foundation for Medical Education and Research). (**b**) schematic. *AFS* anterior fibromuscular stroma, *C* capsule of prostate, *DA* detrusor apron, *DVC* dorsal vascular complex, *ED* ejaculatory ducts, *FTAP* fascial tendinous arch of pelvis, *LA* levator ani muscle, *LAF* levator ani fascia, *NVB* neurovascular bundle, *PB* pubic bone, *PEF* parietal endopelvic fascia, *PF* prostatic fascia, *pPF/SVF* posterior prostatic fascia/seminal vesicles fascia (Denonvilliers' fascia), *PZ* peripheral zone, *R* rectum, *TZ* transition zone, *U* urethra, *VEF* visceral endopelvic fascia. Reprinted [6] with permission

(Fig. 3) [7]. Every zone has its specific architectural and stromal features and specific pathological lesions. The different glandular zones of the prostate can usually be visualised by transrectal ultrasound (Fig. 4) [2].

Peripheral Zone

The peripheral zone comprises the bulk of the glandular tissue (70 %) at the lateral and posterolateral side of the gland. Its ducts drain into the posterolateral recesses of the urethral wall as a double row

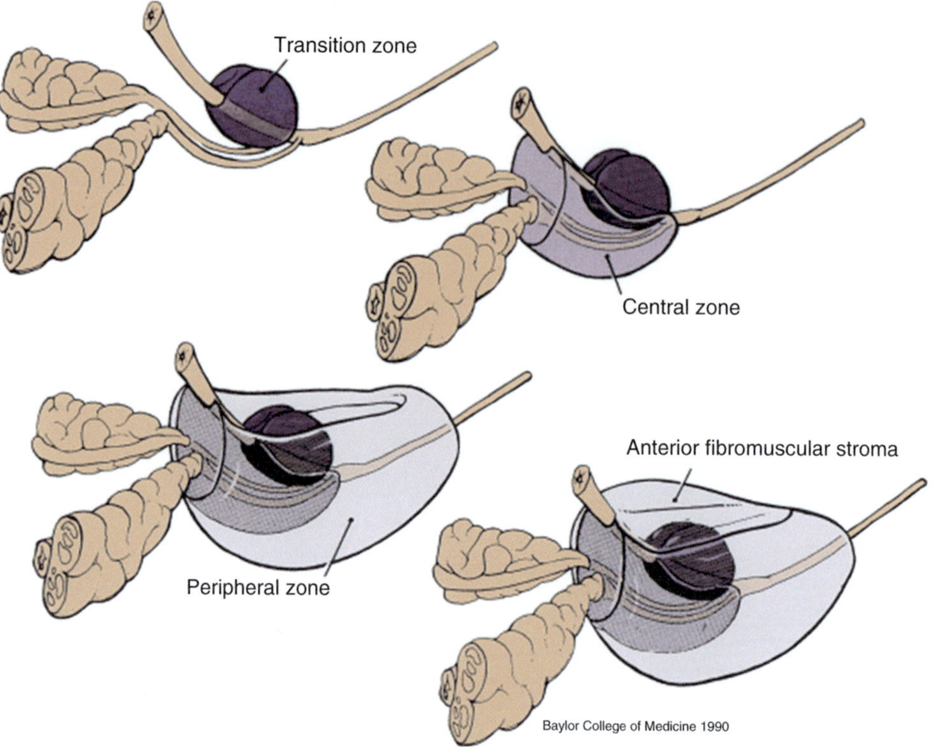

Fig. 3 Zonal anatomy of the prostate as described by J.E. McNeal [7]. Reprinted from [2] with permission

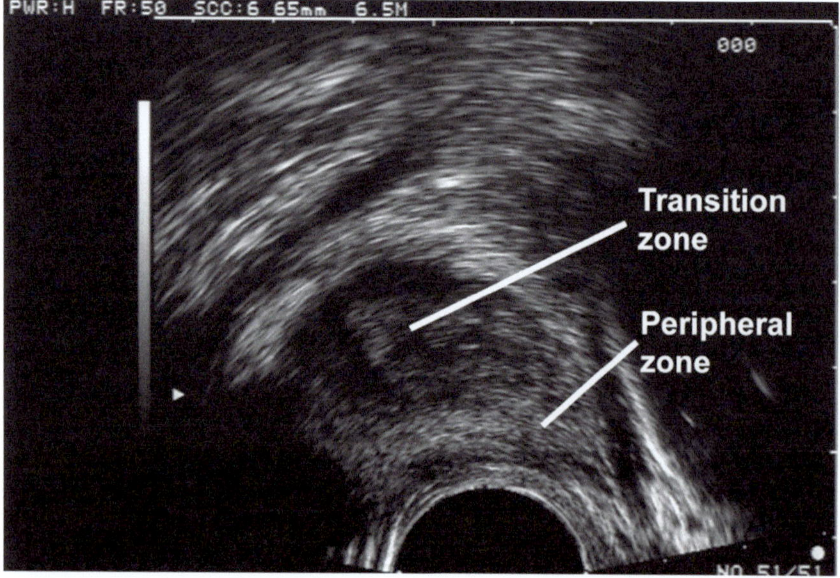

Fig. 4 Ultra sound image. Sagital view of the prostate

extending from the base of the verumontanum to the prostate apex (Figs. 2–4) [2, 7].

This zone is most susceptible region for (chronic) prostatitis. Moreover, it is the site of origin of 70 % of prostatic carcinomas.

Central Zone

The central zone accounts for about 25 % of the volume of the prostate gland. Its ducts arise from a small focus around the ejaculatory duct orifices. These ducts branch directly towards the base of the prostate as a cone around the ejaculatory ducts (Fig. 3). The base of the cone comprises almost the entire base of the prostate. The central zone is quite resistant to inflammation and carcinogenesis. Only 1–5 % of prostate cancers have their origin in this zone, although cancers from adjacent zones may infiltrate it more frequently [2, 7].

Transition Zone

The glandular tissue of the transition zone constitutes only 5–10 % of the prostate gland in early adulthood, but comprises an increasing portion of the gland in ageing men that develop benign prostatic hyperplasia (BPH). The ducts arise at a single point just proximal to the urethral angle that divides the proximal and distal prostatic urethra. The ducts then pass laterally, around the distal border of the preprostatic sphincter, a sleeve of smooth muscle surrounding the proximal prostatic urethra, to travel on its lateral and posterior sides as two independent small lobes (Figs. 2 and 4). A discrete layer of fibromuscular tissue separates the transition zone from the remaining glandular zones, facilitating its visualisation by transrectal ultrasound. The transition zone is the site of origin of BPH and about 20 % of prostate adenocarcinomas arise in the zone [2, 7].

Anterior Fibromuscular Stroma

The anterior fibromuscular stroma is a nonglandular region on the anteromedial aspect of the prostate from the bladder base to the apex, where the stroma blends with the external urethral sphincter. Its lateral margins are continuous with the prostatic capsule (Fig. 5). It is composed of elastin, collagen and smooth muscle, although considerable portions of it may be replaced by glandular tissue in BPH. This zone is very rarely affected by prostate cancer [2, 7].

Seminal Vesicles

The seminal vesicles (SVs) are coiled sacculated tubes of approximately 5 cm long. The tubes are lined by a columnar epithelium and enclosed by a thin layer of smooth muscle. The vesicles lay extraperitoneally at the bladder base, lateral to the termination of the vasa. Each vesicle joins its corresponding vas deferens to form the ejaculatory duct, which transverses the posterior prostate to drain into the verumontanum (Figs. 2 and 6) [2].

The SVs cannot be palpated on digital rectal exam, unless involved by a pathologic process, e.g. invasion of prostate cancer. Seminal vesicle invasion is universally accepted as an adverse prognostic factor. Since SV can be invaded by prostate cancer, standard radical prostatectomy includes "en bloc" resection of the prostate and the SVs. Some recent publications advocated SV-sparing radical prostatectomy for low risk localised prostate cancer, to avoid injury to the pelvic autonomous nerves and improve postoperative recovery of potency and continence [8, 9]. The anatomical evidence for this approach however is unclear: we demonstrated that the nerves surrounding the SVs are mainly sympathetic nerves responsible for ejaculation, rather than parasympathetic cavernous nervous. In our view, seminal vesicle-sparing surgery remains experimental with the potential risk of incomplete oncological resection.

Anatomy of the Pelvic Floor

The male pelvic floor is a complex structure consisting of muscles, fasciae and ligaments that support the visceral organs. It is traversed by the urethra and the rectum and has connections to the bony pelvis, the pelvic organs and the extensive fibro-elastic network in the fat-containing anatomical spaces. Distinct anatomical units of the pelvic floor functionally cooperate to maintain

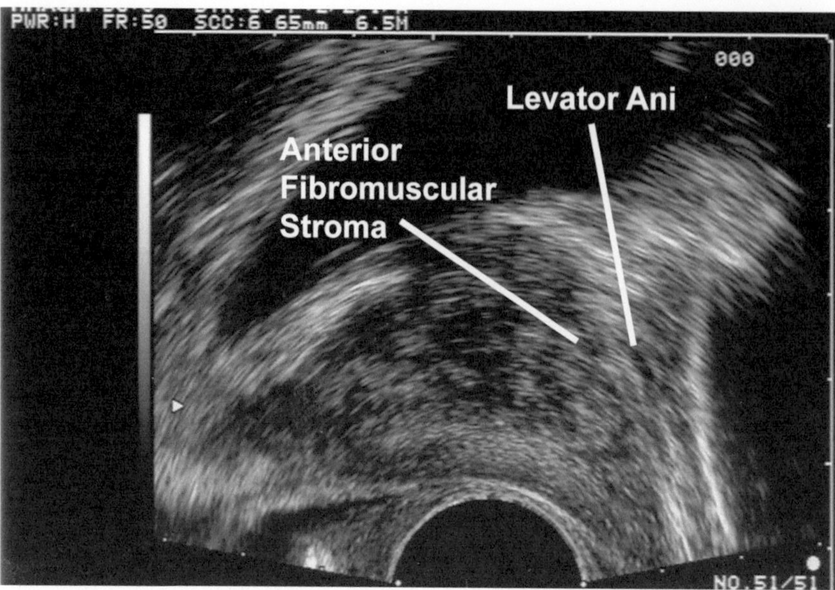

Fig. 5 Ultrasound image. Sagital view

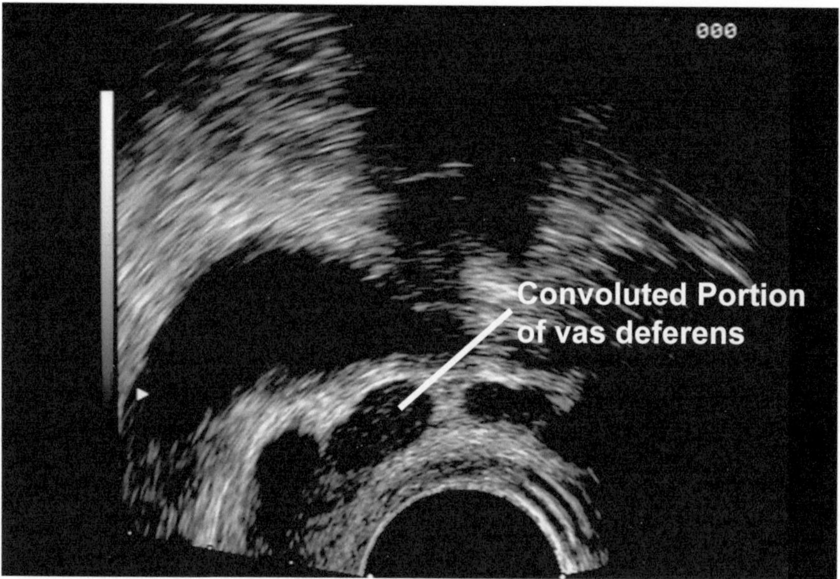

Fig. 6 Ultrasound image using 7.5 MHz probe

continence and to facilitate micturition and defecation [6, 10].

This chapter specifically focuses on the role of the pelvic floor in urinary (patho)physiology, for its role in faecal continence mechanisms readers are referred to the literature [10].

Levator Ani Muscle

The *levator ani* is the largest muscle of the pelvic floor, consisting of different parts (the *pubovisce-ralis, iliococcygeus* and *pubococcygeus* muscles) that originate at the pubic bone, the tendinous arc of the levator ani muscle and the spine of the ischium and sweep down in a series of loops.

The *levator urethrae* or *levator prostatae muscle* constitutes the anteromedial aspect of the pubovisceralis muscle (Fig. 5). It originates at the posterior side of the pubic bone and forms a loop around the prostatourethral junction to insert into the perineal body, between the urethra and the anal sphincter. The *puborectalis* muscle constitutes the main part of the pubovisceralis muscle. It sweeps around the anorectal junction, where it constitutes part of the anal sphincter (for an excellent review see [10]). Contraction of the pubovisceralis muscle lifts and compresses the urethra to stop urine outflow from the bladder. These muscle fibres play an important role in active maintenance of urinary continence. As such it is important to recognise and preserve these muscles during apical prostate dissection [6, 11].

The iliococcygeus and pubococcygeus muscles arise from the pelvic wall and insert into the last two segments of the coccyx and the anococcygeal raphe [10].

Urinary Sphincter

For an excellent review of the anatomical history and current concepts about the urethral sphincter complex, we strongly recommend the review by Dr. M. Koraitim [12].

The male urethral sphincter complex consists of two functional components: an involuntary inner urethral sphincter (IUS) composed of urethral smooth muscle fibres and a voluntary external urethral sphincter (EUS) composed of striated muscle. This sphincter complex surrounds the urethra from the vesical orifice to the distal end of the membranous urethra. Importantly, the urinary sphincter is solely composed of urethral smooth muscle. Bladder smooth muscle fibres do not contribute to the urinary sphincter mechanism.

Inner Urethral Sphincter

The internal urethral sphincter (IUS) also called the lissosphincter, is composed of smooth muscle and elastic connective tissue that completely sur-

round the urethra from the bladder neck to the membranous urethra. The lissosphincter consists of an inner layer of longitudinally oriented fibres surrounded by a wider layer of circular smooth muscle, that is most prominent at the level of the vesical orifice and gets thinner around the proximal urethra (Fig. 7) [11–13].

Functionally, the IUS is responsible for involuntary continence at rest, the so-called passive continence. Involuntary contraction of the circular fibres results in closure of the bladder neck and concentric narrowing of the proximal urethra to provide passive continence. Continence studies after surgery (TURP, prostatectomy [14], urethraplasty [15, 16]) have clearly demonstrated that the full length of the IUS is not mandatory to maintain continence, but there is a crucial minimal length below which incontinence is inevitable. Therefore, careful dissection of the prostatourethral junction and prostatic apex, with maximal preservation of urethral length during radical prostatectomy can contribute to postoperative recovery of urinary continence.

External Urethral Sphincter

The external urethral sphincter (EUS), also called rhabdosphincter consists of striated muscle fibres that largely cover the external side of the IUS. In contrast to the IUS however, the EUS does not completely encircle the urethra, but has an opening on the dorsal side (Fig. 7). In males the EUS has no anatomical connections to the levator urethrae muscle and thus forms a distinct anatomical and functional structure [12, 13].

The rhabdosphincter is most prominent around the membranous urethra and gradually decreases in thickness towards the bladder. The increase in prostate size after puberty causes the muscle fibres to partially atrophy and become more dispersed, with intervening smooth muscle fibres. As such, the superior part of the EUS forms a thin cap on the anterolateral side of the prostate, whereas the inferior part forms a horseshoe-shaped muscle around the membranous urethra. At the infraprostatic level, the thickness of the striated muscle is greater on the

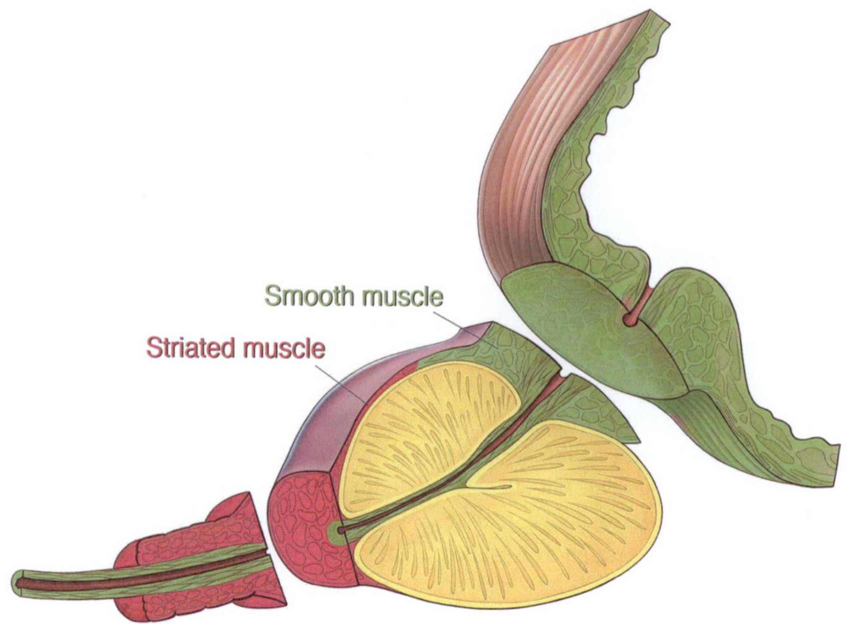

Fig. 7 Urinary sphincter complex

anterior and anterolateral aspect of the sphincter and gradually gets thinner at the posterolateral side. Posteriorly, the circumference of the rhabdosphincter is interrupted by the fibrous median raphe [12, 13].

The rhabdosphincter provides active continence. Contraction of the horseshoe-shaped muscle compresses and angulates the anterior wall of the urethra against the rigid posterior plate formed by the median raphe, Denonvillier's fascia and the rectourethralis muscle [12].

The EUS muscle is composed of both slow (type I) and fast twitch (type II) muscle fibres; with the fast twitch fibres predominating in the infraprostatic part. This allows the EUS to contract quickly and forcefully when the intra-abdominal pressure rises. This contraction can however only be maintained for a short period of time (seconds). In contrast, the lissosphincter that provides involuntary, passive continence cannot contract as strongly but is able to maintain its contraction much longer [12, 17, 18].

The prostatic part of the rhabdosphincter does not play a role in maintaining continence but may play a role in semen propulsion by compression of the prostatic urethra [12].

Fasciae of the Male Pelvis

The pelvic fasciae consist of two components: the endopelvic fascia, which primarily covers the pelvic muscles and the visceral fascia, which covers the pelvic organs and the supplying vessels and nerves [4, 6]. Whereas the endopelvic fascia consists of a condensed layer of collagen fibres, the visceral fasciae consist of connective and fatty tissue that form different layers, which are sometimes difficult to recognise anatomically, with many confusing and conflicting descriptions. Nevertheless, understanding of the fascial investments of the prostate, rectum and levator ani is fundamental for the urologist to perform nerve sparing radical prostatectomy. Various authors have used different terminology to describe the fasciae of the pelvis. In this chapter, we will follow the terminology proposed by Walz et al. in their excellent review of prostate anatomy [6].

The Endopelvic Fascia
The endopelvic fascia is the fascia that covers the pelvic floor. It can be divided in the parietal endopelvic fascia, covering the levator ani muscle, and the visceral endopelvic fascia, covering the

anterior side of the bladder, prostate and rectum. This fascial layer is fused with the anterior fibromuscular stroma of the prostate [6, 19]. The visceral and parietal endopelvic fascia coalesce lateral to the bladder and prostate, forming a whitish line, the *fascial tendinous arch of the pelvis (FTAP)* (Fig. 2). This fascial condensation stretches from the PPL/PVL to the ischial spine. During radical prostatectomy the FTAP needs to be incised to mobilise the prostate. Applying counter traction to the prostate facilitates identification of the fascial reflection between the parietal and visceral endopelvic fascia. This cul-de-sac is easiest to recognise and incise at the base of the prostate, where the space between the levator ani muscle and prostate is larger and the endopelvic fascia is thinner [4, 6, 19].

The Periprostatic Fascia

The term periprostatic fascia (PPF) is used to describe the fascial layers that cover the anterior and lateral surface of the prostate [6]. The PPF does not consist of a single layer of collagenous tissue, but is composed of different layers of connective and dispersed adipose tissue [20]. Importantly, preservation techniques for anatomical dissection often dissolve the adipose tissue, making it hard to recognise these different layers in the dissection room.

The term anterior periprostatic fascia is used for the visceral endopelvic fascia that covers the detrusor apron and dorsal vascular complex on the anterior surface of the prostate (Fig. 2) [6].

The lateral periprostatic fascia enfolds the anterolateral surface of the prostate. It is multilayered and consists of an outer Levator Ani Fascia (LAF) and an inner, usually multilayered Prostatic Fascia (PF) [6]. The layers of the periprostatic fascia form a fascial sheet around the neurovascular bundle on the dorsolateral side of the prostate that is important for the surgeon performing a radical prostatectomy [6, 21, 22]. The PF directly covers the prostatic capsule and fuses with the PPL/PVL and the DVC on the anterior aspect of the prostate. As such the PF runs medial to the NVB. The outer LAF covers the levator ani muscle and runs laterally to the NVB on the dorsolateral aspect of the prostate

(Fig. 2). Posteriorly, this fascia continues as the *Pararectal Fascia* as it separates the levator ani from the rectal wall.

In about half of the patients, the PF and LAF are fused at the anterolateral aspect of the prostate and diverge only at its dorsolateral side, to form a triangular sheet around the NVB, with the medial layer being PF, the lateral layer LAF and the posterior layer Denonvillier's fascia. In the other half, the PF and LAF are not fused, but separated by a thin layer of areolar tissue. In these patients, the fibres of the NVB are dispersed over the lateral surface of the prostate rather than forming a distinct bundle [20].

The Fascia of Denonvilliers

Denovilliers's fascia is an important anatomical landmark for urological and colorectal surgeons. This fascia runs almost vertically between the peritoneal reflection of the rectovesical pouch and the pelvic floor, covering the posterior aspect of the prostate (posterior prostatic fascia) and the seminal vesicles (seminal vesicle fascia) (Fig. 2). Histologically it is composed of dense collagen, smooth muscle fibres, and coarse elastic fibres and varies from a fragile thin layer to a dense, single layered membrane [6, 23].

Denovilliers' fascia separates the prostate from the extraperitoneal rectal wall that is covered by the fatty anterior mesorectum and fascia propria. It is often fused with the prostatic capsule in the midline and is continuous with the central perineal tendon at the prostato-urethral junction. More laterally DF has no significance adherence to the prostatic capsule. It merges laterally with the LAF, herby forming the base of the triangular sheet around the NVB, separating it from the mesorectum. Complete resection of Denonvillier's fascia can be important in to avoidance of positive surgical margins.

The rectal fascia propria is a thin fascial layer (serosa) that is often incorrectly nominated the posterior layer of Denonvilliers fascia. During total mesorectal excision, the plain of dissection should be between Denonvillier's fascia and the fascia propria, to obtain an oncological safe resection while avoiding damage to the neurovascular bundle [23–25].

Detrusor Apron and Pubovesical/Puboprostatic Ligaments

For an excellent review of the anatomy and histology of the detrusor apron, see Myers et al. [26]. Several authors have shown that the bladder smooth muscle does not stop at the vesicoprostatic junction but that superficial, longitudinal smooth muscle fibres of the anterior bladder wall fan out distally covering the anterolateral aspect of the prostate, as the so-called detrusor apron (DA) (Fig. 2). These fibres converge in their path towards the apex as two lateral condensations that attach to the posterior surface of the pubic bone as the pubovesical ligaments (PVL). In small prostates, the detrusor apron forms a thick layer on the anterior surface of the prostate and the relation between the anterior bladder wall and PVL is easily appreciated. As the prostate grows however, the DA gradually gets stretched and the distance between the bladder neck and the pubic attachments of the DA increases. In benign prostatic hyperplasia, the fibrous attachments to the pubic bone seem to be connected to the ventral prostate, without continuity to the bladder and were therefore called puboprostatic ligaments (PPL) [4, 19, 26–28].

The PVL/PPL that support the prostate, urethra and anterior bladder neck are thought to be relevant in anterior stabilisation of the sphincter complex. Several approaches have been described to preserve the PVL/PPL during retropubic or laparoscopic radical prostatectomy in an attempt to improve early recovery of urinary continence [29, 30]. Similarly, a so-called anterior suspension suture is used to restore the anterior stabilisation of the urethra to the posterior pelvic bone ([31, 32] Hurtes, #86). Although there is little evidence, an increasing number of papers try to support a role for the PVL/PPL complex in preservation/restoration of urinary continence after radical prostatectomy.

Vesicoprostatic Muscle

Similar to the anterior detrusor apron, the outer longitudinal fibres of the detrusor muscle continue distal to the posterior vesicoprostatic junction, to form the vesicoprostatic muscle. These fibres fan out between the posterior bladder neck and the insertion of the seminal vesicles and the vasa deferentia. Histologically the vesicoprostatic muscle consists of two layers: on anterior layer of longitudinally oriented muscle fibres that are continuous with the outer layer of the detrusor muscle and a posterior layer that consists of fibroadipose tissue that is continuous with the bladder adventitia [33]. During the so-called Rocco-stitch to repair the posterior suspension mechanism of the rhabdosphincter, the remnant of the transected vesicoprostatic muscle is sutured to the posterior median raphe [34].

Periprostatic Neurovascular Anatomy

Blood Supply to the Prostate and SV

Prostate

The introduction of selective arterial embolisation as an alternative treatment for BPH introduced a renewed interest in the arterial anatomy of the prostate. Although this treatment is still experimental, it has lead to a number of new studies that have improved our insights into the vascular anatomy of the prostate. In addition to dissections on human cadaveric specimens, the newer studies use vascular imaging techniques as arteriography and CT angiography to study the prostatic arteries [35–37].

The prostate receives arterial blood supply from a superior and an inferior prostatic pedicle. The superior pedicle, also called the prostatic artery, provides the main arterial supply to the prostate. This artery divides near the base of the prostate into a medial branch, the *urethral artery* and a lateral branch, the *capsular artery*. Before reaching the prostate, this artery is called the prostatovesical artery and gives a branch to the trigone (the inferior vesical artery) and to the seminal vesicles (Fig. 8) [35, 38].

The medial branches, also called urethral arteries, penetrate the prostatovesical junction posterolaterally, run perpendicular to the urethra and then make a 90° turn to continue parallel to the urethra. These vessels supply the urethra proximal to the urethral crest, the paraurethral glands and the transition zone. These arteries provide the main blood supply to the prostatic adenoma and to the median lobe in BPH [35, 36, 39].

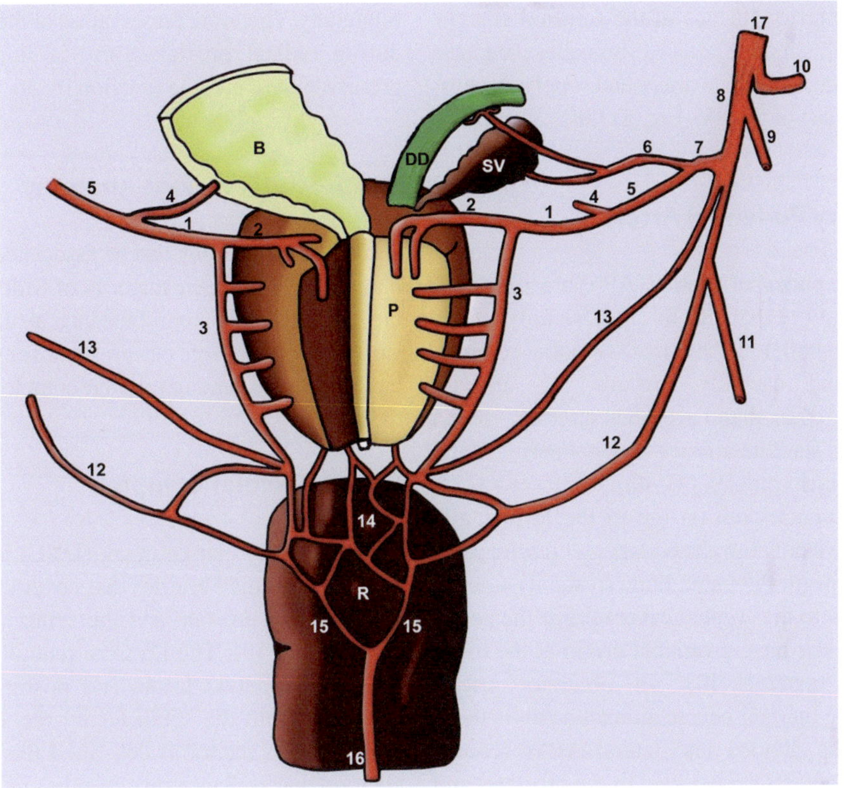

Fig. 8 Arterial blood supply to the prostate 1 sup prostatic pedicle, 2 urethral artery, 3 capsular artery, 4 inf vesical artery, 5 prostatic-vesical artery, 6 vesicle deferential artery, 7 genito-vesical artery, 8 gluteo pudendal trunk, 9 obturator artery, 10 sup gluteal artery 11 inf gluteal artery, 12 IPA 13 middle rectal artery, 14 inf prostatic pedicle 15 sup rectal artery, 17 hypogastric artery B Bladder, DD Deferent Ducts, P Prostate, SV Seminal Vesicle, R Rectum. Adapted from [43] with permission

The lateral branches form the so-called capsular artery. This artery descends caudally to the apex of the gland at the posterolateral side of the prostate, external to the prostatic capsule. Here the cavernous nerves run in close proximity of the capsular artery and the prostatic veins to form the neurovascular bundles. The capsular artery provides perforating branches that pierce the capsule and supply the glandular tissue of the lateral lobes and the distal urethra, where they anastomose with prostatic branches from the inferior pedicle. In about 20 % of cases, the capsular and urethral arteries do not emerge from a common prostatic artery, but from separate vessels.

The origin of the superior prostatic pedicle is very variable. Although it has classically been described as a branch of the internal iliac artery, recent studies have demonstrated that in almost half of the cadaveric specimens, the prostatovesical artery has an alternative origin from the middle rectal artery, the internal pudendal artery (IPA), the obturator artery or an accessory IPA [35, 40].

The inferior prostatic pedicle reaches the posterolateral side of the prostatic apex to form a plexus around the prostatourethral junction, where it anatomises with branches of the capsular arteries. This pedicle receives arterial branches from the IPA and in some cases from the superior, middle or inferior rectal arteries IPA [35, 40].

Seminal Vesicles

Most of the arterial blood supply to the SV is provided by the vesiculodeferential artery, a branch of the superior vesical artery, although its origin may vary along the anterior trunk of the internal iliac. This artery supplies the vas deferens and the anterior surface of the seminal vesicle. Additional, smaller arterial branches originate from the prostatovesical artery and supply the posterior surface of the SV (Fig. 8) [38].

Accessory Pudendal Arteries

Accessory pudendal arteries (APA) are arteries of varying calibre that run in close vicinity of the prostate, parallel to the dorsal vascular complex and extend caudally towards the anterior perineum, other than cavernous arteries, corona mortis and satellite arteries to the superficial and deep vascular complex [41–43].

These arteries run on top of the levator ani, either above or below the endopelvic fascia, passing underneath the pubic bone to supply arterial blood flow to the corpora cavernosa of the penis. These vessels have a variable origin at the internal iliac, external iliac of obturator artery. Depending on their course along the pelvis these arteries are divided into lateral APAs (course along the anterolateral aspect of the prostate) and apical APAs (emerge through the levator ani fibres near the prostatic apex).

These APAs are functionally important because they can tribute significantly to the arterial input of the corpora cavernosa, either unilaterally or bilaterally. Therefore preservation of these arteries during radical prostatectomy is important in preservation of erectile function [6, 36, 41].

Periprostatic Venous Anatomy

Radical prostatectomy can be associated with significant blood loss, the majority of which is attributed directly to venous bleeding at the time of surgery from the large periprostatic veins, particularly the dorsal venous/vascular complex (DVC).

Dorsal Vascular Complex

The dorsal vascular complex (DVC) is a plexus of veins and small arteries that cover the anterior aspect of the prostate and the urinary sphincter (Figs. 9 and 10). The DVC is ventrally covered by the endopelvic fascia and posteriorly it is separated from the sphincter by the sphincter's facia [6, 44]. Santorini described this complex, also known as Santorini's plexus, in 1739 and Walsh and colleagues demonstrated the importance of its careful dissection and ligation during retropubic prostatectomy, providing a bloodless operative field with better recognition of the (peri)prostatic structures [1, 44, 45].

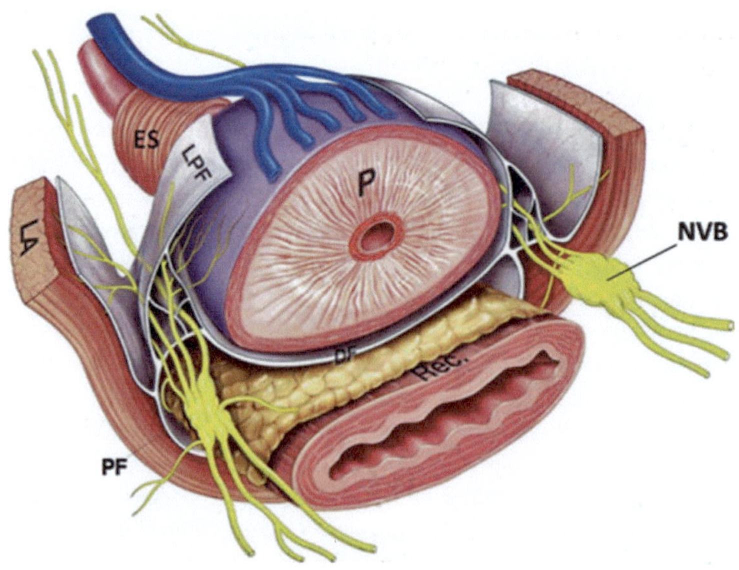

Fig. 9 Dorsal Vascular Complex and neurovascular bundle. P prostate, LA levator ani, LPF lateral prostatic fascia, DF Denonvillier's fascia, rec rectum, PF pararectal fascia

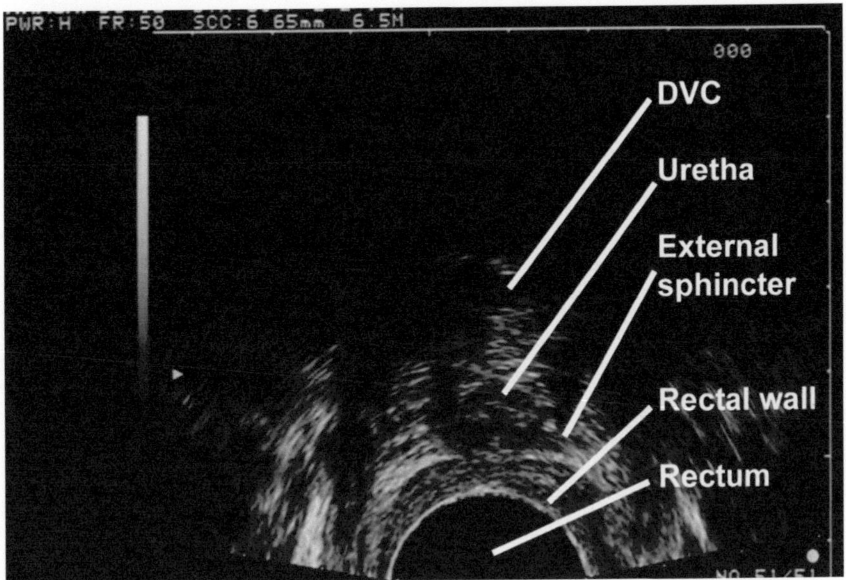

Fig. 10 Ultrasound image. Transverse view. Urethra just distal to prostate apex. 7.5 MHz probe

The DVC receives venous blood from the deep dorsal vein of the penis. After penetration of the urogenital diaphragm, the deep dorsal vein splits in a superficial branch, which travels between the PPL/PVL on top of the endopelvic fascia, and two lateral plexuses. The origin of the small arterial branches is still debated. The DVC continues over the ventral aspect of the prostate and bladder and anatomises with the bladder and lateral prostatic veins [44].

Importantly, the penis has a supralevator and infralevator venous outflow. Ligation of the supralevator outflow in the DVC has no adverse effect on erection, because it does not interrupt the infralevator drainage to the internal pudendal veins [46].

Prostatic Venous Complex

The venous drainage of the prostate is derived mainly from lateral capsular vessels, and to a lesser extent several anteroinferior veins and veins of the vas deferens. The capsular veins drain directly into the lateral plexuses from the DVC that sweep down the sides of the prostate to communicate with the vesical plexuses that drain into the internal iliac vein [45].

Neuronal Structures of the Pelvis

The nerve supply to the pelvic floor and related organs is provided by three sets of peripheral nerves: sacral parasympathetic (pelvic splanchnic nerves), thoracolumbar sympathetic nerves (hypogastric nerves and sympathetic chain) and sacral somatic nerves (pudendal nerves). These nerves contain efferent fibres that control the function of the target organs and afferent fibres that transport information from the organs to the central nervous system.

The Pelvic Plexus

The pelvic plexus or inferior hypogastric plexus constitutes both sympathetic and parasympathetic fibres, together with afferent nerve fibres (Fig. 11).

The sympathetic system regulates the secretary functions of the prostate and SV and controls ejaculation (synchronous contraction of the vas deferens and urethral smooth muscle). These nerve fibres arise from the thoracolumbar segments T10-L2 and pass through the sympathetic chain ganglia, to constitute the superior hypogastric plexus. This plexus splits in a right and left inferior hypogastric nerve that runs down the pelvis and provides sympathetic nerves to the pelvic plexus.

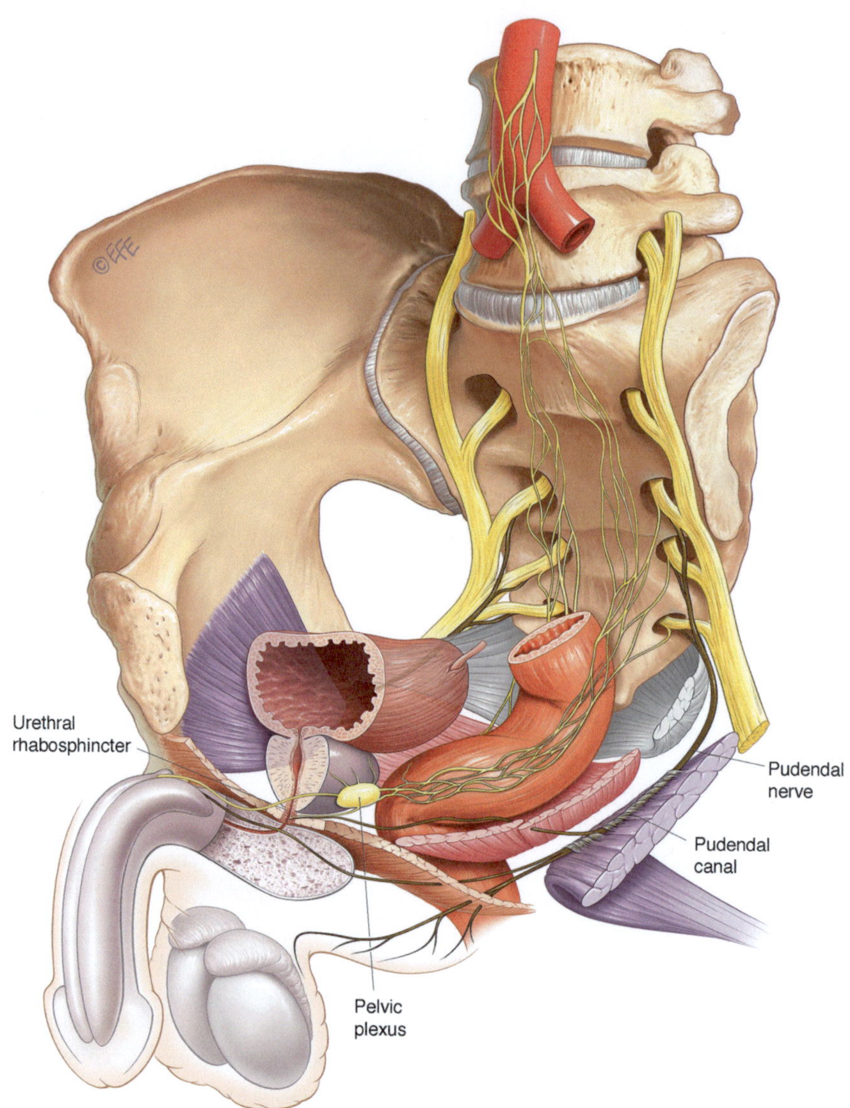

Fig. 11 The pelvic plexus

The sacral parasympathetic outflow enables bladder contraction, relaxation of the urethral lissosphincter and penile erection. Preganglionic fibres originate from the spinal segments S2–S4 and exit from the spinal foramina as pelvic splanchnic nerves and descend anteriorly along the lateral border of the rectum. A part of these parasympathetic nerves continue as nervi erigentes or cavernous nerves to the corpora cavernosa of the penis where day are responsible for vasodilatation and increase arterial blood flow during erection.

The fenestrated pelvic plexus is a retroperitoneal collection of ganglia and nerve fibres located on the lateral surface of the rectum. The plexus runs in a sagittal plane, forming a rhomboid of 3–5.5 cm long and 2.5–5 cm high. It reaches up to 1.5 cm posterior to the rectum to 1 cm superior to the rectovesical pouch of Douglas and is separated from the rectum by the pararectal fascia and 1–2 cm of perirectal adipose tissue (Fig. 9) [22].

The branches of the pelvic plexus form three major projections: (1) anterior, extending across the lateral surface of the seminal vesicle and the inferolateral surface of the bladder; (2) antero-inferior, extending to the prostatovesical junction and obliquely along the lateral surface of the prostate and (3) inferior, running between the rectum and the posterolateral surface of the prostate, forming the neural constituents of the NVB [22].

The neuronal pelvic plexus is closely associated with venous and arterial branches of the inferior vesical vessels. These large vessels mostly run parallel to the lateral surface of the pelvic plexus. The vascular and neural structures generally lay in distinct layers, only to converge at the level of the pelvic plexus projections [22].

The Neurovascular Bundle

The postero-inferior neural branches of the pelvic plexus surrounded by venous and arterial branches of the inferior vesical vessels constitute the neurovascular bundle (NVB) that classically

runs in a groove between the rectum and the posterolateral border of the prostate. In contrast to the original description by Walsh et al., the NVB does not constitute a single nerve fibre, but rather a plexus of fibres, ranging from 6 to 16. On branching from the pelvic plexus these nerves are spread significantly, with up to 3 cm separating the anterior- and posterior-most nerves. The nerves located most anteriorly are intimately associated with the seminal vesicle, coursing along the posterolateral surface, while the nerves located posteriorly run dorsal to the posterolateral verge of the seminal vesicle (Figs. 12 and 13).

Along their track down the prostate, the nerves converge at the mid-prostatic level, forming a more condense NVB, and diverge again when approaching the prostatic apex. The close proximity of the nerves from the NVB to the tip of the seminal vesicles illustrates the importance of gentle dissection of SV during radical prostatectomy to

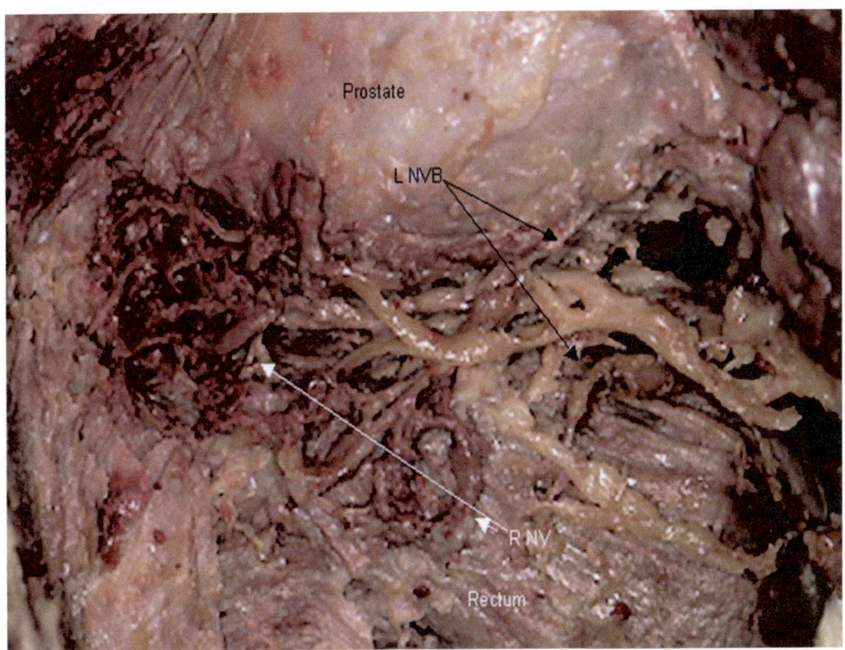

Fig. 12 Cadaveric dissections of the neurovascular bundle. Lateral view of the *LEFT NVB*; the levator ani and lateral pelvic fascia have been excised. The NVB can be seen coursing over the posterolateral surface of the prostate, extending posteriorly to the anterolateral surface of the rectum. The coalescence of the NVB on approaching mid-prostatic level and its divergence to supply neural branches to the levator ani and cavernosal nerves is apparent. The rectum has been displaced posteriorly to varying degrees, exaggerating the distance between the rectum and the prostate. *L NVB* left neurovascular bundle, *R NV* rectal nerves. Reprinted with permission [22]

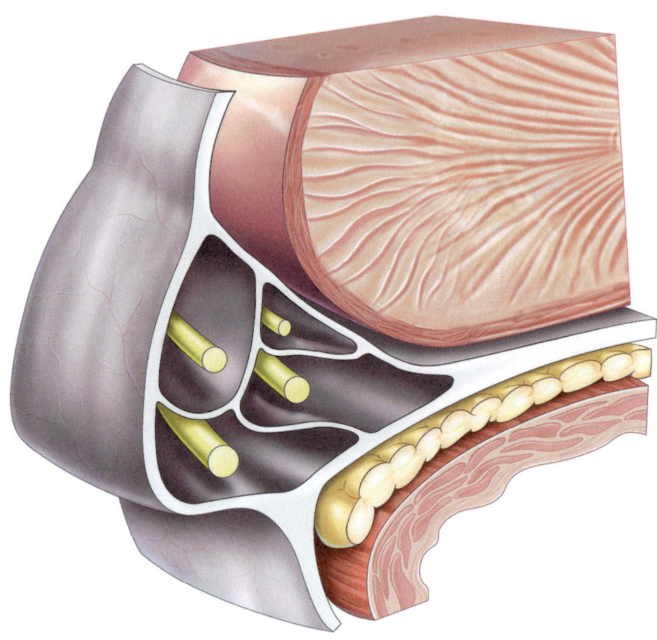

Fig. 13 Fascial compartments of the left neurovascular bundle

improve post-operative continence and potency rates [22].

The nerves of the NVB are intimately associated with vessels branching from the inferior vesical vein and artery. As these vessels course distally toward the prostatic apex numerous terminal branches are given off which, in most cases, mimic the course of the nerves. The nerves running in the NVB not only innervate the corpora cavernosa, but also the rectum, prostate and levator ani musculature. The last three structures also receive a vascular supply from vessels coursing in the NVB. From the apex to the mid-prostate level, arterial and nervous branches supply the anterolateral wall of the rectum. Other nervous branches pass through slit-like openings in the LAF to innervate the superior, middle and inferior segments of the levator ani musculature. The nerves innervating the posterior aspect of the prostate are intimately associated with capsular arteries and veins of the prostate. These structures penetrate the prostatic capsule along its base, mid-portion and apex (Figs. 9 and 14) [22].

The cavernosal nerves (nervi erigentes) and several small vessels pierce the urogenital diaphragm posterolateral to the prostatic apex. At this level the cavernosal nerves divide into numerous small branches that descend along the posterolateral aspect of the membranous urethra, before penetrating the posterior aspect of the corpora cavernosa.

The constituents of the NVB are organised into three functional compartments. The neurovascular supply to the rectum is generally in the posterior and posterolateral sections of the NVB, running within the leaves of Denonvilliers' and pararectal fasciae. The levator ani neurovascular supply is located in the lateral section of the NVB, whereas the cavernosal nerves and the prostatic neurovascular supply descend along the posterolateral surface of the prostate, with the prostatic neurovascular supply most anterior. This functional organisation of the NVB is not absolute, and is less pronounced proximally at the levels of the seminal vesicles and the prostatic base. This description of compartments inside the neurovascular bundle suggests that the synonymous use of

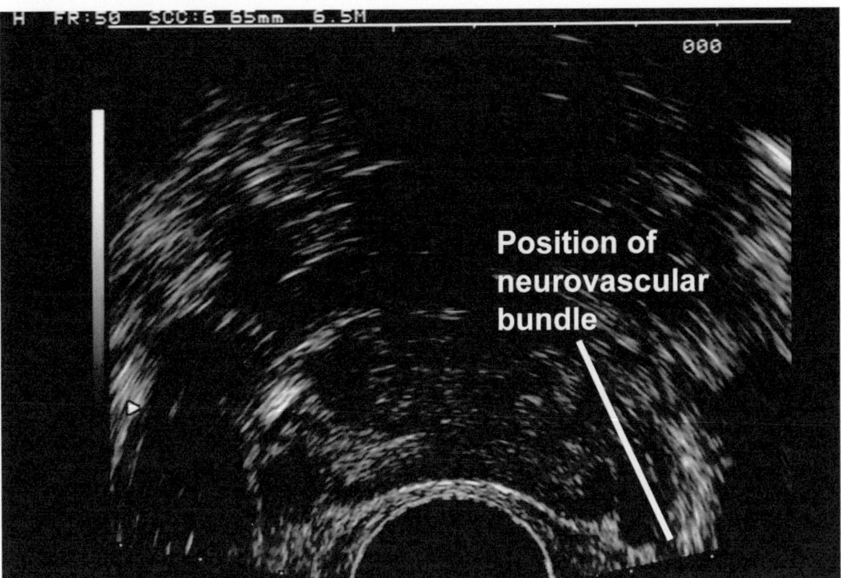

Fig. 14 Ultrasound image. 7.5 MHz probe. The cavernosal nerves (nervi erigentes) and several small vessels pierce the urogenital diaphragm posterolateral to the prostatic apex. At this level the cavernosal nerves divide into numerous small branches that descend along the posterolateral aspect of the membranous urethra, before penetrating the posterior aspect of the corpora cavernosa

NVB and cavernosal nerves is not appropriate (Fig. 13) [22].

This concept of a posterolateral well-defined NVB has recently been challenged. Some authors have described nerve fibres on the anterolateral aspect of the prostate, outside of the NVB, or have characterised a "spray-like" distribution of autonomic nerves at the base and apex of the prostate [47]. It was hypothesised that a proportion of these anteriorly placed nerves are parasympathetic in nature and contribute functionality to the pro-erectile cavernous nerves. Some surgeons have therefore developed a nerve-sparing technique, dubbed the "Veil of Aphrodite" technique [32] to conserve these anterior nerves. Since there was little anatomical evidence to justify this approach, given that the higher placed nerves are most likely destined to innervate the prostatic stroma and not the cavernosal tissue of the penis, we performed a number of dissections at the Royal Melbourne Hospital to characterise the position and nature of the autonomic nerves surrounding the prostate.

We confirmed that autonomic nerve fibres were present on the anterolateral aspects of the prostate between the prostate and lateral prostatic fascia; however, only a small proportion of these were parasympathetic nerves likely to be of functional relevance. At the base, mid-prostate level and apex only 14.3, 18.8 and 23.1 % of the nerves found on the anterior aspect of the prostate were parasympathetic in nature, with the most parasympathetic nerves (69 %, 65 % and 57 %, respectively) being found in the previously defined NVB posterolateral to the prostate. Most of the nerve fibres found on the anterolateral regions examined were sympathetic in nature. These sympathetic nerves innervate the prostatic stroma and the vascular structures in the region and the urethral sphincter. The anteriorly placed parasympathetic nerve fibres are likely to be destined for innervation of the prostatic stroma rather than corpora cavernosa of the penis. We therefore conclude that the anteriorly located parasympathetic nerve fibres have no pro-erectile function. There may however be other explanations for the improved potency outcomes when a high incision of this fascia is performed during nerve-sparing radical prostatectomy. High release of the fascia in this apical region produces less traction on the posterolateral NVB and less thermal damage in this region [21].

Innervation of the External Urethral Sphincter

It is generally accepted that the internal urethral sphincter receives dual autonomic supply via the NVB [48]. The precise innervation of the male urethral sphincter is still a matter of debate. It is well-known that external urethral sphincter receives somatic innervation from the pudendal nerve (Fig. 11) [49–52], but this description may be to simplistic, since preservation of the neurovascular bundle at radical prostatectomy, has been suggested to improve post-operative return to continence [53–55].

The pudendal nerve originates from the S2 to S4 roots of the lumbosacral plexus, with occasional contributions of S5 [49]. It exits the pelvis via the greater sciatic foramen, and re-enters via the lesser sciatic foramen to run in Alcock's canal in the lateral wall of the ischiorectal fossa. It has three terminal branches: the inferior rectal nerve, the perineal nerve and the dorsal nerve of the penis. Pudendal branches to the rhabdosphincter are variable, with conflicting reports of intrapelvic, perineal or dorsal nerve branches [50, 52, 56]. Hollabaugh et al. describe a consistent intrapelvic branch from the pudendal nerve that arises within Alcock's canal in a series of fresh cadaveric dissections [52]. Similarly, a histological study of ten male foetal urethral sphincter specimens demonstrated myelinated nerve fibres running with the unmyelinated fibres from the bladder neck to the rhabdosphincter, suggesting the existence of intrapelvic somatic nerves to the rhabdosphincter. However, the origin of these myelinated fibres could not be determined [57].

There have been descriptions of communication between the pudendal nerve, the nerve to levator ani and the pelvic splanchnic nerve [49, 58]. Given the fine nature of these nerve branches however, traditional anatomical dissections are extremely challenging. An alternative technique using immunohistochemistry of serial sections with three-dimensional reconstruction identified autonomic-somatic communications at three levels: proximal supralevator, intermediary intralevator and distal infralevator [59]. However, other studies have been unable to find any such communications between pudendal and cavernosal nerves [60].

Close proximity of intrapelvic branches of the pudendal nerve may be one explanation for the positive effect of sparing the NVB. Another theory suggests that the effect may be due to preservation of sensory nerves [61]; however, there is no conclusive evidence to explain the neurological mechanism for sphincter weakness following prostatectomy.

Conclusion

Our understanding of male pelvic anatomy has greatly improved in the last few decades. For the urological surgeons, understanding the anatomy of the pelvic organs and the neurovascular structures is of uttermost importance to improve the functional and oncological outcomes of radical prostatectomy. Many of these insights have been acquired during surgery and are still improving thanks to the recent availability of three-dimensional, high-definition video systems. Also the advantages in imaging will contribute to our better understanding of anatomy and (patho)physiology of the male pelvis. Nevertheless, anatomical and histological studies in the dissection lab remain of uttermost importance to confirm or reject the assumptions made during surgery and to deepen insights at the cellular and subcellular levels.

References

1. Walsh PC. The discovery of the cavernous nerves and development of nerve sparing radical retropubic prostatectomy. J Urol. 2007;177(5):1632–5.
2. Brooks JD. Anatomy of the lower urinary tract and male genitalia. In: Kavoussi LR, Novick AC, Partin AW, Peters CA, Wein AJ, editors. Campbell-Walsh urology. 9th ed. Philadelphia: Saunders Elsevier; 2007.

3. Ayala AG, Ro JY, Babaian R, Troncoso P, Grignon DJ. The prostatic capsule: does it exist? Its importance in the staging and treatment of prostatic carcinoma. Am J Surg Pathol. 1989;13(1):21–7.

4. Raychaudhuri B, Cahill D. Pelvic fasciae in urology. Ann R Coll Surg Engl. 2008;90(8):633–7.

5. McNeal JE. Normal and pathologic anatomy of prostate. Urology. 1981;17 Suppl 3:11–6.

6. Walz J, Burnett AL, Costello AJ, Eastham JA, Graefen M, Guillonneau B, et al. A critical analysis of the current knowledge of surgical anatomy related to optimization of cancer control and preservation of continence and erection in candidates for radical prostatectomy. Eur Urol. 2010;57(2):179–92.

7. McNeal JE. The zonal anatomy of the prostate. Prostate. 1981;2(1):35–49.

8. Zlotta AR, Roumeguere T, Ravery V, Hoffmann P, Montorsi F, Turkeri L, et al. Is seminal vesicle ablation mandatory for all patients undergoing radical prostatectomy? A multivariate analysis on 1283 patients. Eur Urol. 2004;46(1):42–9.

9. Secin FP, Bianco FJ, Cronin A, Eastham JA, Scardino PT, Guillonneau B, et al. Is it necessary to remove the seminal vesicles completely at radical prostatectomy? Decision curve analysis of European Society of Urologic Oncology criteria. J Urol. 2009;181(2):609–13. discussion 14.

10. Stoker J. Anorectal and pelvic floor anatomy. Best Pract Res Clin Gastroenterol. 2009;23(4):463–75.

11. Burnett AL, Mostwin JL. In situ anatomical study of the male urethral sphincteric complex: relevance to continence preservation following major pelvic surgery. J Urol. 1998;160(4):1301–6.

12. Koraitim MM. The male urethral sphincter complex revisited: an anatomical concept and its physiological correlate. J Urol. 2008;179(5):1683–9.

13. Wallner C, Dabhoiwala NF, DeRuiter MC, Lamers WH. The anatomical components of urinary continence. Eur Urol. 2009;55(4):932–43.

14. Gudziak MR, McGuire EJ, Gormley EA. Urodynamic assessment of urethral sphincter function in postprostatectomy incontinence. J Urol. 1996;156(3):1131–4. discussion 4–5.

15. Koraitim M, Sabry AA. Mechanism of continence after transpubic urethroplasty. Urology. 1986;27(2):187–90.

16. Koraitim MM, Atta MA, Fattah GA, Ismail HR. Mechanism of continence after repair of posttraumatic posterior urethral strictures. Urology. 2003;61(2):287–90.

17. Tokunaka S, Murakami U, Fujii H, Okamura K, Miyata M, Hashimoto H, et al. Coexistence of fast and slow myosin isozymes in human external urethral sphincter. A preliminary report. J Urol. 1987;138(3):659–62.

18. Elbadawi A, Mathews R, Light JK, Wheeler TM. Immunohistochemical and ultrastructural study of rhabdosphincter component of the prostatic capsule. J Urol. 1997;158(5):1819–28.

19. Myers RP. Practical surgical anatomy for radical prostatectomy. Urol Clin North Am. 2001;28(3):473–90.

20. Kiyoshima K, Yokomizo A, Yoshida T, Tomita K, Yonemasu H, Nakamura M, et al. Anatomical features of periprostatic tissue and its surroundings: a histological analysis of 79 radical retropubic prostatectomy specimens. Jpn J Clin Oncol. 2004;34(8):463–8.

21. Costello AJ, Dowdle BW, Namdarian B, Pedersen J, Murphy DG. Immunohistochemical study of the cavernous nerves in the periprostatic region. BJU Int. 2011;107(8):1210–5.

22. Costello AJ, Brooks M, Cole OJ. Anatomical studies of the neurovascular bundle and cavernosal nerves. BJU Int. 2004;94(7):1071–6.

23. Lindsey I, Guy RJ, Warren BF, Mortensen NJ. Anatomy of Denonvilliers' fascia and pelvic nerves, impotence, and implications for the colorectal surgeon. Br J Surg. 2000;87(10):1288–99.

24. Lindsey I, Warren B, Mortensen N. Optimal total mesorectal excision for rectal cancer is by dissection in front of Denonvilliers' fascia (Br J Surg 2004; 91: 121–123). Br J Surg. 2004;91(7):897.

25. Lindsey I, Warren BF, Mortensen NJ. Denonvilliers' fascia lies anterior to the fascia propria and rectal dissection plane in total mesorectal excision. Dis Colon Rectum. 2005;48(1):37–42.

26. Myers RP. Detrusor apron, associated vascular plexus, and avascular plane: relevance to radical retropubic prostatectomy—anatomic and surgical commentary. Urology. 2002;59(4):472–9.

27. Myers RP, Goellner JR, Cahill DR. Prostate shape, external striated urethral sphincter and radical prostatectomy: the apical dissection. J Urol. 1987;138(3):543–50.

28. Walsh PC. Radical prostatectomy, preservation of sexual function, cancer control. The controversy. Urol Clin North Am. 1987;14(4):663–73.

29. Poore RE, McCullough DL, Jarow JP. Puboprostatic ligament sparing improves urinary continence after radical retropubic prostatectomy. Urology. 1998;51(1):67–72.

30. Asimakopoulos AD, Annino F, D'Orazio A, Pereira CF, Mugnier C, Hoepffner JL, et al. Complete periprostatic anatomy preservation during robot-assisted laparoscopic radical prostatectomy (RALP): the new pubovesical complex-sparing technique. Eur Urol. 2010;58(3):407–17.

31. Tewari AK, Bigelow K, Rao S, Takenaka A, El-Tabi N, Te A, et al. Anatomic restoration technique of continence mechanism and preservation of puboprostatic collar: a novel modification to achieve early urinary continence in men undergoing robotic prostatectomy. Urology. 2007;69(4):726–31.

32. Menon M, Shrivastava A, Kaul S, Badani KK, Fumo M, Bhandari M, et al. Vattikuti Institute prostatectomy: contemporary technique and analysis of results. Eur Urol. 2007;51(3):648–57. discussion 57–8.

33. Dorschner W, Stolzenburg JU. A new theory of micturition and urinary continence based on histomorphological studies. 3. The two parts of the musculus sphincter urethrae: physiological importance for continence in rest and stress. Urol Int. 1994;52(4):185–8.

34. Rocco F, Carmignani L, Acquati P, Gadda F, Dell'Orto P, Rocco B, et al. Restoration of posterior aspect of rhabdosphincter shortens continence time after radical retropubic prostatectomy. J Urol. 2006;175(6): 2201–6.

35. Bilhim T, Pisco JM, Rio Tinto H, Fernandes L, Pinheiro LC, Furtado A, et al. Prostatic arterial supply: anatomic and imaging findings relevant for selective arterial embolization. J Vasc Interv Radiol. 2012;23(11):1403–15.

36. Bilhim T, Tinto HR, Fernandes L, Martins Pisco J. Radiological anatomy of prostatic arteries. Tech Vasc Interv Radiol. 2012;15(4):276–85.

37. Carnevale FC, Antunes AA, da Motta Leal Filho JM, de Oliveira Cerri LM, Baroni RH, Marcelino AS, et al. Prostatic artery embolization as a primary treatment for benign prostatic hyperplasia: preliminary results in two patients. Cardiovasc Intervent Radiol. 2010;33(2):355–61.

38. Clegg EJ. The arterial supply of the human prostate and seminal vesicles. J Anat. 1955;89(2):209–16.

39. Pisco J, Campos Pinheiro L, Bilhim T, Duarte M, Rio Tinto H, Fernandes L, et al. Prostatic arterial embolization for benign prostatic hyperplasia: short- and intermediate-term results. Radiology. 2013;266(2):668–77.

40. Fernandes L, Rio Tinto H, Pereira J, Duarte M, Bilhim T, Martins Pisco J. Prostatic arterial embolization: post-procedural follow-up. Tech Vasc Interv Radiol. 2012;15(4):294–9.

41. Secin FP, Karanikolas N, Touijer AK, Salamanca JI, Vickers AJ, Guillonneau B. Anatomy of accessory pudendal arteries in laparoscopic radical prostatectomy. J Urol. 2005;174(2):523–6. discussion 6.

42. Secin FP, Touijer K, Mulhall J, Guillonneau B. Anatomy and preservation of accessory pudendal arteries in laparoscopic radical prostatectomy. Eur Urol. 2007;51(5):1229–35.

43. Garcia-Monaco R, Garategui L, Kizilevsky N, Peralta O, Rodriguez P, Palacios-Jaraquemada J. Human cadaveric specimen study of the prostatic arterial anatomy: implications for arterial embolization. J Vasc Interv Radiol. 2014;25(2):315–22.

44. Power NE, Silberstein JL, Kulkarni GS, Laudone VP. The dorsal venous complex (DVC): dorsal venous or dorsal vasculature complex? Santorini's plexus revisited. BJU Int. 2011;108(6):930–2.

45. Reiner WG, Walsh PC. An anatomical approach to the surgical management of the dorsal vein and Santorini's plexus during radical retropubic surgery. J Urol. 1979;121(2):198–200.

46. Benoit G, Droupy S, Quillard J, Paradis V, Giuliano F. Supra and infralevator neurovascular pathways to the penile corpora cavernosa. J Anat. 1999;195(Pt 4):605–15.

47. Tewari A, Takenaka A, Mtui E, Horninger W, Peschel R, Bartsch G, et al. The proximal neurovascular plate and the tri-zonal neural architecture around the prostate gland: importance in the athermal robotic technique of nerve-sparing prostatectomy. BJU Int. 2006;98(2):314–23.

48. Gosling JA, Dixon JS. The structure and innervation of smooth muscle in the wall of the bladder neck and proximal urethra. Br J Urol. 1975;47(5):549–58.

49. Akita K, Sakamoto H, Sato T. Origins and courses of the nervous branches to the male urethral sphincter. Surg Radiol Anat. 2003;25(5-6):387–92.

50. Narayan P, Konety B, Aslam K, Aboseif S, Blumenfeld W, Tanagho E. Neuroanatomy of the external urethral sphincter: implications for urinary continence preservation during radical prostate surgery. J Urol. 1995;153(2):337–41.

51. Strasser H, Ninkovic M, Hess M, Bartsch G, Stenzl A. Anatomic and functional studies of the male and female urethral sphincter. World J Urol. 2000;18(5): 324–9.

52. Hollabaugh Jr RS, Dmochowski RR, Steiner MS. Neuroanatomy of the male rhabdosphincter. Urology. 1997;49(3):426–34.

53. Srivastava A, Grover S, Sooriakumaran P, Tan G, Takenaka A, Tewari AK. Neuroanatomic basis for traction-free preservation of the neural hammock during athermal robotic radical prostatectomy. Curr Opin Urol. 2011;21(1):49–59.

54. Wei JT, Dunn RL, Marcovich R, Montie JE, Sanda MG. Prospective assessment of patient reported urinary continence after radical prostatectomy. J Urol. 2000;164(3 Pt 1):744–8.

55. Burkhard FC, Kessler TM, Fleischmann A, Thalmann GN, Schumacher M, Studer UE. Nerve sparing open radical retropubic prostatectomy—does it have an impact on urinary continence? J Urol. 2006;176(1): 189–95.

56. Shafik A. A study of the continence mechanism of the external urethral sphincter with identification of the voluntary urinary inhibition reflex. J Urol. 1999; 162(6):1967–71.

57. Karam I, Droupy S, Abd-Alsamad I, Uhl JF, Benoit G, Delmas V. Innervation of the female human urethral sphincter: 3D reconstruction of immunohistochemical studies in the fetus. Eur Urol. 2005;47(5):627–33. discussion 34.

58. Song LJ, Lu HK, Wang JP, Xu YM. Cadaveric study of nerves supplying the membranous urethra. Neurourol Urodyn. 2010;29(4):592–5.

59. Alsaid B, Moszkowicz D, Peschaud F, Bessede T, Zaitouna M, Karam I, et al. Autonomic-somatic communications in the human pelvis: computer-assisted anatomic dissection in male and female fetuses. J Anat. 2011;219(5):565–73.

60. Strasser H, Klima G, Poisel S, Horninger W, Bartsch G. Anatomy and innervation of the rhabdosphincter of the male urethra. Prostate. 1996;28(1):24–31.

61. Michl UH, Lange D, Graefen M, Huland H. Re: intraoperative nerve stimulation with measurement of urethral sphincter pressure changes during radical retropubic prostatectomy: a feasibility study. C. P. Nelson, J. E. Montie, E. J. McGuire, G. Wedemeyer and J.T. Wei. J Urol, 169: 2225–2228, 2003. J Urol. 2004;171(1):359. author reply.

Basic Physics of Diagnostic Ultrasound

Ernest J. Feleppa

The development of small, easy-to-operate ultrasonic imaging systems has led to the widespread use of ultrasound to visualize anatomic structures during clinical examinations and surgical procedures. These systems provide clinicians with high-definition, real-time images that facilitate transcutaneous, endoscopic, and intraoperative visualization and evaluation. To interpret ultrasonic images effectively and to apply the information they provide properly in the emergency room, endoscopic suite, or operating room, the clinician can benefit from an understanding of some of the basic physics of ultrasonography. This chapter briefly presents key principles of ultrasound that have a direct bearing on medical applications of ultrasound. More-comprehensive discussions of ultrasonic imaging are available in various other technical, scientific, and engineering publications [1–12].

Fundamental Concepts

Sound is a vibration that propagates through a medium and transports mechanical energy. It consists of alternating high- and low-pressure regions in the direction of propagation. These alternating high- and low-pressure regions represent waves; the regions are sometimes termed *regions of compression* and *regions of rarefaction,* respectively. Because the compressions and rarefactions cause the medium to move forward and backward in an oscillatory manner parallel to the propagation direction, the waves are termed *longitudinal waves*; occasionally, the term *compression wave* is used. In contrast, waves that have oscillatory medium movement perpendicular to the propagation direction, such as ocean surface waves, are termed *transverse waves*. All waves can be characterized by their wavelength, frequency, and propagation velocity, which are related by the equation

$$c = v\lambda \tag{1}$$

where c is the propagation speed, v is the oscillation frequency, and λ is the wavelength. The mechanical properties (e.g., "rigidity") of the propagation medium determine c; the source of the sound determines v; and λ simply equals c/v. The propagation speed is measured in units of distance per unit of time, e.g., meters per second (m/s) or millimeters per microsecond (mm/μs). Frequency is the rate at which rarefactions or compressions pass a point in space; it is measured in units of cycles per second or Hertz. The inverse of the frequency is termed the *period, T*; the period is commonly used to specify wave properties and is measured in units of time, e.g., microseconds (μs). Frequency and period generally do not change as a wave propagates through

E.J. Feleppa, Ph.D., F.A.I.U.M., F.A.I.M.B.E. (✉)
Biomedical Engineering Laboratory, Lizzi Center for
Biomedical Engineering, Riverside Research,
156 William Street, 9th Floor, New York,
NY 10038, USA
e-mail: efeleppa@riversideresearch.org

C.R. Porter and E.M. Wolff (eds.), *Prostate Ultrasound: Current Practice and Future Directions,*
DOI 10.1007/978-1-4939-1948-2_4, © Springer Science+Business Media New York 2015

Table 1 Attenuation coefficients and speed of sound of various tissues

Tissue type	Attenuation (dB/MHz-cm)	Sound speed (m/s)	Reference
Aqueous humor (human)	0.10	–	[13]
Blood (human, heparinized)	0.22	1,542	[15]
Bone (human, femur)	25.6	3,375	[15]
Breast (human, *in vivo*)[a]	0.28–0.63	–	[15]
Breast (human, *in vivo*)[a]	1.7	–	[16]
Choroidal melanoma (human, *in vivo*)	0.90	–	[15]
Fat (dog, omentum, *in vivo*)	–	1,459	[15]
Fat (human, subcutaneous, *ex vivo*)	0.64	–	[15]
Liver (human, *ex vivo*)	0.64	–	[15]
Ocular lens (human)	2.0	–	[13]
Uterus (human, *in vivo*)	0.22–0.44	–	[15]
Vitreous humor (human)	0.10	–	[13]

[a]Note the wide range of published values for breast-tissue attenuation. See the cited references for a discussion of the methodologies [13–16]

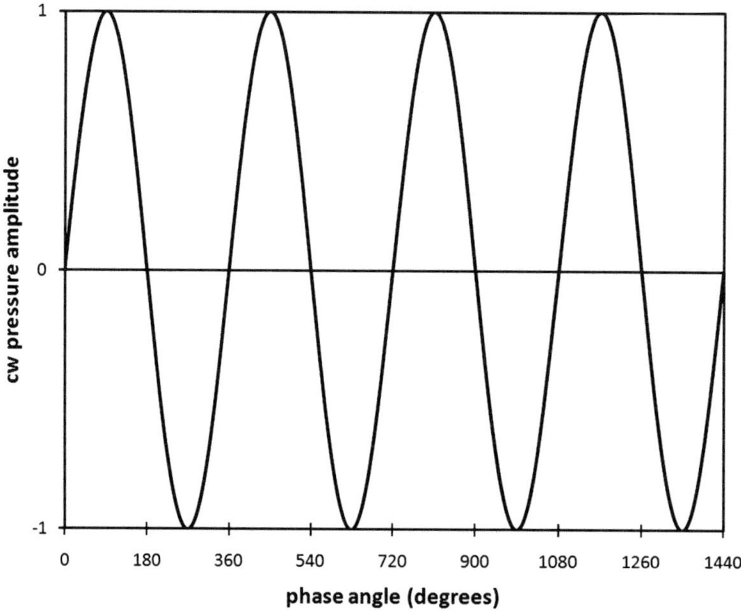

Fig. 1 A continuous wave (cw). A four-cycle portion of a simple, continuous, sinusoidal signal with uniform amplitude

one or several different media. The wavelength is the distance between two adjacent rarefactions or compressions or any adjacent points of like "phase"; it is measured in units of distance, e.g., meters (m) or microns (μm). The speed of sound ranges from about 340 m/s in air to more than 6,000 m/s in granite and glass. In tissue, sound speed is close to that of water, i.e., approximately 1,500 m/s; it varies with tissue type, and ultrasonic instruments typically use a fixed assumed value of 1,540 m/s for the sound propagation speed in tissue. Speed-of-sound values for some tissues are shown in Table 1.

Figure 1 illustrates how the pressure amplitude of a simple, sinusoidal, continuous wave (cw) varies with time or with distance. The figure shows the pressure amplitude, A, the wavelength, λ, and the phase angles of the wave.

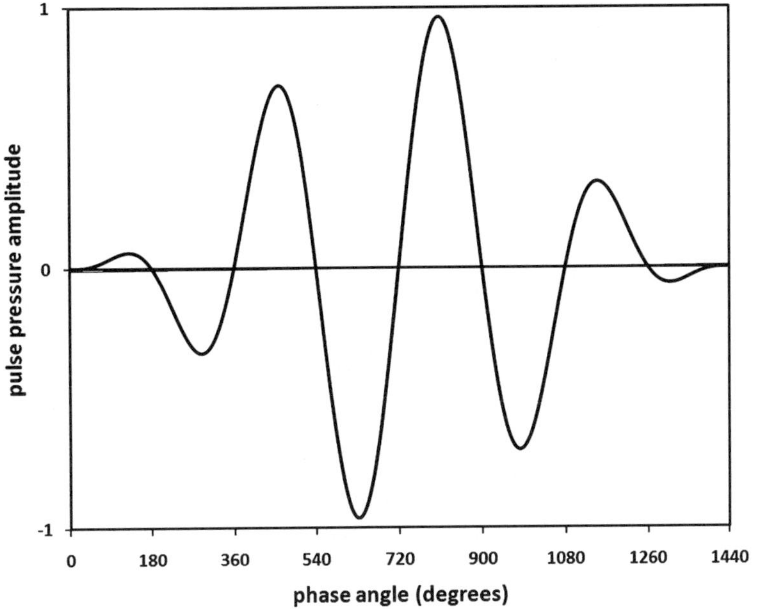

Fig. 2 A pulse wave. Four cycles of a modulated sinusoidal signal illustrate a pulse used for imaging

The frequency range to which the human ear responds is 20–20,000 Hz. For a propagation speed in air of 340 m/s, this frequency range corresponds to a wavelength range of 17 m to 17 mm. Most conventional diagnostic ultrasound instruments operate in the frequency range of 1.5–15 million cycles per second or megahertz (MHz). Assuming a propagation speed in tissue of 1,500 m/s, this frequency range corresponds to a wavelength range of 1.0–0.1 mm. General-purpose instruments tend to employ frequencies ranging from 3 to 10 MHz; frequencies below 3 MHz and above 10 MHz tend to be used only in special-purpose instruments. Intraoperative or endoscopic (endoluminal) instruments can use higher frequencies ranging from 5 to 15 MHz because attenuation (discussed later) is less of a limiting factor than it is in percutaneous applications.

An important variable that affects many propagation phenomena is acoustic impedance. The acoustic impedance, z, is defined as

$$z = \rho c \qquad (2)$$

where ρ is the mass density of the propagation medium and c is the speed of sound.

Ultrasonic imaging systems transmit brief bursts of ultrasonic energy commonly termed *pulses*. These pulses contain one or a very few complete cycles of the ultrasound signal. Brief pulses are also short in terms of their length in space. For example, a 10-MHz signal that spans two full cycles, i.e., two wavelengths of sound, has an overall length of 300 μm (0.3 mm) in a medium with a sound speed of 1,500 m/s, which approximates conditions in soft tissue.

Figure 2 illustrates how the pressure amplitudes of sinusoidal waves vary with time; the variation with distance is the inverse (left to right) of the depicted curves. Figure 2 shows the shape of a typical transmitted diagnostic-ultrasound pulse.

Imaging ultrasound uses very brief (therefore, short) ultrasonic pulses for a variety of reasons, such as resolution, that are discussed below in the section describing imaging phenomena. These very brief signals conventionally are characterized by a nominal frequency. However, because of the brevity of these signals, they do not consist of a single frequency; rather, they consist of a continuous distribution of frequencies over a usable frequency range or *band*, and the center of

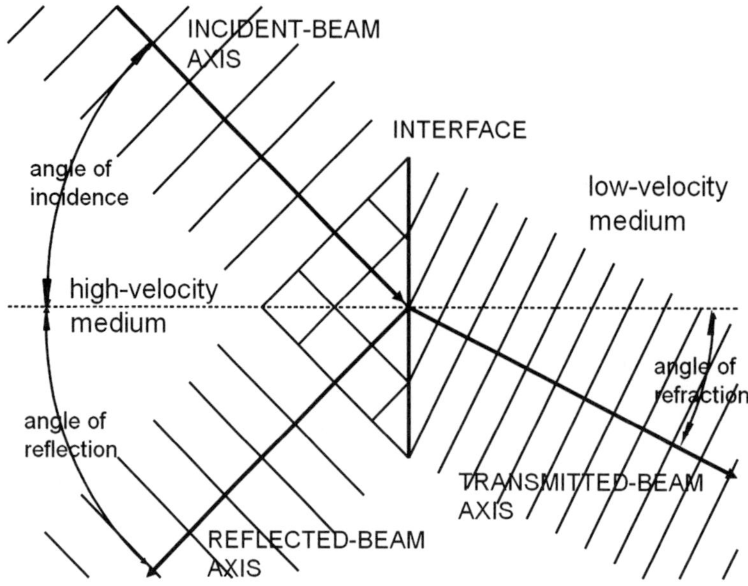

Fig. 3 Reflection and refraction at an interface. The incident wave is specularly reflected at a reflection angle equal to the incident angle and is transmitted at a refraction angle that depends upon the sound-propagation speeds of the two media

the band defines the nominal frequency of the signal. Only a very long signal (compared to the period of the wave) can properly be defined by a single frequency. A brief pulse consisting of one or a very few cycles of sound is termed a *broadband signal*. Usable bandwidth affects many properties of ultrasonic imaging systems, including axial spatial resolution (i.e., resolution in the propagation direction) and Doppler resolution, as discussed later in this chapter.

The propagation of alternating high- and low-pressure regions within a medium corresponds to the transport of energy through the medium. The energy is proportional to the square of the pressure amplitude of the wave. The intensity of the wave is defined as the power density, i.e., power over a unit of area, and power density typically is expressed as watts per square centimeter (W/cm^2).

In addition to being characterized by its amplitude, a wave can be characterized by its phase, which is expressed in terms of angular units, i.e., degrees or radians ($360° = 2\pi$ rad, i.e., 1 rad is approximately 57.3°). If the phase of a sinusoidal signal is considered to be zero when the pressure is increasing through zero, then the phase is 90° at the positive-pressure maximum, 180° as the pressure decreases through zero, 270° at the negative pressure maximum, and 360° as the pressure increases again through zero, as shown for the cw case in Fig. 1. (Pressure is defined here in relation to ambient pressure, i.e., the pressure in the medium. Absolute pressure never can be less than zero). Note that 360° corresponds to one full wavelength. Waves can be characterized in space by contours of constant phase; these contours are termed *wavefronts*. The wavefronts of ocean waves are curves parallel to the surface and perpendicular to the direction of propagation at any point; the wavefronts of ultrasonic waves are surfaces in three dimensions and also are perpendicular to the direction of propagation at any point. The schematic depictions of wave propagation in this text show waves in terms of their wavefronts, e.g., in Figs. 3, 4 and 5.

Propagation Phenomena

Like all waves, ultrasonic waves are affected by the following propagation phenomena: refraction, reflection and transmission, scattering, absorption, attenuation, dispersion, interference,

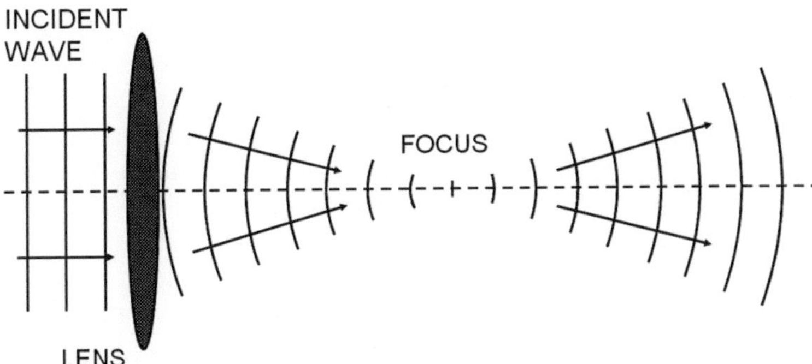

Fig. 4 Refraction by a lens. Refraction at the lens surface causes the wave to converge to a focal point and then diverge beyond the focal point

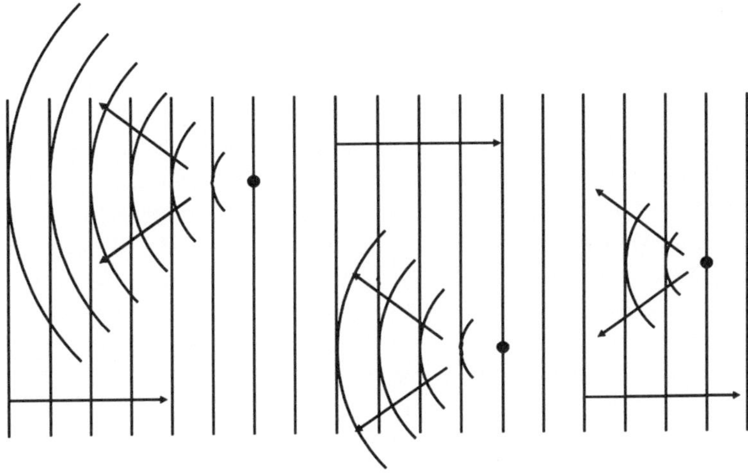

Fig. 5 Backscattering. The incident ultrasound wave is redirected by scattering particles; the portion that is redirected back toward the source is termed the *backscattered* wave

and diffraction. Clinicians must understand how these phenomena affect the propagation of ultrasonic waves in order to understand the principles underlying ultrasound image formation.

Refraction

If a wave passes from a medium with one propagation speed into a medium with a different propagation speed, and if the direction of propagation is not perpendicular to the interface between the two media, then the direction of propagation changes as the wave passes from the first medium into the second. The propagation direction is more nearly perpendicular to the interface in the lower-velocity medium, as illustrated in Fig. 3.

Refraction provides a means of focusing waves by using lenses. The curved surface of a spherical lens causes the propagation direction to change more for regions of the wave that pass through the peripheral portions of the lens than for those that pass through the central portions. As shown in Fig. 4, this effect can be exploited to concentrate the wave of a broad beam into a narrow focal region. The relationship between the refracted and incident beam angles is

$$\sin\theta_2 = (c_2 / c_1)\sin\theta_1 \qquad (3)$$

where θ_1 and θ_2 respectively are the angles of the incident and refracted propagation directions relative to the perpendicular to the interface between the two media, and c_1 and c_2 are the sound speeds of the incident and refracted waves. Note that if $c_2 = c_1$, then no change occurs in the direction of propagation at the interface. Similarly, if the incidence is normal, i.e., if the beam is perpendicular to the interface and $\sin\theta_1 = 0$, then $\sin\theta_2 = 0$, then again, no change occurs in the direction of propagation at the interface. If $c_2 > c_1$ and the value of $(c_2/c_1)\sin\theta_1$ equals 1, then the refracted wave does not penetrate the interface; it is totally reflected at the interface. The angle at which this occurs is termed the *critical angle* for total internal reflection, and it can occur at the lateral walls of cysts or the surfaces of bones, as discussed in the section on ultrasound propagation in tissue. At any angle of incidence beyond the critical angle, all wave energy is reflected, as described in the next section.

Refraction along the propagation path in tissues can degrade the quality of images, either by causing an imaged structure to be displaced from its actual position or by randomly perturbing the uniform propagation properties of an ultrasound beam thereby "blurring" and distorting imaged structures. This effect can be minimized by orienting the transducer beam perpendicular to the tissue interfaces causing the refraction; so called phase aberrations caused by refraction are discussed further in the section describing imaging phenomena. Phase aberration is the subject of considerable research; however, a discussion of the methods of minimizing it is beyond the scope of this chapter.

Reflection and Transmission

Reflection is the partial reversal of the propagation direction of a wave incident on a smooth interface between media with different acoustic impedances. The smoothness of the surface is defined with respect to the wavelength of the incident wave; a smooth surface has irregularities on a scale far smaller than a wavelength. Reflection by objects that are smooth compared to a wavelength is termed *specular*; reflection by objects that are not smooth compared to a wavelength is termed *diffuse*.

As shown in Fig. 3, reflection reverses the direction of the incident propagation component perpendicular to the interface, but it does not change the propagation component parallel to the interface. In specular reflection, the angle of propagation of the reflected wave with respect to the perpendicular to the surface is the negative of the angle of the incident wave. (An analog to specular ultrasonic reflection is the reflection of light from a mirror.) In diffuse reflection from a rough surface, i.e., where surface irregularities are larger than a fraction of a wavelength, most of the reflected energy may be concentrated about the propagation direction of specular reflection, but a significant proportion of the reflected energy randomly propagates at other, slightly different angles. (Reflection of light from a matte surface is analogous to diffuse ultrasonic reflection.)

The pressure amplitude, A_2, of a specularly reflected wave is

$$A_2 = A_1 (z_2 - z_1) / (z_2 + z_1) \qquad (4A)$$

where A_1 is the incident pressure amplitude and z_2 and z_1 are the acoustic impedances of the two media and z_1 is the impedance of the medium where the wave originates. The reflection coefficient, R_I, is

$$R = I_2 / I_1 = (A_2 / A_1^2) = ((z_2 - z_1)^2 / (z_2 + z_1)^2) \qquad (4B)$$

where I_2 is the *intensity* (i.e., the square of the amplitude) of the reflected wave and I_1 is the intensity of the incident wave. Because energy is conserved, the wave that continues through the reflecting interface, i.e., the transmitted wave, contains all the energy of the incident wave minus the energy of the reflected wave. Therefore, the transmission coefficient, T_I, is

$$T = I_3 / I_1 = A_3^{\,2} / A_1^{\,2} = (1 - R)$$
$$= 1 - (z_2 - z_1)^2 / (z_2 + z_1)^2$$
$$= 4z_1 z_2 / (z_2 + z_1)^2 \qquad (4C)$$

and the pressure amplitude, A_3, of the transmitted wave is

$$A_3 = 2A_1 (z_1 z_2)^{1/2} / (z_2 + z_1) \qquad (4D)$$

Note that if either z_1 or z_2 is far greater than the other, i.e., a very strong impedance mismatch exists, then $R \to 1$, $A_2 \to A_1$, $A_3 \to 0$, and nearly all incident ultrasound is reflected while almost none is transmitted. A good example of this would be the strong reflections at the surface of bone or an air-filled space such as the lung. Alternatively, if $z_1 = z_2$, i.e., if no impedance mismatch exists, then $T = 1$, $A_3 = A_1$, and $A_2 = 0$, and all incident ultrasound is transmitted while none is reflected. An example of this would be the transmission of the sound wave inside a simple cyst. A simple cyst has no internal signal because it is uniform liquid and so its impedance properties remain uniform, and consequently no scattering or reflection of the sound wave occurs. Also, note that in total internal reflection, described in the section on refraction, $R = 1$ and $T = 0$.

Scattering

Scattering is the random redirection of energy out of an incident wave; it results from the interaction of the incident wave with scattering entities that are small compared to the wavelength of the incident ultrasound. The scattering entities are called *scatterers*, and in tissue, the actual scatterers may be blood vessels, collagen fibers, microscopic pockets of necrosis, individual or aggregated melanocytes, foam cells, platelet aggregates, or other microscopic tissue constituents or simply spatial variations in the velocity of propagation or density of the tissue (i.e., variations in acoustic impedance). Depending upon the size, shape, and orientation of the scatterers, scattering can redirect energy uniformly in all directions, or it can redirect energy primarily in the same direction as the incident propagation (termed forward scattering) or in the reverse direction (termed *backward scattering* or *backscattering*), as shown in Fig. 5. In most cases, backscattered energy provides the signals utilized in ultrasonic image formation. The amount of backscattered energy depends upon the size, shape, concentration, and relative acoustic impedance of the scatterers. The relative acoustic impedance, Q, is the impedance of the scatterers compared to their surroundings and can be expressed as

$$Q = (z_s - z_m) / (z_s + z_m) \qquad (5)$$

where z_s is the scatterer impedance and z_m is the impedance of the surrounding medium. The amount of energy that is backscattered increases as scatterer size, concentration, and the square of relative acoustic impedance increase. However, backscattering is most strongly dependent on scatterer size. (Note the similarity of the expression for relative acoustic impedance in Eq. (5) to the expression describing reflection in Eqs. (4A and 4B).

Because scattering causes energy to be redirected out of the forward-propagating wave, it reduces the total energy carried by the wave in the forward direction. The loss of energy in the forward-propagating wave is termed *attenuation* and it consists of absorption as well as scattering components.

Absorption

As an acoustic wave propagates through a medium, the alternating regions of high and low pressure cause vibrating movement to occur in the medium. Friction among vibrating elements within the medium generates heat. This converts acoustical to thermal energy; it reduces the acoustic energy in the ultrasound beam and dissipates it as heat within the medium. This phenomenon is termed *absorption*.

Attenuation

Absorption is a major cause of energy reduction in an ultrasound wave. However, reflection and scattering redirect acoustic energy from the wave propagating through a medium and contribute to the loss of energy propagated in the forward direction by the incident wave. The reduction of energy caused by the combination of absorption and scattering is termed *attenuation*. Attenuation can be described by the equation

$$A_2 = A_1 e^{-\alpha(x_2 - x_1)} \tag{6A}$$

where A_2 and A_1 are the pressure amplitudes at positions x_2 and x_1 (and where $x_2 > x_1$) and a is the frequency-dependent attenuation coefficient, commonly expressed as decibels (dB) per MHz-cm. (A decibel is a logarithmic expression of a ratio, e.g., 20 log (A_2/A_1) expresses the ratio of pressure, A_2, to pressure, A_1, in decibels. If A_2 is half of A_1 then 20 log $(A_2/A_1) = -6$ dB. Similarly, 10 log (I_2/I_1) expresses the ratio of intensity, I_2, to intensity, I_1, in decibels. If I_2 is half of I_1, then 10 log $(I_2/I_1) = -3$ dB.)

Attenuation increases with increasing ultrasound frequency. In tissue, attenuation increases approximately linearly with frequency, and α, the attenuation coefficient of Eq. (6A), is more-rigorously expressed as

$$\alpha(v) = \alpha_0 v^p \tag{6B}$$

where α_0 is the attenuation coefficient at 1 MHz, v is the frequency, and the exponent, p, is 1 if the frequency dependence is linear. In tissue, the value of p typically is very close to, but not exactly equal to, 1, and different tissues may exhibit different values of p. Interestingly, the value of p for water is approximately 2, i.e., the relatively very low attenuation coefficient of water at frequencies near 1 MHz quadruples when the ultrasound frequency doubles to 2 MHz.

The attenuation coefficients for tissues range from an insignificant value of <0.1 dB/MHz-cm for cystic and aqueous structures up to 2.0 dB/MHz-cm for the lens of the eye. Most solid soft tissues have attenuation coefficients in the range of 0.4–0.7 dB/MHzcm; some examples are shown Table 1 [13–16]. Because of the frequency dependence of attenuation, ultrasonic imaging of structures that lie deep within the body requires lower frequencies than those required for imaging structures that are near the surface or that are accessible intraoperatively or endoscopically. As discussed below, spatial resolution improves as frequency increases, but a judicious choice must be made between resolution and penetration depth when selecting an optimal ultrasound frequency for a specific imaging application.

Dispersion

Dispersion is not considered to be a significant phenomenon in medical ultrasonic acoustics, although it is quite important in optics. Dispersion is the separation of different frequency components of a propagating wave as a result of differences in propagation velocities for different frequencies. As an example, the spectrum produced by a prism and the chromatic aberration produced by a lens result from the fact that blue light propagates at a slower speed in the prism than red light and therefore is more strongly refracted.

Interference

When one part of a wave is made to be coincident with another part of a wave, e.g., through refraction or reflection, the combination of the two waves results in the algebraic summation of the pressure amplitudes of the waves. This phenomenon is termed *interference*. Recall that pressures in acoustic waves can be negative as well as positive; therefore, in some regions of space, interfering waves can combine to produce higher positive or negative pressures and in others they can cancel and produce reduced pressure. Interference that produces higher positive or negative pressures is called constructive interference; interference that reduces the pressure is called destructive interference. Because interference occurs over a volume, cancellation of out-of-phase waves

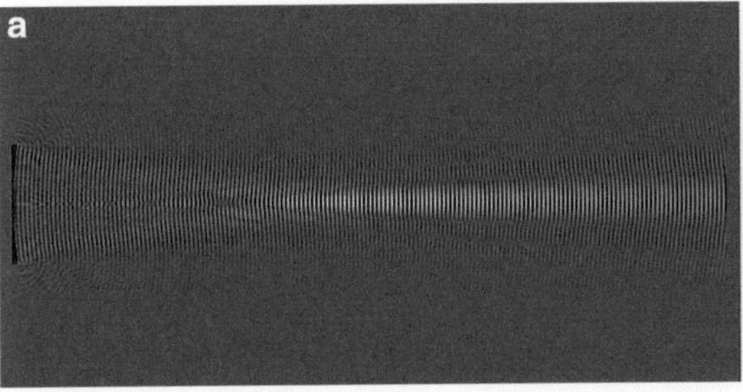 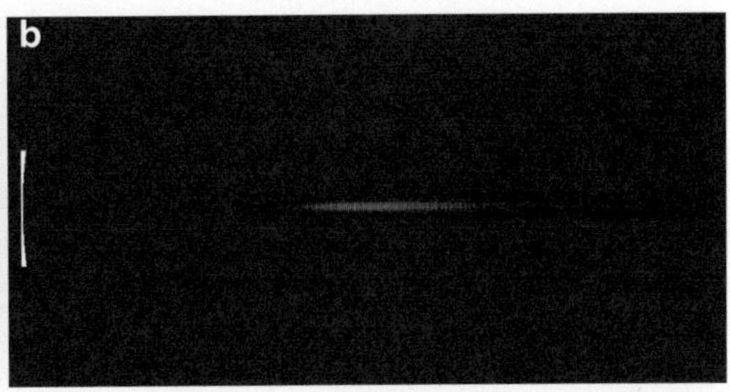

Fig. 6 Focused cw field generated by a spherically curved transducer. A continuously radiating transducer with an 8-mm aperture and a 32-mm radius of curvature generates the 5-MHz ultrasound field shown in the plane containing the transducer axis. Note the complex pattern proximal to the focus and the apparent peak values closer to the transducer than to the geometric (32-mm) focus. (**a**) Pressure-amplitude distribution (ambient pressure is *gray*, positive pressure is *light*, and negative pressure is *dark*). (**b**) Intensity distribution

(destructive interference) in one region of space is balanced by reinforcement of in-phase waves (constructive interference) in another region of space so that energy is conserved.

When a wave maintains a predictable and stable relationship over time or throughout space among the phase values at different points in the wave, it is termed a *coherent wave*. If interference occurs with a coherent signal, the pattern of constructive and destructive interference is stable. The light produced by lasers and the sound produced by medical ultrasonic imaging systems are two examples of coherent signals. The classic interference phenomenon associated with ultrasonic imaging is *speckle*, which is discussed below in the section on imaging.

Diffraction

If the distribution of ultrasonic energy over a surface in space is known, then the distribution of energy can be predicted over any other surface by considering every point on the first surface to be a source of a new wave. The wave emanating from each point interferes with the waves emanating from all other points to produce the new distribution of energy.

The propagation of waves in accordance with this phenomenon is termed *diffraction*; diffraction determines the distribution of wave energy accurately and is not subject to the limitations of simple geometric optics or acoustics, which assume that wave propagation can be defined by rays (straight lines). Diffraction more-realistically takes into account the complex distribution of energy in the acoustical waves generated by medical ultrasonic instruments, as illustrated in Figs. 6 and 7.

Figures 6 and 7 depict the ultrasonic pressure amplitudes and intensity distributions of ultrasound fields in accordance with strict diffraction phenomena, but that are not predicted by geometric optics. The dimensions are equivalent to those of a spherically curved transducer having an 8-mm aperture diameter and 32-mm radius of curvature generating a 5-MHz wave. These figures are computer-generated distributions of pressure amplitudes and intensity in a plane containing the axis of the transducer, i.e., a line drawn perpendicular to the concave surface of the transducer though the center of the transducer. Figures 6a and 7a show pressure amplitude distributions; Figs. 6b and 7b show intensity distributions. Figure 6 shows the pattern produced by a continuous wave. The focus, where the highest pressure amplitudes and intensity values occur, is slightly closer to the transducer than to the geometric focus. Note the clear patterns of constructive and destructive interference that occur in the *near field* between the transducer and the focal region Please note that the focus is where all the energy converges in the figure. Also note the patterns of pressure and intensity lateral to the central axial region; these distributions of energy are termed *side lobes* and are distributions

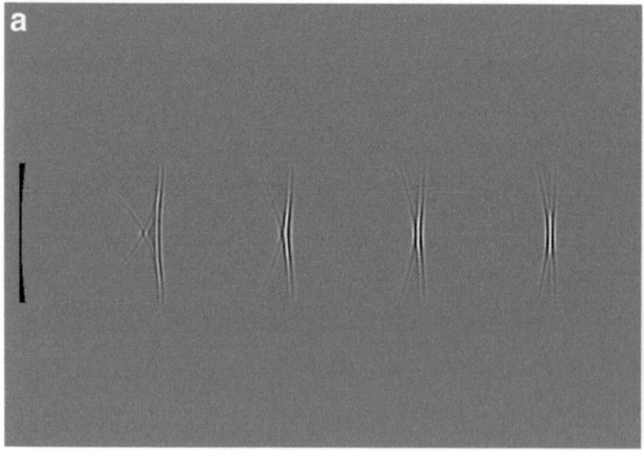
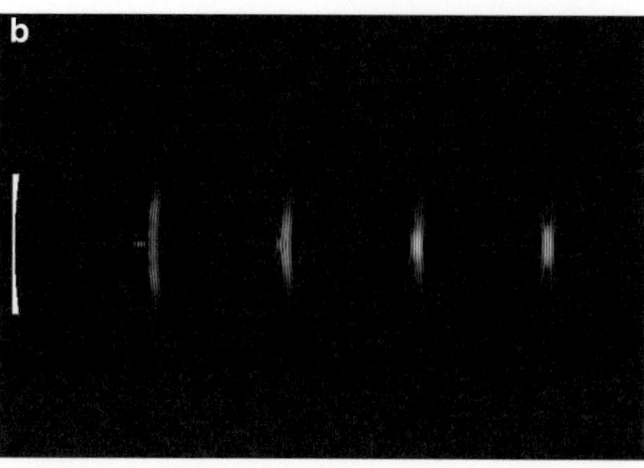

Fig. 7 Focused pulsed-wave fields generated by a spherically curved transducer. A spherical transducer equivalent to that of Fig. 6 generates the 5-MHz pulses shown in the axial plane; the pulses are "idealized" in a manner equivalent to the pulse depicted in Fig. 2. Note the gradual beam convergence to the symmetrical fourth pulse, which is located at the geometric focus; however, the third pulse actually displays the highest pressure-amplitude and intensity. (**a**) Pressure-amplitude distribution (ambient pressure is *gray*, positive pressure is *light*, and negative pressure is *dark*). (**b**) Intensity distribution

of energy coaxial with the central or main lobe This pattern is defined by Eq. (9) below. Figure 7 shows four nearly ideal pulses as they propagate from the spherically curved transducer. Note the arc-shaped patterns of energy distributed well outside the edges of the central pulse, and for the pulses nearest to the transducer, behind the pulse; these are termed *edge effects*, and are not significant in the continuous wave of Fig. 6 because, in the continuous wave train, they are canceled by subsequent portions of the wave. The edge effects are produced by the edge of the transducer and are not to be associated with edging artifacts that occur from a combination of reflection and refraction when sound waves strike a curved surface.

Imaging Phenomena

This section discusses imaging phenomena in terms of the following five topics: generation, propagation, and detection of ultrasonic waves; resolution; scanning methods; image-display methods; and image properties. For the clinician, interpretation of ultrasonic images requires an understanding of these topics. Health care providers may need to make decisions rapidly based on ultrasonic images generated in real-time; these decisions, which often are based upon the physician's subjective interpretation of images have an impact on the patient's outcome. Therefore, the clinician must be able to evaluate the information displayed on the monitor of the scanner expeditiously and accurately.

Generation of Ultrasonic Waves

Ultrasonic imaging instruments generate very brief (in time) pulses of ultrasound pressure to produce very short (in space) pressure perturbations in the propagating medium. Short pressure perturbations are necessary to achieve good resolution in the propagation direction, termed the *axial* or *range* dimension.

Ultrasound units used in clinical practice employ piezoelectric elements to generate and sense ultrasound signals; piezoelectric materials change their size when subject to a voltage and generate a voltage when subject to a pressure change. The means of generating acoustic pulses for ultrasonic imaging is illustrated schematically in Fig. 8. Generation of an acoustic pulse begins with electronic generation of a voltage pulse of brief duration. Modern instruments may generate voltage pulses that are "shaped" in time to maximize the efficiency of ultrasonic pulse generation. For example, while some systems may generate a simple "rectangular" pulse, more-sophisticated systems may generate a bipolar,

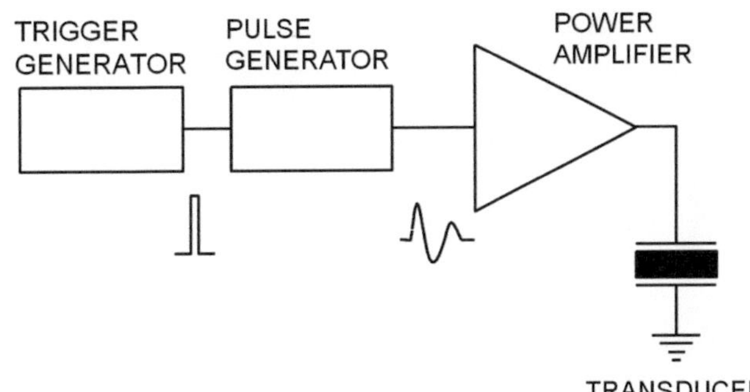

Fig. 8 Generating an ultrasound pulse. Control signals (e.g., from position sensors or timing circuits) produce a trigger voltage that is converted to a voltage pulse. The voltage pulse is amplified and applied to a piezoelectric element that generates an ultrasound pulse

sinusoidal pulse with a shape that matches the desired sinusoidal acoustic signal.

The voltage pulse is applied to a transducer consisting of one or several piezoelectric elements. (The use of multiple piezoelectric elements is discussed in the section addressing scanning methods.) A transducer is any device that converts electrical to mechanical energy or vice versa, e.g., a solenoid, a loud speaker, a strain gauge, a microphone, or in the case of ultrasound, one or more piezoelectric elements.

A piezoelectric transducer changes its thickness when a voltage is applied; this thickness change is a mechanical phenomenon that generates a pressure change at the surface of the transducer in contact with a propagating medium. If a continuous, sinusoidal voltage is applied, then the pressure change at the surface of the transducer also is continuous and sinusoidal. If the applied voltage is a brief pulse, then the voltage pulse causes the transducer to change thickness immediately and then to resonate briefly (like a struck bell or chime) at its natural resonance frequency, which is determined by its thickness and by the velocity of sound propagation within it. To obtain a brief ultrasonic pulse, a transducer must be damped to minimize its reverberation time. Damping is provided by using a backing material that absorbs sound. This material is placed in acoustic contact with the rear surface of the piezoelectric element and, in a high-quality transducer, reduces the acoustic pulse duration to slightly more than one period of the resonant frequency of the element.

A flat transducer generates a plane wave, i.e., a wave in which regions of the same phase define a plane at its surface. This is intuitively obvious, since the pressure pulse is generated along the flat surface of the transducer. However, because of diffraction, the wave is truly planar only immediately at the transducer surface. As the wave propagates away from the transducer, new waves are generated at every point on the wavefront, and the new waves generated at the edges of the original wave lead to spherical waves emanating outward from the propagation axis. Accordingly, the beam produced by a plane transducer is essentially planar, but actually is quite complex near the transducer, particularly at its periphery; eventually, at some distance from the transducer, diffraction leads to the formation of an approximately spherical wave that appears to originate from a point source. The fact that the planar transducer appears to be a point at distances far greater than the transducer aperture (diameter) may be intuitively apparent. The region where the beam is complex, but approximates a plane wave, is termed the *near field* (or *Fresnel region*); the region where it approximates a spherical wave is termed the *far field* (or *Fraunhofer region*). The range, L, at which the near field transitions to the far field is given by the equation

$$L = d^2 / 4\lambda \qquad (7)$$

where d is the diameter of aperture of the piezoelectric element.

In the far field, the beam width, B_u, where the intensity is 3 dB below (i.e., 50 % of) the intensity at the center of the beam, is given by the equation

$$B_u = \lambda z / d \qquad (8)$$

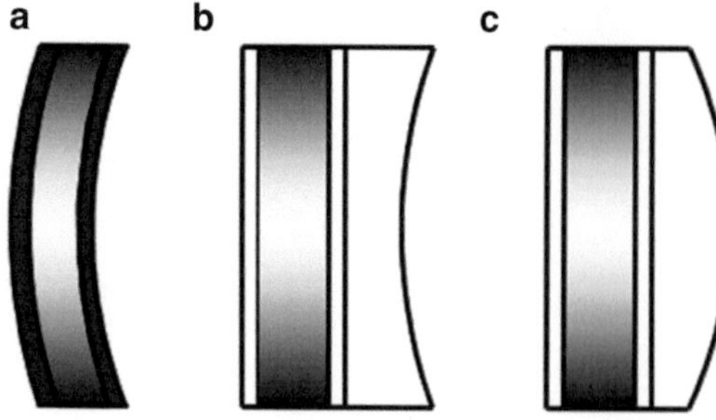

Fig. 9 Focusing an ultrasound beam. The shape of the wavefront can be made spherical by (**a**) shaping the transducer; (**b**) using a concave lens with a high speed of sound; or (**c**) using a convex lens with a low speed of sound

where z is the distance from the transducer to the point at which B_u is calculated. (Note that z must be greater than L for this equation to apply.) Clearly, the spreading beam generated by a planar transducer is too broad to be useful in imaging. Narrow beams are required to provide image resolution in a direction perpendicular to the beam axis; this direction is termed the *radial* or *cross-range* dimension. (Resolution is discussed later in this section.)

Narrow beams are formed by using focused transducers. Focused, single-element transducers may employ spherically curved piezoelectric elements or planar elements with lenses, as shown in Fig. 9. While simple geometric considerations would predict beam convergence to an infinitesimal width in the focal region, diffraction actually leads to a finite beam width in the focal zone and, in addition, forms concentric, secondary beams around the central beam. The central beam is termed the *main lobe* and the concentric beams outside the main lobe are termed *side lobes*. In the focal zone, the diameter, B_f, of the main lobe to the radial point the intensity is 3 dB below its central value, is given by the equation

$$B_f = \lambda F / d \tag{9}$$

where d is the diameter or aperture of the piezoelectric element and F is the distance from the surface of the spherically curved transducer or acoustic center of the lens to the center of the focal zone. (Note that for a curved transducer, $F = R$ where R is the radius of curvature. Also note that F/d is the *f-number* of the transducer element,

equivalent to the *f*-number of a lens.) As this equation shows, shorter wavelengths (i.e., higher frequencies) give narrower beams at the focus for a given transducer geometry. A typical transducer may have an *f*-number of 4; then, if the frequency is 10 MHz, the wavelength is 150 μm, and the focal-zone beamwidth is 600 μm or (0.6 mm), according to Eq. (9). For a given frequency, increasing the aperture or decreasing the focal length decreases the focal-zone beam width. A major trade-off in specifying the focusing properties of the transducer involves the choice between the width of the beam at the focus and the length of the focal zone. If frequency is not changed, then decreasing the ratio F/d, i.e., decreasing the f-number, narrows the beam in the focal zone but also shortens the distance over which the beam is sharply focused; increasing the ratio F/d broadens the beam but lengthens the distance over which the beam is narrow.

A second trade-off in specifying transducer properties involves the choice between a focal zone size and penetration depth. If transducer geometry is kept constant, increasing the frequency shortens the pulse and reduces the size of the focal zone; however, because attenuation is proportional to frequency, the depth of penetration of the ultrasound beam is reduced. For these reasons, ophthalmic systems, which examine small structures and are not significantly affected by attenuation in the vitreous humor, use high frequencies (in the range of 10–15 MHz). Breast systems, which examine structures within a few centimeters or so of the surface through a medium consisting of skin, a thin layer of subcutaneous fat, connective fibrous tissue, and glandular tissue, tend to use intermediate frequencies (in the range of 5–8 MHz). Abdominal systems, which examine deeply lying structures such as the kidneys, liver, and pancreas through several centimeters of subcutaneous and other fat layers, muscle layers, and visceral organs require lower frequencies (in the range of 3–5 MHz). Intraoperative and endoscopic ultrasound systems do not need to traverse body-wall tissues and can utilize moderately high frequencies (in the range of 5–10 MHz) to obtain improved resolution. (See the discussion of resolution later in this section.)

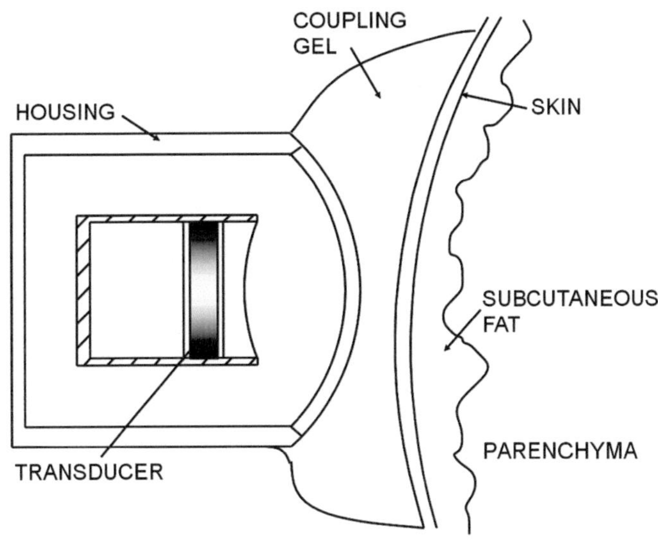

Fig. 10 Refractive and reflective interfaces. The ultrasound-transmitted and echo-signal pulses pass through several interfaces outside and within the body (e.g., surfaces of the transducer lens, transducer-housing surfaces, skin, and subcutaneous layers)

Propagation of Ultrasonic Pulses in Tissue

As the ultrasound pulse generated by the piezo-electric element propagates from the element, it may first pass through a coupling medium within the transducer housing, a membrane or capsule layer at the face of the transducer housing, a coupling medium (such as a saline water bath or gel) between the transducer and tissue, and finally tissue; this is schematically illustrated in Fig. 10. In transcutaneous applications, the propagating beam first encounters skin and subcutaneous layers, and is relatively strongly refracted and reflected at the surfaces it encounters. Similar reflections and refractions may occur in intraoperative or endoscopic applications, but in some cases, the surface layers that cause the relatively strong, complex, transcutaneous reflections and refractions are absent.

Once the ultrasound pulse enters tissue, it is subject to scattering at every change of impedance—even microscopic changes with scale sizes on the order of a few tens of microns, depending on the ultrasonic wavelength. The granular microstructure of tissue typically represents continuously changing impedance; therefore, ultrasound passing though tissue is effectively being scattered continuously in all directions. Differences in microstructural tissue architecture cause the scattering to differ somewhat from tissue to tissue, and to be markedly different at organ surfaces and at interfaces between tissues. The relatively uniform scattering within homogeneous tissue, such as liver parenchyma, leads to the relatively even texture pattern presented on an ultrasound image. In contrast, the relatively abrupt differences in impedance at the interfaces between tissues cause reflections or strong scattering and lead to image features that permit the visualization of tissue boundaries and internal organ structure.

As the pulse propagates through tissue, scattering, reflection, and absorption reduce its energy; therefore, less energy is backscattered or reflected from tissues distal to the transducer than from tissues proximal to the transducer. If the pulse encounters a structure with higher attenuation than the adjacent tissues, then tissue distal to the high-attenuation structure receives less ultrasonic energy than tissue distal to adjacent tissues; this effect is termed *shadowing*. However, if the pulse encounters a structure with less attenuation than the adjacent tissues, such as a cyst, then tissues distal to the low-attenuation structure receive more ultrasonic energy than adjacent tissues; this effect is termed *anti-shadowing* or *posterior enhancement*. Calcifications and calculi are examples of tissue constituents that cause extreme shadowing; cancerous lesions commonly produce moderate shadowing. Cysts, large vessels, and ducts are examples of structures that cause anti-shadowing or posterior enhancement. In addition, the smooth, curved surfaces of cysts and vessels and the significant difference in propagation velocity inside and outside their borders often produce strong refractive effects; such refractive effects are visible as complex patterns of artifactual shadowing and enhancement distal to the lateral boundaries of cysts and vessels. Because of the extreme difference in the impedance of bone and soft tissue, the surfaces of bone cause extreme refractive and reflective effects. Little ultrasonic energy penetrates bone from soft tissue because of reflection, and the energy that propagates past the surface is strongly refracted and attenuated, so that bone typically presents a very bright proximal surface and severe shadowing.

Detection of Ultrasound

Virtually all contemporary ultrasonic instruments use the piezoelectric elements in a transducer to receive as well as to transmit ultrasound. Any propagation event, such as scattering or reflection, that redirects the ultrasonic pulse back along its initial path leads to an echo signal impinging upon the piezoelectric elements of the transmitting transducer.

When ultrasonic energy returns to the piezoelectric elements, the high- and low-pressure regions of the incident train of pulses impinging on the elements deform the piezoelectric material in an oscillatory manner, causing it to generate an oscillatory voltage. Hence, the ultrasonic echo signal incident upon the piezoelectric element is converted to an electrical signal. The voltage of this signal is proportional to the average pressure across the entire face of the receiving piezoelectric element; therefore, if the wavefront impinges on the element at an angle, the average pressure across the element may be very low. Although pulses of 200 V or more are used to generate acoustic waves, the relatively small amount of

energy returning to the transducer from tissue results in echo-signal voltages of a few millivolts (mv) or less. As a consequence, the electronics that receive, amplify, and process the echo-signal voltages face the difficult task of withstanding the very-high-voltage pulses needed to generate ultrasonic pulses, recovering from those high voltages, and processing very-low-voltage signals derived from the ultrasonic echoes. (The time available for recovery is very brief; the echo signal from a distance of 7.5 mm arrives at the transducer approximately 10 µs after the transmitted pulse is generated.)

The returning ultrasonic echo signals from tissue consist of high- and low-pressure regions. Therefore, the echo-signal voltage generated by the piezoelectric element is positive and negative (i.e., bipolar), with amplitude and phase properties matching those of the received ultrasonic signal. This bipolar voltage signal is termed the *radiofrequency* (*RF*) *signal*.

The RF signal is not suitable for a display; it is converted into a display signal termed the *video* or *envelope signal*. Traditional ultrasonic systems generate the signal displayed on the monitor in four steps: (1) amplify the echo-signal voltage as it is generated by a piezoelectric element; (2) rectify it so that it is a unipolar signal (either all positive or all negative); (3) smooth it to produce the video signal representing the envelope of the received RF signals; and (4) further amplify the video signal, typically applying greater amplification to low-amplitude signals than to high-amplitude signals thereby "compressing" the signal so that a greater range of signal amplitudes can be accommodated within the dynamic range of the display system. The video signal determines the brightness of pixels in the image that represents the ultrasound scan. The sequence of steps leading to traditional video-signal generation is depicted schematically in Fig. 11.

Most modern instruments convert the RF echo-signal voltages to digital signals and generate their video signals digitally. This approach is particularly useful in systems that employ array transducers, as discussed below.

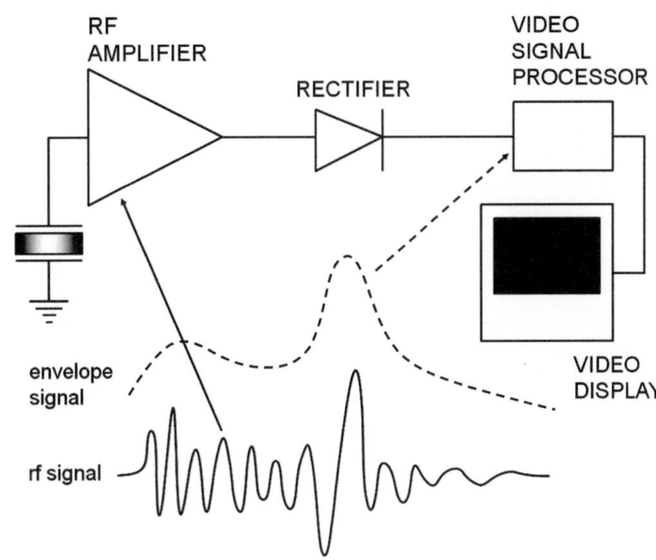

Fig. 11 Receiving an ultrasound pulse. Returning, echo-signal, pressure pulse trains impinge on a transducer, which generates a weak oscillatory (positive and negative) voltage signal. The weak echo-signal voltage is amplified, rectified (to make an all-positive or all-negative envelope signal), and further processed and amplified (typically with compression) to produce the video signal that controls pixel brightness in the image

Image Resolution

Resolution is a very important property of imaging systems. It is properly defined as the *minimal distance* between two imaged objects at which the two objects can be determined to be separate objects. Strictly speaking, *lower* resolution is superior to *higher* resolution according to this definition. However, popular usage has tended to reverse this terminology. This semantic confusion can be prevented by using the terms *finer*, *superior*, and their equivalent to describe resolution that permits closer-spaced objects to be distinguished.

Axial or *range resolution* refers to the ability of an ultrasonic imaging system to distinguish two objects that are at different distances or ranges from the transducer along the beam axis. Under these conditions, the two objects are insonified by the same transmitted pulse; they are separated from each other only in the direction of the beam axis. As indicated above, axial resolution depends on the pulse duration, but as a simple, practical approximation for a modern high-definition (low-resolution) instrument, the minimal practical pulse length is 1.5 cycles, i.e., the spatial pulse length is approximately 1.5λ. Therefore, resolution can be considered to be 1.5 times the wavelength of the pulse generated at the resonant frequency of the transducer. For a 10-MHz ophthalmic system, a propagation velocity of 1,500 m/s results in a wavelength of 150 μm and therefore an axial resolution of approximately 1.5×150 μm $= 225$ μm. A 20-MHz system has a wavelength of 75 μm and therefore an axial resolution of approximately 113 μm. While these guidelines are practical for real systems, theoretical limits are approximately half the values determined from these guidelines; for example, a 10-MHz system theoretically could have a resolution as fine as 112 μm, and a 20-MHz system theoretically could have a resolution of 56 μm.

Radial, *lateral*, or *cross-range resolution* refers to the ability of an ultrasonic imaging system to distinguish between objects that are at the same distance from the transducer and are separated in a direction perpendicular to the beam axis within the plane of the scan. As discussed in the next section, scanning is performed by sequential ultrasonic pulses that are displaced from each other either angularly or linearly. If the two objects are so close together that adjacent beams cannot distinguish them, then they are not resolved. If they are sufficiently far apart that adjacent beams can distinguish them, then they are resolved. For practical purposes, the beam width defined by Eq. (9)

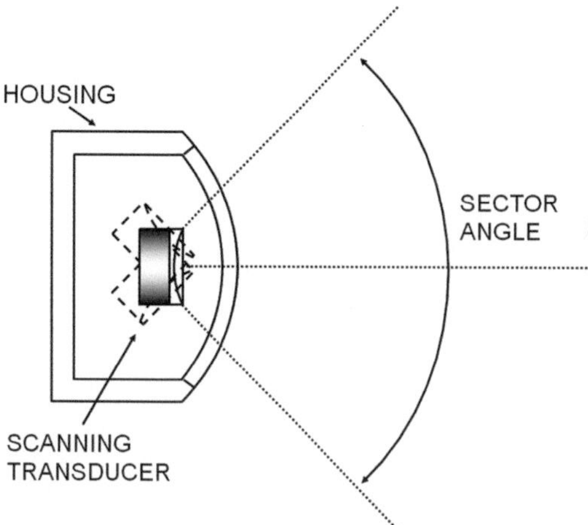

Fig. 12 Mechanical sector scan. A transducer sweeps back and forth over a well-controlled sector angle as it transmits and receives ultrasound at small, fixed, angular increments within the large sector angle

specifies the best possible lateral resolution for an ultrasonic imaging system. Equation (9) gives the beam width of a focused beam at its minimal value, i.e., its value at the focus. Proximal and distal to the focus, the beamwidth is greater; therefore, the lateral resolution is poorer. The guideline applies only in the focal zone and requires the beam spacing to be close enough for beam separation not to exceed the beam width at the focus. If this latter requirement is not satisfied, two objects separated in the lateral direction by a distance equal to the beamwidth would be insonified only by one beam and therefore could not be resolved in the lateral direction.

Scanning Methods

A transducer consisting of one or more piezoelectric elements transmits an ultrasonic pulse as a focused wave that propagates along a known path. As echoes return from the scatterers and reflecting surfaces along that path, the video signals derived from the ultrasonic echo signals are displayed on a monitor along a line corresponding to the propagation path. The transducer then transmits a second focused wave along a path adjacent to the path of the previous wave. The video signals derived from the echoes returning from the second path are displayed in the proper position adjacent to those of the previous path. By rapidly repeating this process typically 100 or more times in 1/30 s or less, a real-time image is generated that consists of 100 or more scan lines or vectors over the scanned plane.

Traditional ultrasonic imaging instruments and many modern instruments operating at frequencies higher than 10 MHz, e.g., ophthalmic scanners, utilize a transducer consisting of a single focused piezoelectric element. This single element scans a plane by mechanical movement of the transducer. Typically, the mechanical scanning movement is angular, so that the scan involves a sector covering between 45° and 120°. Transducers used to scan blood vessels from within the vessel lumen may produce a scan covering 360°, but these are specialized, very-high-frequency, catheter-housed transducers. A typical mechanical sector-scanning arrangement is schematically illustrated in Fig. 12, and an example of a sector scan image is shown in Fig. 13. Figure 13 shows a *transverse* or *axial* scan of a cancer-containing prostate gland, with the rectal wall at the apex of the sector and showing the gland as a roughly circular, isoechoic region bounded by a hyperechoic capsule. The gland itself contains a moderately hyperechoic region proximal to the urethra and a moderately hypoechoic region adjacent to the rectal wall that corresponds to the peripheral zone. This image is typical of a cancer-containing prostate gland because the lesion is not detectable; the peripheral zone tends to be hypoechoic in normal as well as cancerous glands.

Within the past decade, transducers consisting of several, small, closely spaced piezoelectric elements have been employed in medical instruments. Such transducers may consist of as few as 50 or as many as 200 elements arranged in a row and are termed *linear arrays*. The assembly consisting of the transducer, its associated electronics components, housing, lenses, and so on is termed a *probe*. Linear arrays are focused to a line parallel to the long dimension of the array by a lens or element curvature, as illustrated in Fig. 14. This focus is fixed and is termed the *mechanical* or *elevation focus*. The focusing of transmitted waves in the plane that contains the

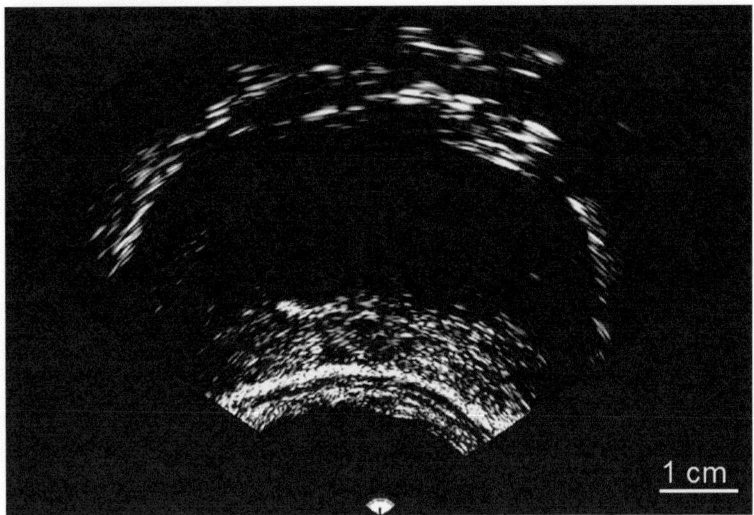

Fig. 13 Sector-scan image of a human prostate. A transrectal probe was used to acquire this transverse scan of a cancer-containing prostate; the lesion is not visible. Acoustical coupling was provided by a water-filled latex sheath in contact with the rectal mucosa. The gland is the central circular region with a hyperechoic boundary; the rectal wall is at the apex of the sector

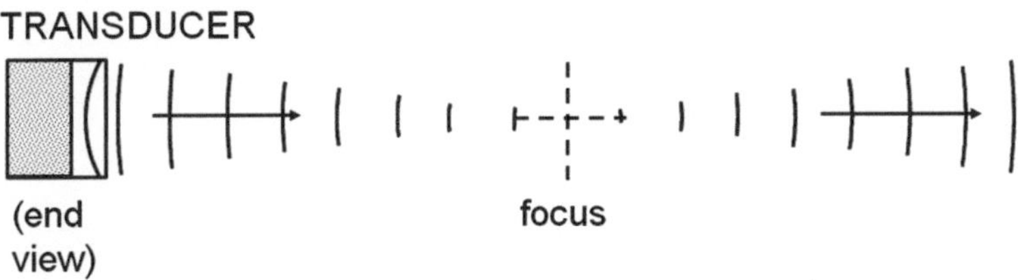

Fig. 14 Elevational aspect of a linear array. The end view of a linear-array transducer shows the fixed "elevation" focus determined by curving the elements or using a lens

long dimension of the array is performed by delaying the pulses sent to central elements compared to the pulses sent to peripheral elements; this delay is controlled electronically and has the effect of curving the transmitted wave as if it were generated by a curved or lensed transducer, as shown in Fig. 15a. The focusing in this plane is electronically variable and is termed the *scan-plane* or *azimuthal focus*. Because the curvature is controlled electronically, it can be adjusted by the operator to suit the depth of tissue being examined. In addition to delaying the pulses sent to the central elements compared to those sent to the peripheral elements, the delay can be linearly varied from one end of the array to the other. The effect of the linear delay is to tilt the transmitted wave and thereby to propagate it at an angle.

By varying the angle of the transmitted wave, the linear array can scan a plane in a sector-like sweep. Alternatively, the transmitted wave can be generated by a subset of the elements available for transmission, as illustrated in Fig. 15b. This subset can be shifted along the array for a sequence of transmitted waves, which results in a linear scan consisting of a set of parallel scan lines.

Received signals from the peripheral elements of an array can be delayed with respect to those of the central signals. This delay can be decreased with time as received signals return from a single transmitted pulse. By changing the delay over time, the transducer can be dynamically focused at the range from which signals are returning. Figure 16 shows how the delay can be controlled to put the received signals from different elements

Fig. 15 Azimuthal aspect of a linear array in transmission mode. (**a**) Transmission using the entire array focuses the beam by delaying the pulses sent to the central elements relative to those sent to the peripheral elements; changing the delay changes the transmit focal distance. (**b**) Transmission using only selected elements shifts the beam across the face of the array

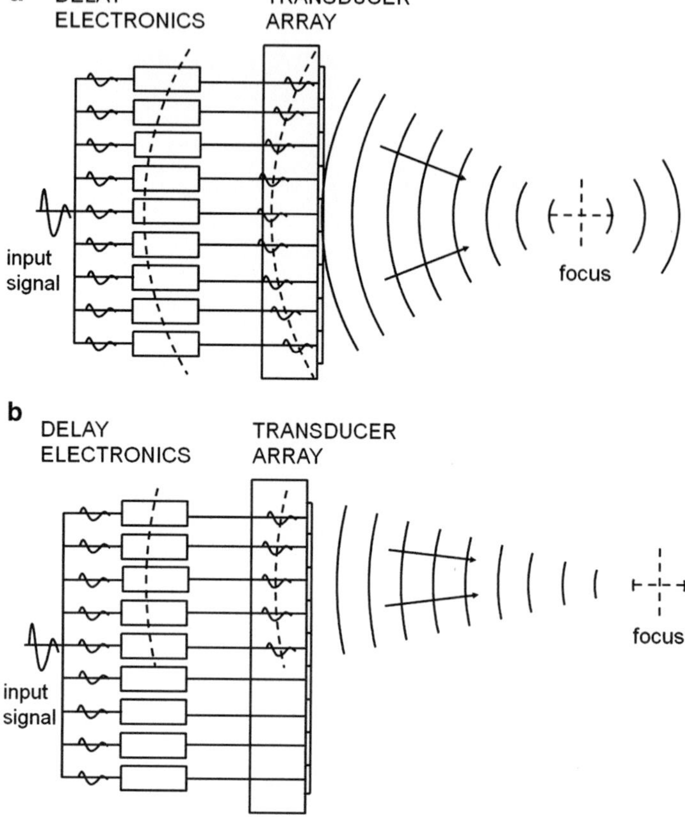

Fig. 16 Azimuthal aspect of a linear array in receive mode. Focusing in receive mode can be dynamic. (**a**) A short focal distance is used for early echoes from near scatterers by applying a relatively large delay for signals from central compared to lateral elements. (**b**) As time passes, the relative delay is reduced to allow the focus to recede. In addition, a subset of elements can be used to displace the receive axis laterally (just as selected elements can be used to shift the transmitted beam axis laterally, as shown in Fig. 15b)

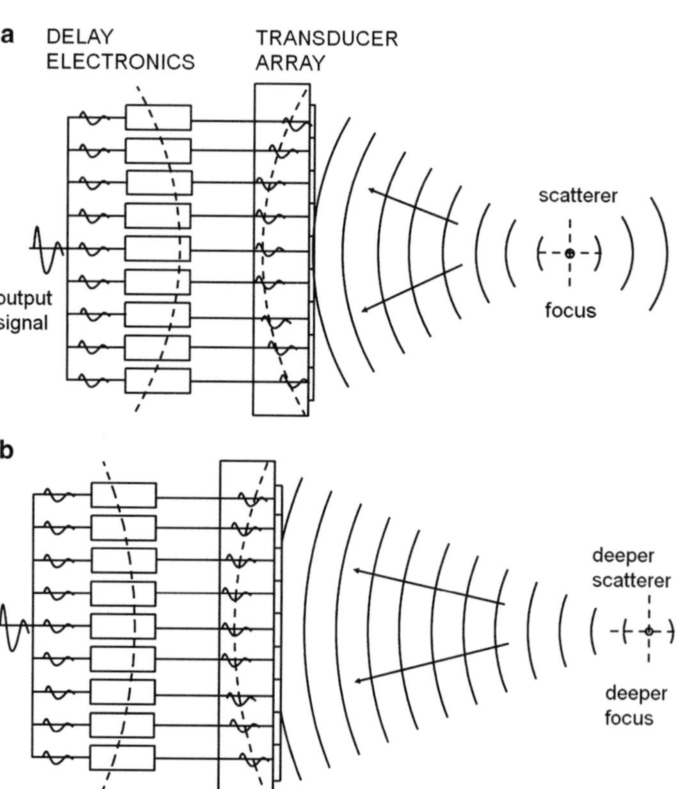

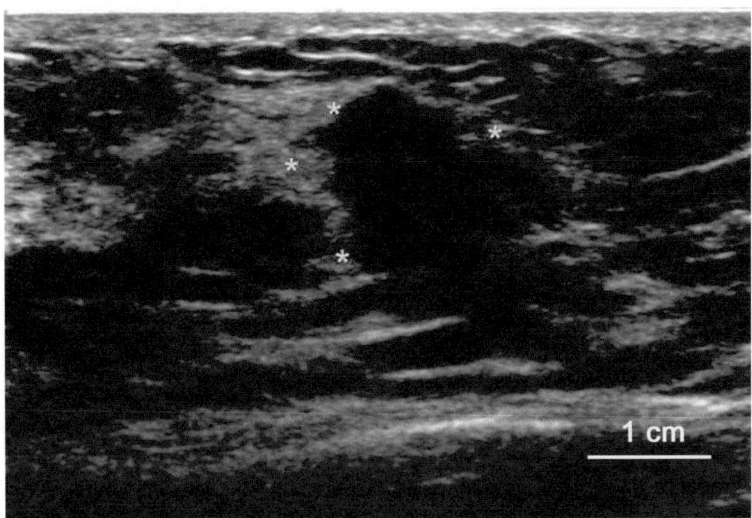

Fig. 17 Linear-scan image of a breast lesion. A linear-array probe was placed on the skin of the breast to acquire this image; the 2-cm lesion is an invasive ductal carcinoma, as discussed in the text. Acoustical coupling was provided by a gel. The 128 constituent scan lines are parallel as a result of shifting the subset of transmitting and receiving elements along the array for each pulse

in phase for nearer scatterers (Fig. 16a) and more-distant scatterers (Fig. 16b). Consequently, received signals can be optimally focused over the full useful range of the transducers. As in the case of transmission, the delay applied to the received signals also can be varied linearly from one end of the array to the other to provide an angular sweep of received signals corresponding to the angular sweep of transmitted waves. Alternatively, a subset of receiving elements can be used and the subset can be displaced along the array with each transmitted pulse to provide a linear sweep.

Figure 17 shows a linear-array scan of a breast containing an invasive ductal carcinoma approximately 2 cm in diameter. This example is somewhat unusual because of the strong refraction effects at the lateral margins of the lesion and the moderate anti-shadowing effect distal to the lesion; however, it is typical of breast carcinoma because of its internal heterogeneity and lobulated margins.

Image-display Methods

Modern, ultrasonic medical imaging instruments feature *B-mode* images that display maps of echo-signal amplitude on a monitor with gray-scale, pixel-brightness values that are a function of the video signal. As stated above, video signals typically are compressed versions of the rectified and "smoothed" envelope signals derived from the original RF echo signals; compression logarithmically enhances the details depicted by low-amplitude echo signals by increasing their dynamic range while reducing the dynamic range of high-amplitude echo signals. Color encoding of B-mode images is a rarely employed alternative to gray-scale encoding. When color encoding is used, it most often is done in quantitative research images, e.g., in the quantitative-ultrasound methods discussed elsewhere in this book.

B-mode images are the successor to now virtually clinically obsolete A-mode displays, which are oscilloscope traces of the RF or video signal along a given propagation axis. Although B-mode images are universal, A-mode displays continue to be utilized in certain specialized clinical applications requiring very accurate biometry, e.g., in ophthalmic applications involving measurement of globe or anterior-chamber dimensions.

C-mode images are not used clinically, but sometimes they are utilized in research to examine thin, excised biological specimens or nonbiological materials. C-mode images display the amplitude of sound reflected from a base plate after the beam has traversed the specimen; the specimen is scanned in a raster pattern by a beam perpendicular to the specimen and base-plate surfaces. C-mode images sometimes use range-gating to capture and display echo signals from a plane that is parallel to the base plate but within the specimen. Most typically, this is done in research applications where 3-D image data are displayed as three orthogonal planes as an operator "dials" through the 3-D image volume.

M-mode images depict echo amplitude along a single spatially fixed scan line. The scan-line position typically is adjusted using a B-mode display. A single scan line is repeatedly displayed as a function of time, and each new scan line is added to the end of the set, while all other scan lines are laterally displaced and the oldest scan line is dropped. Therefore, the presentation appears to move laterally while echo patterns move vertically as movement in the range direction occurs in the body. M-mode images can be very useful for depicting movements quantitatively as a function of time. Perhaps the best-known application is echocardiography, in which M-mode displays are used to evaluate valvular or heart-wall motion. Doppler images, a fifth category of ultrasonic images, are discussed at the end of this chapter.

Image Controls

Contemporary instruments typically provide many controls allowing the operator to optimize the image in terms of personal preferences regarding visualization of anatomic structure. These controls are provided to adjust overall image brightness and contrast as well as receiver gain as a function of range. Overall brightness can be changed by changing the transmitted-pulse power or by changing the receiver gain and bias levels; many instruments provide means of controlling pulse power as well as receiver gain. An additional control, and perhaps the one most-often used, is termed *time-gain control* (*TGC*) or *time-varying gain* (*TVG*). This control increases the gain during the time that the echo signals from a single transmitted pulse are being received from increasing ranges. The increase in receiver gain as a function of echo-signal range is intended to counter the effects of attenuation, i.e., to provide higher gain for signals returning from deeper (more distal) regions. Because attenuation within an organ varies, TGC may be controlled in several (e.g., 10 or more) steps covering the useful range of a transducer. Alternatively, gain may be controlled in terms of near gain, far gain, the length of the near and far regions, and the distance between them. The means of setting TGC vary from manufacturer to manufacturer and even may differ from model to model within the same manufacturer's product line.

The operator must set all controls in an ultrasonic imaging instrument with care to ensure that a visually enhanced image does not exclude information by inappropriately setting overall gain or TGC. Excessive pulse power or receiver gain can saturate the receiver amplifier or the display, or it can overload the receiver amplifier to such an extent that it cannot recover in time to properly amplify echo signals originating near the transducer. Too little gain or excessive contrast can result in images that appear to be sharp and crisp, but that actually lose information present in extremely low- or high-level signals. Some instruments have a threshold control to mask the display of noise (arising either in the instrument electronics or in the environment). With experience, the appearance of low-level signals in an image can be distinguished from noise, and gain and threshold controls can be set so that noise is not displayed yet low-level signals are retained in the image. At the same time, contrast should be set so that desired high-level signals do not saturate the amplifiers or the display. Often, both criteria cannot be met simultaneously. In these cases, the desired information may not reside in the low-level and high-level signals simultaneously. If it does, then gain can be increased and decreased alternately to permit visualization of both signal-level extremes.

Image Properties

The properties of ultrasonic images depend on all the considerations summarized above. The clinically oriented chapters in this book provide ample discussion and specific examples of image properties and of the clinically relevant information to be derived from image features. This section briefly reviews some salient features of images that are important for proper image interpretation.

Attenuation and Diffraction

Attenuation and diffraction tend to cause changes in image brightness with range. The skilled operator can correct for this effect by judicious use of TGC. When the TGC is set to a fixed value (i.e., constant as a function of range), an image of a uniformly scattering target such as tissue or phantom is moderately bright near the transducer and increases in brightness as range increases until maximal brightness occurs at the focal distance; past the focus, the brightness decreases with range. The increase in brightness with range proximal to the focus, i.e., in the near field, occurs because beam intensity increases as the beam cross section decreases with range and because the spherical shape of the waves backscattered from small scatterers better matches the acoustic surface of the transducer. Usually these effects outweigh the effect of attenuation in the near field; however, past the focus, attenuation and the reduction in beam intensity with increasing beam diameter are dominant, and image brightness decreases with range.

Beamwidth Artifact

A beamwidth artifact also makes the apparent cross-range size of scatterers appear to increase in the far field at a uniform rate because, distal to the focus, each scatterer intercepts the wide beam in several adjacent beam positions; in contrast, the same size scatterer closer to the focus may intercept the beam in only one beam position. A similar effect occurs in the near field, but may not be as pronounced as the far-field effect, depending on the scanning geometry.

Speckle Artifact

When multiple small scatterers are present in an insonifying pulse, then the scattered waves from separate scatterers interfere. The pattern of interference is random because the spacing between scatterers varies randomly. In one small location, interference may be constructive and may form a bright spot in the image; in an adjacent region, it may be destructive and may form a dark spot. In the overall image, the resulting interference pattern gives the effect of grains of sand spread over the imaged structures. The grainy texture is termed *speckle*. Although speckle contains information on scatterer statistics, it is generally considered to be an image-degrading artifact. Much research effort is being directed toward developing effective methods of minimizing it without losing true detail. Much of the "texture" in conventional images such as those of Figs. 13 and 17 is speckle artifact. Standard methods of reducing speckle include spatial compound scanning, in which the image is generated by combining images obtained from different transducer locations, and simple spatial blurring of conventional images. Both methods can cause a significant degradation of resolution, and refraction encountered in the compound-scanning method often poses difficult problems in registering the combined component images.

Artifactual Echoes

When a strongly reflecting object (e.g., bone surface, calcification or bubble) exists in a scan plane, then its strong echoes can be reflected from the transducer surface back into the tissue where they can again be reflected by the strongly reflecting object. These multiple reflections create artifactual echoes repeating into the imaged tissue beyond the reflecting object and appearing as deeper, distorted versions of the object. Eventually, attenuation reduces the multiple echoes to an insignificant level. In extreme cases, the timing of the transmitted pulses may cause the multiple artifactual echoes to appear closer to the transducer than the primary echo. The appearance of a second, weaker echo mimicking a primary echo anywhere in the image, but typically distal to the primary echo at twice its range, should alert the operator to the possibility of a multiple-reflection artifact.

Reverberation Artifact

A closely related artifact, termed *reverberation* artifact, occurs when the reflections occur between two closely spaced reflectors within tissue, e.g., the two strongly reflecting surfaces of a thick membrane. Reverberation artifact causes multiple occurrences of an imaged structure to appear immediately distal and adjacent to the reflecting surfaces.

Doppler Methods

Doppler methods sense and present information on moving constituents of the body, most typically, flowing blood. A thorough discussion of Doppler methods is beyond the scope of this chapter, but some operationally useful concepts are summarized below. (Reference [12] is a recent publication that discusses Doppler and other flow-measurement methods in depth.)

Most often, the moving constituent of interest is blood in large arteries; arterial blood moves at velocities high enough to be sensed easily by ultrasonic Doppler technology. However, when the velocity of flow is small in a direction parallel to the ultrasound beam or when the vessel lumen is small, Doppler methods may be inadequate to sense flow.

Basic Doppler Concepts

Doppler methods sense motion based on the change in frequency experienced by a wave that is backscattered or reflected from a moving object. Such objects may be the erythrocytes in a blood vessel, the wall of a blood vessel, the wall of the heart, tissues adjacent to the wall of a blood vessel, and so on. The change of frequency, Δv, is given by the simple equation

$$\Delta v = v_{\mathrm{D}} - v_0 = 2v_0 S\left(\cos\varphi\right)/c \qquad (10)$$

where v_0 is the incident frequency, v_{D} is the Doppler-shifted frequency, S is the speed of the scattering object, and φ is the angle between the direction of object movement and the axis of the ultrasound beam, as illustrated in Fig. 18. The term *Doppler frequency* is applied to the variable Δv. The signal having this frequency is termed the *Doppler signal*. Note that the angle φ is 0° when the incident ultrasound beam is propagated in the same direction as the blood velocity and 180° when the blood is flowing directly toward the transducer. Therefore, $\cos\varphi$ and Δv can have positive or negative values, and the sign of Δv can be sensed and displayed in a manner that indicates flow toward or away from the transducer.

The difference signal in a Doppler system is produced by electronically combining the transmitted and received Doppler-shifted echo signals. The resulting signal contains each of the component (transmitted and received) signals, a signal with a frequency that is the sum of the component-signal frequencies, and a signal with a frequency that is the difference of the component-signal frequencies. A filter blocks the component and frequency-sum signals, leaving only the frequency-difference signal, i.e., the Doppler signal, with the frequency, Δv, given by Eq. (10). In the

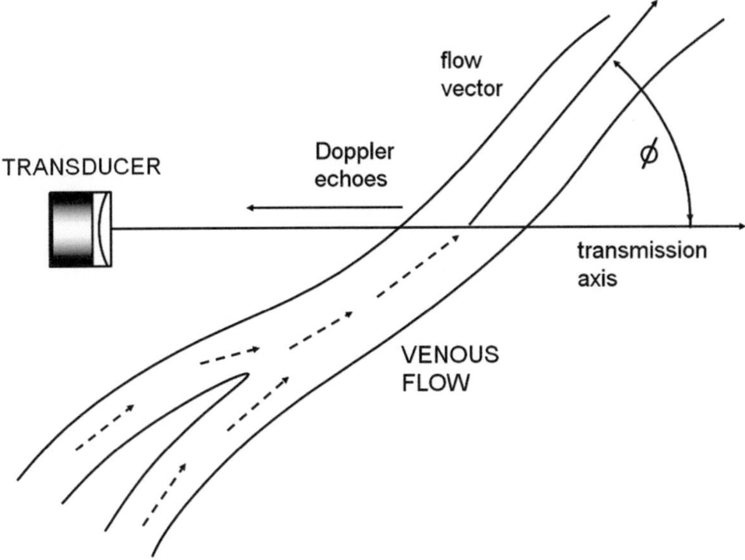

Fig. 18 Geometry of Doppler imaging. Flow in a vein is illustrated showing the direction of flow, the direction of ultrasound propagation from and back to the transducer, and the angle, φ, between the flow and ultrasound directions as defined in Eq. (10)

case of a flowing fluid such as blood, the backscattered signal results from impedance differences between suspended particulate scatterers such as single and aggregated erythrocytes in blood and the surrounding plasma. Because velocity varies across the vessel (whether flow is laminar or turbulent) and across the beam, the backscattered signals contain a range of Doppler-shifted frequencies. The amplitude of the Doppler-shifted echo signals is dependent on the scattering strength of the scatterers and the volume of the beam intersection with the moving fluid or tissue.

When the component of velocity perpendicular to the beam is extremely low, the Doppler signal cannot be distinguished reliably from the primary backscattered signal. The frequency threshold for acceptance of Doppler signals is adjustable by the operator in all modern systems. Because one of its major uses is to permit visualization of blood flow without artifact from vessel-wall motion, this threshold control is commonly termed the *wall filter*, and the threshold value is typically expressed in terms of Hertz, e.g., 50 Hz. Note that according to Eq. (10), a 50-Hz threshold in a 5-MHz system with a beam axis at 60° to the flow axis is $S = \Delta vc/2v_0\,(\cos\varphi) = 1.5$ cm/s.

Flow information often is presented in an image. In order to estimate velocity with reasonable accuracy, the frequency of the incident ultrasonic wave should be well defined, i.e., the bandwidth of the pulse should be narrow, and the pulse duration should be long enough to include several cycles of the insonifying signal. This requirement conflicts with the requirement for brief pulses needed for axial resolution. *Therefore, a system cannot be operated as a high-definition B-mode instrument and as a Doppler instrument simultaneously.* Doppler imaging systems use pulses containing several cycles of sound to provide adequate sensitivity and velocity resolution while still allowing presentation of flow information in images having reasonable axial spatial resolution. Assuming a relatively rectangular envelope from the pulse of a transmitted signal in a Doppler imaging system, the axial resolution, δ, is approximately

$$\delta = c\tau = n\lambda \qquad (11)$$

where τ is the pulse duration and n is the number of cycles in the pulse. In the case of a high-quality, i.e., well-damped, B-mode imaging system, n is approximately 1.5; in a Doppler system, *n* may be 5 or higher. *Therefore, the axial spatial resolution of a B-mode system is far superior to that of a Doppler imaging system.*

The earliest Doppler systems did not present flow information in images. Instead, they provided an audible Doppler signal derived from the difference between the transmitted and received signals. Since this difference produces a Doppler signal in the frequency range to which the human ear responds, the signal provides flow information in a form that is easy to interpret in a qualitative manner. These simple systems have very high Doppler-signal resolution, but they do not provide any range solution; they utilize a continuously transmitted signal, and the operator manipulates the transducer based on the audible signal and external anatomic landmarks to aim the beam at a vessel of interest. Because these systems use continuously transmitted waves, they are termed *continuous-wave-* or *cw-Doppler systems.*

Doppler Display Methods

Because the information available in cw-Doppler systems cannot be displayed in an image, pulsed-Doppler technologies were developed to allow well-defined visualization of the distribution of flow in a scan plane. As stated above, the number of sound cycles needed to provide appropriate Doppler signals is large compared to the number of cycles needed for good spatial resolution. However, modern instruments provide a reasonable compromise between the conflicting requirements for spatial resolution and Doppler information, and many allow the operator to switch from optimized B-mode imaging to optimized Doppler imaging.

Current clinical instruments employ the following three methods for displaying flow or blood-tissue-motion information visually: duplex Doppler, color Doppler, and power Doppler. Figure 19 shows an example of each type of Doppler image.

Duplex Doppler does not image flow directly; rather, it provides a conventional B-mode image in conjunction with an image of a Doppler-signal spectrum. Using a high-quality B-mode image as a guide, the operator manipulates the probe and selects a scan line that passes through a vessel or other region of interest. The operator then selects a segment of the scan line from which to analyze Doppler echo signals. The selected segment, termed the *sample volume*, is highlighted on the B-mode display. The instrument computes the spectrum of the Doppler signal derived from the operator-selected scan-line segment. The operator can manipulate the probe and can move the scan plane and the sample volume within the scan plane so that the Doppler signal is obtained from a vessel or even a portion of a vessel of interest. Although flow information is not displayed in a spatial map over the scan plane, a quantitative depiction of flow over a small, well-defined region is provided. Furthermore, the operator can move the sample volume through the entire imaged volume, deriving an excellent sense of the three-dimensional distribution of flow. The Doppler-spectrum display shows frequency on the vertical axis, time on the horizontal axis, and spectral amplitude as brightness. Flow toward the transducer is displayed above the time axis, and flow away from the transducer is shown below the axis. In addition, duplex-Doppler instruments typically also provide an audible Doppler signal. An example of a duplex-Doppler image is shown in Fig. 19a. The display of the time-varying Doppler spectrum, combined with a high-quality B-mode image and an audible signal, conveys a great deal of diagnostically useful information in a quantitative manner.

Color Doppler presents flow or motion information as color encoding superimposed upon a gray-scale B-mode image. Red depicts flow toward the transducer and blue depicts flow away from the transducer. Color Doppler has been available in commercial instruments for many years and is perhaps the most popular current method of depicting flow. It provides a real-time spatial display of flow using color to indicate direction and brightness to indicate flow magnitude. However, it is subject to a great deal of artifact, and the display controls, particularly the wall-filter and persistence controls, need to be set with care to minimize wall motion

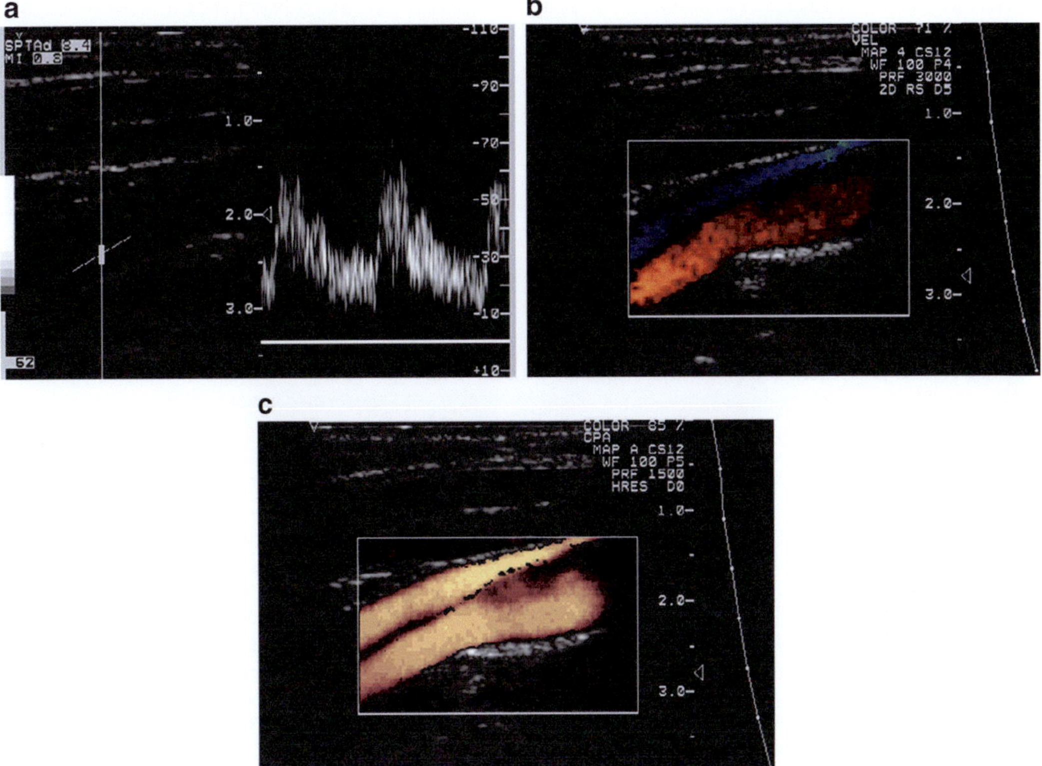

Fig. 19 Doppler images of the carotid artery. (**a**) Duplex Doppler image showing (on the *left*) a reference B-mode image with a small, white, user-controlled, rectangular region of interest within the carotid artery at the intersection of a long, vertical, white line defining the ultrasound beam axis and a short, angled, white line defining the flow axis; and showing (on the *right*) the Doppler-shift frequency indicating pulsatile flow toward the transducer. (**b**) Color Doppler image showing carotid-artery flow toward the transducer in *red* and jugular-vein flow away from the transducer in *blue*. (**c**) Power Doppler image showing flow in the carotid artery and jugular vein in orange; pixel brightness indicates the level of backscattered energy in the flowing regions

and other effects that degrade flow-image quality and accuracy. Fortunately, many color-Doppler instruments also provide duplex-Doppler outputs for applications requiring fine resolution. An example of a color-Doppler image is shown in Fig. 19b.

Power Doppler is rapidly increasing in popularity. It depicts regions of motion with an orange color; direction and velocity are not depicted. The image color encodes movement, typically in flowing blood, with an intensity that depends on the power of the Doppler signal. By displaying the power in the Doppler signal as a function of position in the scan plane, a major improvement is possible in distinguishing the Doppler signal from noise; in effect, the sensitivity to motion is dramatically increased at the cost of eliminating velocity information. The resulting image is semiquantitative in terms of total Doppler-signal power but not in terms of flow parameters. However, power-Doppler instruments typically include color-Doppler capabilities as well. Consequently, they provide power-Doppler displays that depict regions of flow in a dramatic easy-to-visualize manner that is free of many of the artifacts associated with color Doppler while also providing the traditional Doppler images that have proven to be so valuable clinically. An example of a power-Doppler image is shown in Fig. 19c.

Acknowledgments I thank Lippincott, Williams, and Wilkins of Philadelphia, for their permission to base this chapter on a previously published chapter in *Ultrasound for Surgeons*, edited by Machi and Sigel and published by Igaku-Shoin of New York and Tokyo in 1997; Lippincott, Williams, and Wilkins currently owns the copyright to *Ultrasound for Surgeons*. I also thank Roslyn Raskin for her invaluable assistance in preparing the manuscript, particularly for her meticulous proofreading. The prostate image of Fig. 13 was obtained in the course of research supported in part by NIH Grant R01CA135089 administered by the National Cancer Institute. The Doppler images of Fig. 19 were provided by Tina Nack, MPE, RVT, RDMS, Supervisor, Vascular Laboratory, Division of Diagnostic Ultrasound, Department of Radiology, Thomas Jefferson University and the Jefferson Ultrasound Research and Education Institute in Philadelphia.

References

1. Feleppa EJ, Lizzi FL. Ultrasonic imaging in medicine. Imaging Q. 1988;3:4–6.
2. Shung K, Thieme G, editors. Ultrasonic scattering in biological tissues. Boca Raton, PL: CRC Press; 1993.
3. Ferrari LA, editor. Proceedings of the SPIE international symposium on pattern recognition and acoustical imaging. Bellingham, WA: International Society of Optical Engineering; 1987.
4. Thijssan JM, Mazeo V, editors. Ultrasonic tissue characterization and echographic imaging. Nijmegen, the Netherlands: University of Nijmegen Press; 1986.
5. White D, Lyons EA, editors. Ultrasound in medicine. New York: Plenum Press; 1978.
6. Hussey M. Basic physics and technology of medical diagnostic ultrasound. 2nd ed. New York: Elsevier; 1985.
7. Kremkau FW. Diagnostic ultrasound: principles, instrumentation, and exercises. Orlando, FL: Grune & Stratton; 1984.
8. Kempczinski RF, Yao JS. Practical non-invasive vascular diagnosis. Chicago: Year Book Medical; 1982.
9. Wells PNT. Biomedical ultrasonics. London: Academic; 1977.
10. White DN, editor. Ultrasound in medical diagnosis. Kingston, ON: Ultramedison; 1976.
11. Wells PNT, editor. Physical principles of ultrasonic diagnosis. New York: Academic; 1969.
12. Jensen JA. Estimation of blood velocities using ultrasound. New York: Cambridge University Press; 1996.
13. Begui ZE. Acoustic properties of refractive media of the eye. J Acoust Soc Am. 1954;26:365–8.
14. Goss SA, Johnston RL, Dunn F. Compilation of empirical ultrasonic properties of mammalian tissues. J Acoust Soc Am. 1978;64:423–57.
15. Goss SA, Johnston RL, Dunn F. Compilation of empirical ultrasonic properties of mammalian tissues, II. J Acoust Soc Am. 1980;68:93–108.
16. Berger G, Laugier P, Thalabard JC, et al. Global breast attenuation: control group and benign breast diseases. Ultrason Imaging. 1990;12:47–57.

Advanced Prostate Imaging: Correlating Prostate Anatomy with MRI and MRI/Ultrasound Fusion

Adnan Ali, Bachir Taouli, and Ashutosh K. Tewari

Introduction

Prostate cancer (PCa) is the most common non-cutaneous malignancy among men in the USA and Europe. An estimated 238,590 new cases of PCa were diagnosed and 29,720 people died of the disease in the USA in 2013 [1, 2]. Widespread use of prostate specific antigen (PSA) as a biomarker for prediction of PCa has led to a dramatic shift towards early detection of organ-confined disease in a younger patient population [3, 4]. Currently, transrectal ultrasound (TRUS) guided biopsy is considered the preferred method for PCa detection following abnormal PSA or DRE. However, using this approach, up to 30 % of cancers can be missed. This is because PCa is a multifocal and histologically heterogeneous disease, and TRUS guided biopsy is limited in

PCa characterization and detection. Therefore, there is a need for improving PCa detection and characterization of tumor aggressiveness.

In recent years, magnetic resonance imaging (MRI) has been more frequently used for treatment planning of PCa patients, mainly for preoperative staging. It is also being used for detection of PCa in patients with negative TRUS guided biopsy and high serum PSA. Earlier use of prostate MRI relied on T1- and T2-weighted images (T2WI), which have limited sensitivity and specificity. Multiparametric MRI, which includes newer functional sequences such as diffusion weighted imaging (DWI), dynamic contrast-enhanced MRI (DCE-MRI) and magnetic resonance spectroscopic imaging (MRSI), provides additional information that has significantly improved the detection and characterization of PCa lesions.

In this chapter, normal MRI anatomical characteristics, components of multiparametric endorectal MRI and its utility in PCa detection, current biopsy practices and their limitations are highlighted. New biopsy techniques based on multiparametric MRI are also described.

A. Ali, M.B.B.S.
Department of Urology, Icahn School of Medicine, Mount Sinai Hospital, New York, NY 10029, USA
e-mail: dr.adnanali@hotmail.com

B. Taouli, M.D.
Department of Radiology, Icahn School of Medicine, Mount Sinai Hospital, 1176 Fifth Avenue, MC Level, Box 1234, New York, NY 10029, USA
e-mail: bachir.taouli@mountsinai.org

A.K. Tewari, M.D., M. Ch. (✉)
Department of Urology, Icahn School of Medicine, Mount Sinai Hospital, 1425 Madison Avenue, 6th Floor Suite L6-50, New York, NY 10029, USA
e-mail: ashtewari@mountsinai.org

Normal Prostate Gland Anatomy

The normal anatomy of the prostate gland and its relationship to its neighboring organs and tissue planes has been well described in the earlier anatomy chapter in this book. The prostate

C.R. Porter and E.M. Wolff (eds.), *Prostate Ultrasound: Current Practice and Future Directions*, DOI 10.1007/978-1-4939-1948-2_5, © Springer Science+Business Media New York 2015 is located inferior to the bladder, superior to the urogenital diaphragm, posterior to the pubic symphysis, and anterior to the rectum. The base is contiguous with the bladder neck superiorly. The apex is continuous with the striated urinary sphincter and is directed inferiorly against the urogenital diaphragm. The position of the gland in reference to the pubic arch above and the rectum is below is important when considering imaging modalities. *Endorectal coil MRI provides a window of access to the gland parenchyma; in essence, MRI is able to utilize functional sequencing to exploit the potential differences in gland cellular architecture, thereby maximizing the potential to improve diagnostic capabilities.*

3 T Multiparametric Endorectal Magnetic Resonance Imaging (3 T mp-eMRI) of Prostate

3 T mp-eMRI consists of two or more functional MRI sequences to supplement the anatomical information provided by T2WI acquired by placing a receiving endorectal coil in the patient's rectum. The functional sequences include diffusion-weighted imaging (DWI), dynamic contrast-enhanced MRI (DCE-MRI), and, less frequently, MR spectroscopic imaging (MRSI). These functional sequences provide information about tissue microstructure, microvascular density, capillary perfusion, and metabolite concentrations. The addition of these sequences to T2WI can help distinguish between benign prostatic pathology, such as prostatitis, hemorrhage, atrophy, scarring, and benign prostatic hyperplasia, and effects of radiation therapy, cryotherapy, or hormonal therapy from prostate cancer. T1WI is sensitive to the presence of postbiopsy hemorrhage and is also useful in demonstrating extraprostatic anatomy, such as NVB, enlarged lymph nodes, and bone lesions [5].

The 3 T mp-eMRI has higher signal-to noise ratio (SNR) when compared with a 1.5 T MRI. Although, the number of protons aligned along the magnetic field at 3 T is twice that of 1.5 T, the realized gain in SNR is usually 1.5–1.8 times due to technical limitations [6]. Nevertheless, this higher SNR can be used to improve the spatial resolution or decrease the acquisition time [7]. The increased spatial resolution has the potential to improve lesion detection and characterization. The decreased acquisition time leads to reduced motion artifacts. However, the use of 3 T MRI requires a comprehensive understanding of the safety hazards related to the use of high-magnetic field strength for imaging. Currently, the latest FDA guideline considers clinical imaging with static magnetic field up to 8 T as a "nonsignificant risk" to the patient [8].

The use of endorectal coil in addition to the external pelvic phased array coil is currently controversial. Since the endorectal coil is placed a few millimeters away from the prostate, the amount of signal available for image generation is increased. This increased signal availability is most advantageous at 1.5 T, whereas the higher overall SNR makes the endorectal coil usage less certain at 3.0 T [9]. However, the additional use of endorectal coil at 3.0 T improves the sensitivity of MRI due to increased spatial resolution, excellent SNR, and clear anatomical demarcation of lesions in relationship to the prostatic capsule [10, 11].

Imaging Sequences

T2-Weighted Imaging

High resolution fast spin-echo T2-weighted images acquired in axial, sagittal and coronal planes are optimal for assessing prostate morphology, margins and internal structure. To obtain high resolution images, a small field of view with thin sections is generally used. There has been some interest in developing 3D T2WI, which may decrease acquisition time by removing the need for coronal and sagittal acquisitions. With the use of endorectal coil, sensitivity and specificity of T2WI for prostate cancer detection varies widely, ranging from 77 to 91 % and 27 to 61 %, respectively [12, 13]. Without the use of endorectal coil, the sensitivity and specificity for prostate cancer detection are 45 % and 73 %, respectively [14].

Diffusion-Weighted Imaging

Diffusion-weighted imaging (DWI) utilizes pulse sequences sensitive to diffusion of water molecules at the cellular level. DWI makes use of the constant random movement of water molecules known as "Brownian motion", this motion depends on the kinetic energy of the molecules and is temperature dependent. However, in biological tissues, the movement of water molecules is not truly random and is affected by cell organization, density, microstructure and microcirculation. Also, chemical interactions of water with cell membranes and macromolecules affect diffusion properties. Therefore, the water diffusion is referred to as "apparent diffusion".

DWI relies on the application of paired diffusion weighted gradients to protons. When there is no motion of water molecules, they acquire information from the first diffusion gradient and will subsequently be refocused by the second diffusion gradient with no net change in signal. They will appear bright on DWI due to the application of the additional gradient. However, with movement of molecules, the information gathered from the first gradient will not be completely refocused by the second subsequent gradient, producing a loss of signal that appears as areas of signal loss. Changing the amplitude of gradients varies the sensitivity of diffusion weighting sequence to water molecule motion for a given set of DWI images, which is referred to as its b-value. Typically at least two b-values are acquired, a 0 s/mm^2 combined with a second, high b-value of 1,000 s/mm^2 or greater. The information acquired from two different b-values can be used to generate an apparent diffusion coefficient (ADC) map. On the ADC map, an area with restricted diffusion appears to have low signal intensity as opposed to the native diffusion images.

It is important to realize that DWI permits a mechanism for evaluation of tumors. As in most solid tumors the movement of water molecules is restricted in the extracellular space by the higher density of hydrophobic cellular membranes. On the other hand, in necrotic or cystic areas, the movement is unrestricted. Therefore, DWI provides us with distinct functional quantitative information that reflects integrity of cellular membranes, cellular density, and extracellular space [15]. ADC is inversely correlated to Gleason score and is helpful in differentiating between low, intermediate and high-risk Gleason scores [16]. DWI also improves PCa detection when combined with T2WI, with described sensitivity and specificity of 89 % and 91 %, respectively [17]. As a caveat, it is worthwhile to note that changes in the movement of water molecules occurs in conditions other than malignancy and can be found in benign processes as well.

Dynamic Contrast Enhanced Imaging

Dynamic contrast enhanced imaging provides information about tissue vascularity and flow. It assesses the microvascular changes, such as blood flow, density, and capillary perfusion, for detection of PCa lesions [18–20]. This is performed by acquiring dynamic 3D T1-weighted sequences every 3–10 s for 4–6 min after intravenous administration of gadolinium based contrast agent, which distributes between plasma and extravascular extracellular space (EES). The injected gadolinium chelates have an increased signal on T1WI as it causes T1 shortening. Changes in signal intensity over a period of time allow measurement of gadolinium concentration and indirectly provide information about tissue vascularity. The determination of rate of exchange of contrast between plasma and EES is based on pharmacokinetic models and can be measured quantitatively using pharmacokinetic parameters K^{trans} and k_{ep} [21, 22]. K^{trans} is the forward volume transfer constant and represents permeability multiplied by capillary surface area. k_{ep} is the reverse reflux rate constant between extracellular space and plasma.

DCE-MRI data can be interpreted in three ways: qualitative, semiquantitative, and quantitative. Qualitative interpretation is the visual analysis of DCE-MRI images for rapidly and intensely enhancing lesions. The semiquantitative interpretation requires calculation of parameters to characterize the shape of a time-intensity curve, such as wash-in, washout, peak enhancement and area under the curve at 60 s. The quantitative interpretation is based on pharmacokinetic models (such as the modified Tofts model) and calculation of K^{trans} and k_{ep}. The qualitative method is simple, but is prone to inter reader variability, while the semiquantitative and quantitative methods require dedicated software for interpretation and can be time consuming. Currently, the superiority of one interpretation method over the others has not been established. There are several commercial software packages that can be used to quantify these metrics in real time.

Prostate cancer lesions in peripheral zone on DCE show elevated K^{trans} and k_{ep} in comparison to normal peripheral zone. However, in the transition zone, BPH nodules are also characterized by neovascularization. Therefore, BPH and prostate cancer demonstrate similar characteristics on DCE-MRI [23]. The sensitivity and staging accuracy for detecting tumors are improved by the addition of DCE-MRI to T2WI. The sensitivity and accuracy for detection of prostate cancer in peripheral zone on color coded DCE-MRI maps overlaid on T2WI are 96 % and 97 %, respectively, as determined in a previous study [14].

Magnetic Resonance Spectroscopic Imaging

Magnetic resonance spectroscopic imaging (MRSI) assesses metabolic information by analyzing the relative concentrations of metabolites in the cytoplasm and extracellular space commonly performed with three-dimensional chemical shift imaging, which are then overlaid on T2 images. Water, lipids, choline, citrate, lactate, creatine, and amino acids are the molecules that can be studied with MRSI. Normal prostatic tissue is unique in the body and characterized by high citrate levels of about 500 times higher than blood plasma levels. It is an important intermediary in the Krebs cycle [24]. In prostate cancer, the concentration of citrate and choline is changed. Citrate level decreases and choline level increases [25]. The

decreased citrate level is assumed to be due to the altered intermediate metabolism in Krebs cycle, which occurs due to the down regulation of zinc uptake transporter ZIP1, leading to decreased zinc levels, increased mitochondrial aconitase activity, increased citrate oxidation, and ultimately decreased citrate level [26]. The increased choline level is less understood and is thought to be associated with high turnover of phospholipids in the cell membranes of prostate cancer cells [27]. On MRSI, the spectral peaks of choline and creatine are inseparable, thus prostate cancer on MRSI is characterized by an increased ratio of choline+creatine to citrate (CC/Ci) [28, 29].

Currently, prostate MRSI is challenging and time consuming and is not usually included in clinical MRI protocols for detection of prostate cancer. Chronic prostatitis in the PZ and BPH in the TZ can have identical ratios to cancerous tissue, resulting in false positive results.

The Need for Standardization

The additional information provided by different multiparametric scans requires an approach for combining the findings from different scans into a comprehensive, single standardized reporting format. Such standardization could help simplify and enable broader consistent adoption of the mpMRI. This would help reduce discrepancies in interpretation of the different scans, which are common with small low grade lesions.

Recently, such comprehensive guidelines were provided by the European Symposium on Urogenital Radiology (ESUR) for the acquisition, interpretation and reporting of multiparametric MRI. A standardized reporting system was detailed in the report known as PI-RADS (Prostate Imaging Reporting and Data System) [10]. Using PI-RADS, each lesion can be assigned a score from 1 to 5 for each sequence (T2WI, DWI, DCE, and MRSI) based on its characteristics in the different scans. In addition to the PI-RADS score for the probability of a significant lesion, extra-prostatic extension was also suggested to be scored on a five point scale.

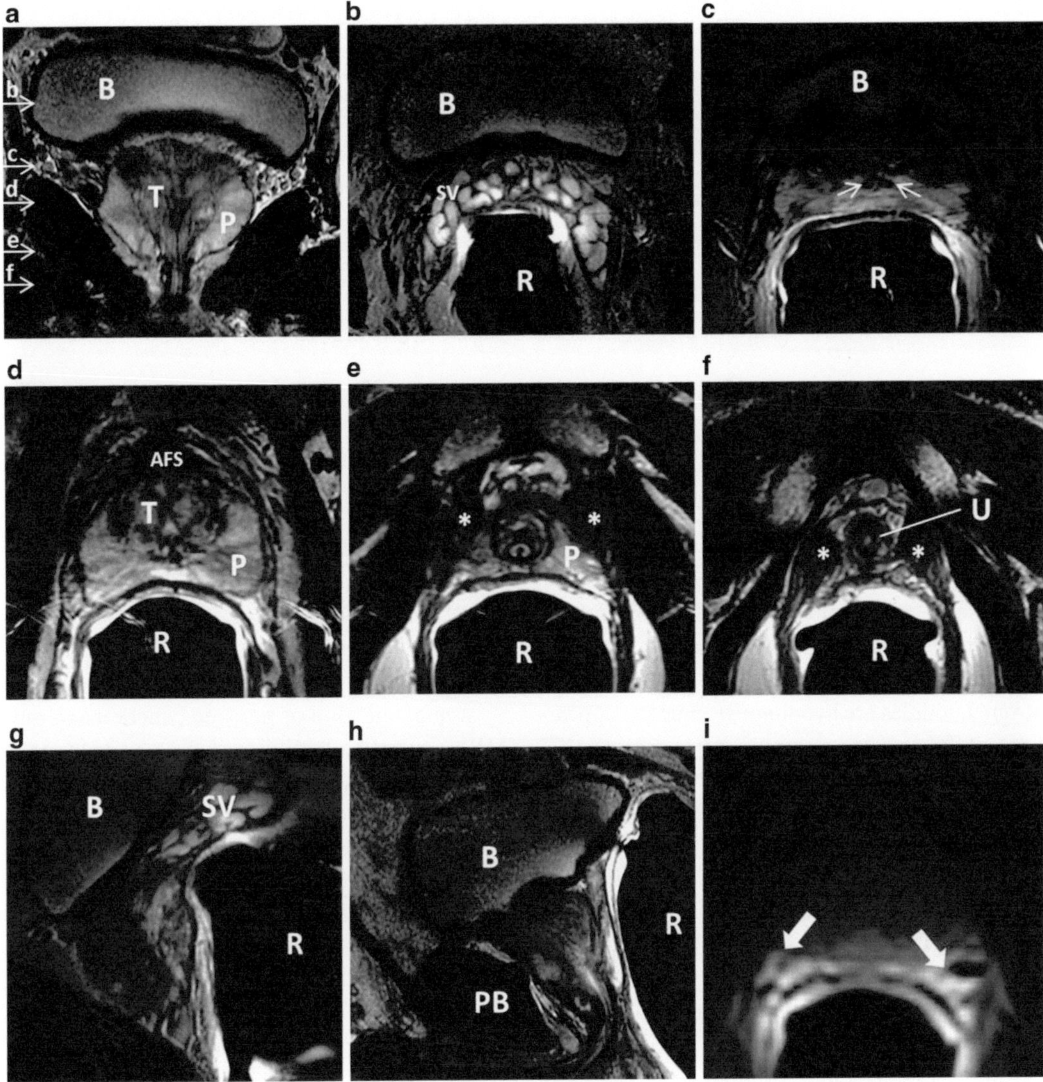

Fig. 1 Normal prostate zonal anatomy demonstrated with FSE T2 weighted endorectal 3 T MRI. (**a**) Coronal image (the *letters* along with the *arrows* correspond to the level of slices used in images **b–f**), (**b**) axial image at the level of seminal vesicles, (**c**) the base of prostate (*white arrows* show ejaculatory ducts), (**d**) mid gland, (**e**) apex, (**f**) membranous urethra (**g**) parasagittal and (**h**) midsagittal. (**i**) T1 weighted image demonstrating a homogenous intermediate signal, white arrows point to neurovascular bundles. *B* urinary bladder, *T* transition zone, *P* peripheral zone, *SV* seminal vesicles, *R* rectum with endorectal coil, *AFS* anterior fibromuscular stroma, *asterisk* levator ani muscle, *U* urethra, *PB* pubic bone

Normal Anatomy

On T1WI, the normal prostate has homogenous intermediate signal intensity. The NVB's have high signal intensity and are located posterolaterally on either side of the prostate. The zonal anatomy cannot be demonstrated using this sequence. This sequence is used for detection of post-biopsy hemorrhage.

T2WI is the most ideal sequence for demonstration of zonal anatomy (Fig. 1). On T2WI, the peripheral zone (PZ) is normally hyperintense surrounded by a decreased signal intensity capsule. A clearly demarked capsule is visible from

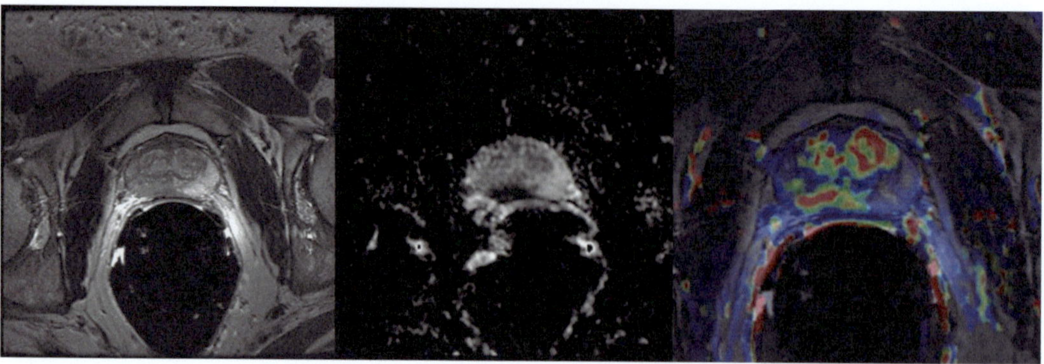

Fig. 2 Localization of prostate cancer using multiparametric MRI combining T2WI, DWI and DCE. (**a**) T2 weighted image shows hypointense lesion in right peripheral zone (*arrow*). (**b**) Corresponding ADC map shows restricted diffusion with low ADC in tumor compared to normal peripheral zone. (**c**) A color coded map obtained with DCE-MRI overlaid on T2WI shows marked enhancement in the same region, as well as hypervascularity in central gland

the base to mid portion and less consistently at the apex, which is often devoid of capsule. Glandular nodules in TZ are hyperintense while stromal nodules are hypointense, thus the appearance of TZ is heterogeneous. Anterior to the TZ lies the hypointense fibromuscular stroma. The prostatic apex is bordered by NVB posteriorly

Role of 3 T mp-eMRI in Prostate Cancer

Multiparametric MRI of prostate using a high field strength magnet can provide pertinent information about location, volume, aggressiveness and staging of prostate cancer. These findings can then be used for biopsy guidance and can also help substantially in making informed decisions regarding the choice for optimal management of PCa.

Localization and Tumor Volume Estimation

Accurate detection of the exact location of cancer within the prostate contributes significantly to patient care. It has been found that using any two functional sequences in addition to T2WI improves detection; however the addition of a third functional sequence to improve prostate cancer detection is uncertain [30]. Using all three functional sequences (DWI, DCE-MRI and

MRSI) in addition to T2WI has been shown to achieve a positive predictive value of 98 % in experienced hands [31] (Fig. 2).

While detection of prostate cancer using mp-MRI is mostly effective for large and high grade tumors, sensitivity for small Gleason 6 tumors as well as sparse tumors (malignant tissue intermixed with more than 50 % normal PZ tissue) has been shown to be lower [31, 32]. Moreover, careful interpretation of mp-MRI should be done in patients with multiple negative biopsies and increasing PSA levels for tumors in the TZ and those located anteriorly, as these areas are less frequently sampled during TRUS biopsy. T2WI findings supporting the presence of TZ tumors include homogenous low signal intensity, ill-defined margins, lack of capsule, interruption of surgical pseudocapsule (TZ to PZ boundary of low signal intensity), lenticular shape and invasion of the urethra or anterior fibromuscular stroma [33]. Nevertheless, for detection of TZ lesions the sensitivity and specificity of mp-MRI is 88 % and 86 %, respectively [35]. Tumor detection may be hampered by post-biopsy hemorrhage (Fig. 3), leading to over or underestimation of tumor presence and extent. A delay of 6–8 weeks is recommended between biopsy and MRI [35–37]. This prolonged hemorrhage may be attributed to high levels of citrate in the prostate, which has anticoagulant properties [38].

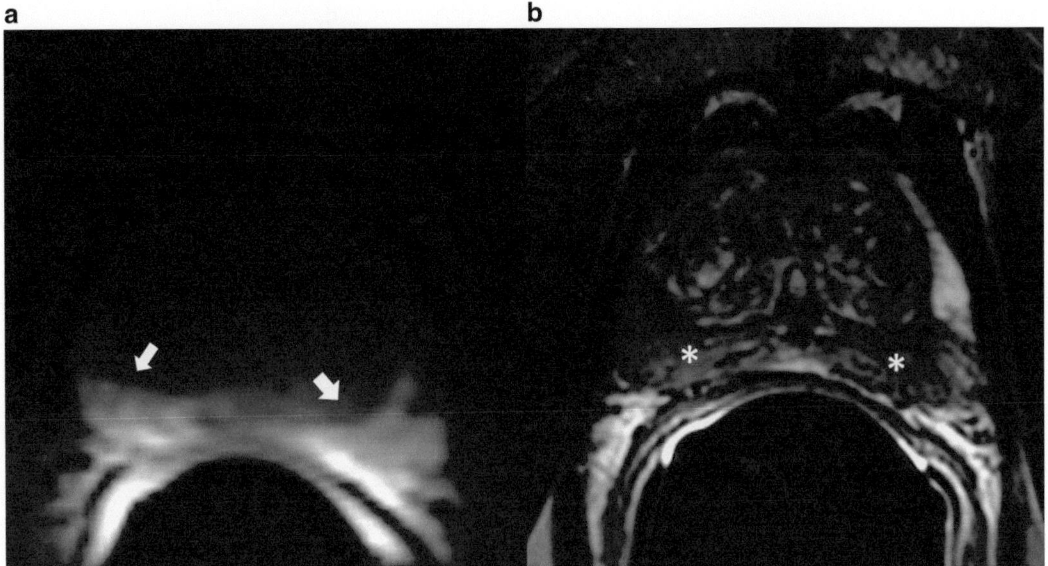

Fig. 3 Post-biopsy hemorrhage (**a**) T1 weighted image showing hyperintense areas (*arrows*) in the peripheral zone. (**b**) T2 weighted image shows hypointense (*aster-* *isk*) lesions in the same region. This is indicative of post-biopsy hemorrhage

Also, tumor volume estimation by multiparametric MRI has been shown to closely correlate with histopathological findings following radical prostatectomy. Such information about the spatial location along with the tumor volume may become important for evolving concepts of focal treatments with directed brachytherapy.

Aggressiveness

Characterization of biological aggressiveness of detected lesions is ideal for clinical decision making. An inverse correlation has been widely reported between the Gleason score and ADC values from DWI. The ADC values in addition to characterization of aggressiveness can also be helpful in assessing interval change in a tumor. However, as there is substantial inter-patient variation in ADC values of normal PZ, it has been recently shown that when the background ADC values of benign PZ are taken into consideration, there is a significant improvement in the ability to discriminate among different Gleason scores.

DCE-MRI quantitative parameters have not been shown to correlate with tumor grade or vascular growth factor (VEGF) expression as a molecular marker of angiogenesis [39].

Meanwhile, MRSI has been found to have higher sensitivity of 89.5 % for detection of Gleason 8 and above tumors compared with a sensitivity of 44.4 % for Gleason 6 tumors [40].

Staging

The use of endorectal coil in conjunction with pelvic coil regardless of the magnetic field strength has been proven to be superior for the assessment of extraprostatic extension when compared to use of pelvic coil alone (Fig. 4). Criteria for detecting extraprostatic extension includes NVB asymmetry, gross tumor surrounding the NVB, a tumor-capsule interface of more than 1 cm, obliteration of the rectoprostatic angle, irregular or speculated margin and a breach of the capsule with direct evidence of tumor extension. Seminal vesicle invasion is demonstrated on T2WI as focal low signal-intensity seminal vesicle, enlarged low signal-intensity seminal vesicles or ejaculatory ducts, obliteration of the angle between the prostate and SV and direct extension of tumor from prostate base into the SV. Accuracy of MRI in prostate cancer staging has been shown to range from 54 to 93 %, which has led to concerns about inter-observer variability.

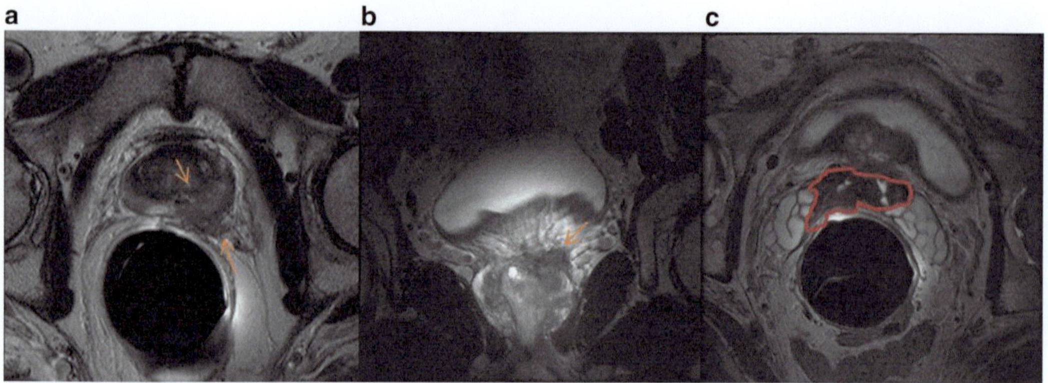

Fig. 4 Prostate cancer with extraprostatic extension. (**a**) Axial and (**b**) coronal T2 weighted images demonstrate extraprostatic extension in the left lateral base invading left neurovascular bundle. There is also seminal vesicle invasion (marked in *red*) as seen on axial T2WI obtained more superiorly (**c**)

MRI and CT have shown equivocal efficacy for lymph node metastasis, with both having low sensitivity. Recently, MRI with lymphotropic superparamagnetic iron oxide nanoparticles has shown considerable promise in occult lymph node metastases detection.

Prostate Biopsy: Current Status and Limitations

Grey scale TRUS guided systematic needle biopsy is currently the accepted standard for histologic prostate cancer diagnosis in men considered at high risk for prostate cancer on the basis of DRE and PSA findings. Hodge et al. first described the sextant prostate sampling technique using ultrasound, in which six samples were obtained, three from each left and right lobes in equally spaced regions from apex, mid and base along a parasagittal line drawn midway between the lateral border and the midline of the prostate gland [41]. To improve the diagnostic yield the sextant technique has undergone modifications with inclusion of more cores. Biopsies with 8, 10 or 12 cores from PZ have resulted in improved prostate cancer detection [42, 43]. The concept of increasing numbers of cores has been taken further with saturation biopsies, in which 20 or more cores are obtained. Saturation biopsy does not offer an additional benefit as an initial biopsy technique, but it may serve as a follow-up

strategy in patients with negative initial biopsy findings and increasing PSA. Sampling of TZ has been controversial, with a few studies claiming benefit while others have concluded that it is of limited benefit [42, 44, 45].

The regular grey-scale TRUS biopsy has limited specificity and sensitivity for prostate cancer detection as it is unable to detect isoechoic neoplastic lesions. Therefore, grey scale US does not have the ability to differentiate a significant proportion of prostate cancers from normal-appearing parenchyma. Alternative US modalities and approaches have been employed to try to correct this defect in grey scale US imaging, including color Doppler, Power Doppler with and without intravenous contrast administration, and sonoelastography [46]. Advanced US techniques have been addressed in this book, including techniques such as quantitative US and sonoelastography. Many of these techniques are still limited in use and it is fair to say that none of these alternative techniques have demonstrated sufficient sensitivity in every day clinical use to justify its substitution for the standard technique [47].

The ability to perform US via a transrectal approach is an obvious advantage in terms of acquiring high resolution grey scale images. Prostate biopsy in patients who have undergone a complete proctocolectomy and diverting ileostomy must be done using alternative approaches. The most commonly used is the transperineal approach. Alternative approaches in this patient

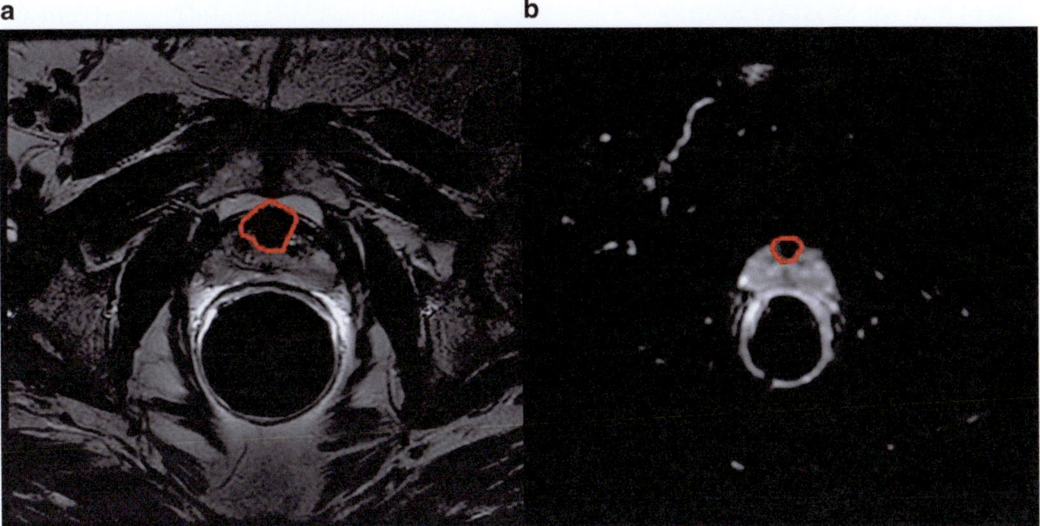

Fig. 5 Anterior tumor. (**a**) Homogenously hypointense lesion seen on T2 weighted image in the anterior portion of the central gland with (**b**) corresponding low ADC values as seen on ADC map

group include image-guided (computed tomography, ultrasound, or MRI) transperineal biopsy or transurethral resection of the prostate, with its limitation of obtaining tissue mostly from the TZ [48–50]. Transperineal prostate biopsy utilizing transrectal ultrasound guidance will be addressed later in the book in the chapter on Prostate Biopsy and Prostate Cancer Staging.

Limitations of Grey Scale Ultrasound and the Transrectal Approach to Prostate Biopsy

There are several factors which limit the effectiveness of prostate cancer diagnosis by TRUS biopsy.

1. Serum PSA is one of the triggers for prostate biopsies, the other being positive DRE. PSA is an imperfect biomarker for the detection of prostate cancer and leads to unnecessary biopsies. Many benign conditions, such as benign prostatic hyperplasia, acute or chronic prostatitis, also cause elevation of PSA. Also, when the accepted threshold of 4 ng/mL is used for defining abnormal serum PSA, 15 % of cases are found to have prostate cancer with a serum PSA level of 4 ng/mL or less [52].

2. TRUS biopsy has a low sensitivity ranging from 39 to 52 %, although its specificity is approximately 80 % [52]. Due to high false negative rates, repeat biopsies are required. The rate of prostate cancer detection ranges from 22 to 28 % on initial biopsy. This falls to 10–17 % at second biopsy and 5–15 % at third biopsy [52–54].

3. Sampling errors and inability to localize clinically significant lesions by transrectal ultrasound results in inaccurate Gleason score following TRUS biopsy. Upgrading of Gleason score in prostatectomy specimens occurs in 25–42 %, while downgrading occurs in 14 % of cases [55].

4. 21 % of tumors are located in the anterior part of the prostate (Fig. 5) [56]. Utilization of transperineal approaches for biopsy has demonstrated that significant anterior based tumors may be diagnosed. The anterior part of the prostate is under sampled when biopsies are performed by a transrectal approach. In patients who underwent MRI guided biopsy after a previous negative TRUS guided biopsy, anterior tumors were found in 47–57 % of cases [54, 57]. Similarly, in patients undergoing transperineal prostate biopsy with TRUS guidance anterior tumors were found in 17 % of men who had undergone prior transrectal approaches [58].

Use of MRI for Prostate Biopsy

The above listed limitations of TRUS guided biopsy accentuates the need for alternative image guided systems capable of detecting, localizing and targeted sampling of regions indicative of prostate cancer. Detection of prostate cancer utilizing mp-MRI, which has a sensitivity ranging from 60 to 96 %, offers a major improvement over transrectal ultrasound, which has a reported sensitivity of 39–52 % [52, 59]. The following are the different techniques used for MRI guided biopsies.

Cognitive Fusion

In a cognitive fusion biopsy, significant lesions that appear on previously reviewed MRI are targeted during TRUS guided biopsy. Such sampling of targeted lesions in addition to the systematic biopsy does appear to yield improved accuracy. However, it is subject to potential human error in overlaying MRI findings over real-time TRUS.

MRI Guided Biopsy

In MRI guided biopsy, targeted sampling of the prostate is done under real-time MRI. This has been made feasible due to the relative decrease in the time required to perform MRI, development of MRI-compatible biopsy needles and targeting mechanisms, and advanced visualization tools for guiding and verifying needle placement.

MRI guided biopsy is performed in low-field strength open systems or in closed-bore 1.5 or 3 T MRI [53, 54, 60, 61]. Low-field strength modalities offer easy access to the patient, while closed-bore systems have a higher SNR allowing increased spatial resolution. Transperineal and transgluteal approaches have been used utilizing the open MRI platform, while a transrectal approach has been used in most studies with a closed-bore MRI platform. Using MRI guidance for prostate cancer detection yields rates of cancer detection ranging from 38 to 59 % [52, 54, 61, 62]. The disadvantages of this method include increased expenses, as two MRI scans are required, and the time required; the reported duration has varied from 30 to 90 min [54].

Robot-assisted MRI guided biopsy is currently under evaluation for use in guided biopsies and it may increase the accuracy of needle placement in the prostate gland. The robot is constructed of nonmagnetic and dielectric materials, which allows it to be fully operational in a magnetic resonance imaging suite. In recent years, various MRI-compatible robotic intervention systems have been introduced. The first commercially available robot assisted MRI guided system (Innomotion; Innomedic, Herxheim, Germany) was recently evaluated in a cadaver study for MRI guided transgluteal biopsies [63].

MRI-US Fusion Biopsy

MRI-US fusion offers an alternative to targeted prostate biopsies. The fusion of two imaging modalities is due to advances in coregistration of previously acquired MRI and real-time TRUS. The techniques for fusion were primarily developed for brachytherapy. The early systems were limited by prostate motion, resulting in loss of accuracy. Since then other techniques have been developed to overcome this problem.

In MRI-Fusion biopsy, first a multiparametric endorectal MRI is done; the studies are then loaded into software that allows the radiologist to mark the prostate gland and the regions of interest for biopsy in different slices and views of the MRI, known as segmentation (Fig. 6). This information is then loaded onto the device. The second step involves real-time MRI-TRUS fusion to create a three-dimensional real-time reconstruction of the prostate on which the aiming and tracking of biopsy site is done. This technique can be done in an outpatient setting under local anesthesia within a few minutes. Currently five devices approved by the FDA are available for MRI-TRUS fusion biopsy. The Artemis device (Eigen, GrassValley, California, USA) has a mechanical arm with ultrasound transducer probe and is capable of tracking and recording biopsy locations.

The real-time fusion on Artemis steps are as follows:

1. Scan—Using an ultrasound system connected to the Artemis, a 360° scan of the prostate is done. The Artemis converts the conventional

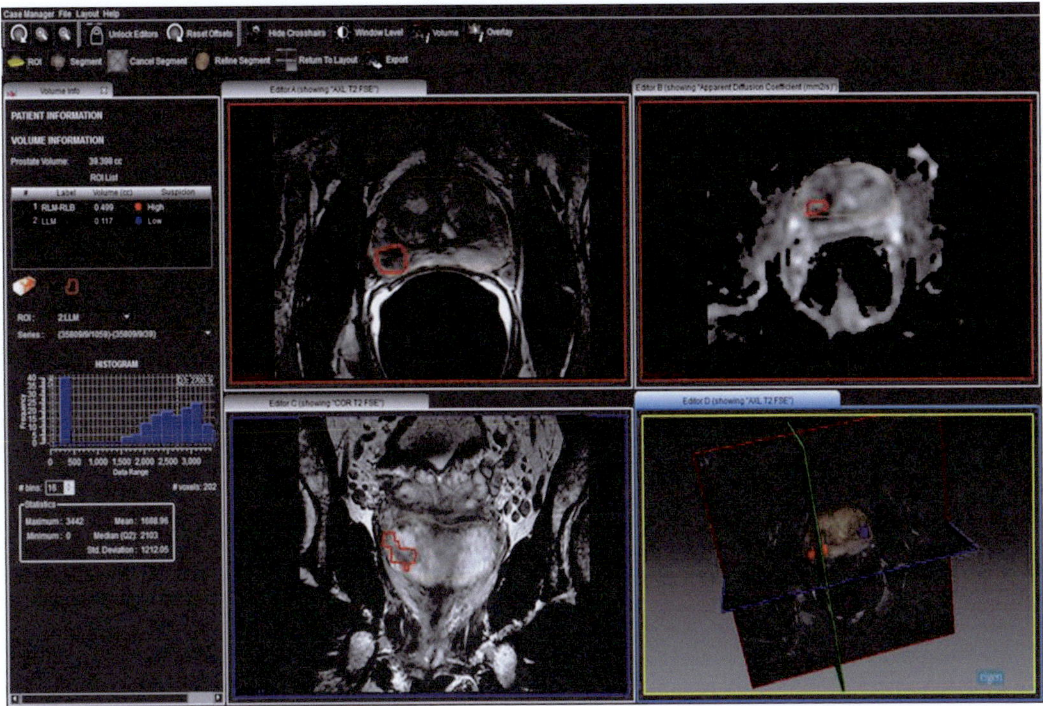

Fig. 6 A screenshot from ProFuse software showing a segmented prostate with a region of high suspicion for prostate cancer marked on the right base to mid gland showing restricted diffusion on the corresponding ADC map. Also a three dimensional model of the prostate with the regions marked is shown

two dimensional ultrasound scan into real-time 3D along with views in different planes—coronal, transverse, and sagittal. Image segmentation computes prostate gland boundaries and volume.

2. Plan—The planning module allows any of the following plans:

   (a) MR-TRUS Fusion—Segmented data of the prostate gland obtained from MRI with marked regions of interest on multiparametric-MRI is loaded onto Artemis before the procedure. During the procedure non-rigid registration is done with mapping of regions of interests from MRI to TRUS and overlaid in real-time. Regions of interest to biopsy are selected.

   (b) Conventional 6-core or 12-core plans are computed and fitted to gland shape (Fig. 7a).

   (c) Custom plans, if defined, can be fit to a candidate prostate shape.

   (d) Revisit plan for a patient with a previous procedure on active surveillance—Maps from previous biopsies are loaded into current prostate shape. It uses gland boundaries from previous and current procedures to incorporate any changes in gland shape and size. This plan can be used to revisit a positive core from a previous procedure to monitor disease progression in cases of active surveillance.

3. Biopsy—Irrespective of the plan chosen, using real-time biopsy needle tracking capabilities, Artemis allows accurate needle placement for targeted biopsy of regions and stores the location of biopsy sites. This allows for precise future resampling of biopsy sites in active surveillance patients (Fig. 7b).

4. Report—Generates report with images from biopsy procedure including measurements made during the biopsies, such as linear measurements, prostate volume, etc. The report

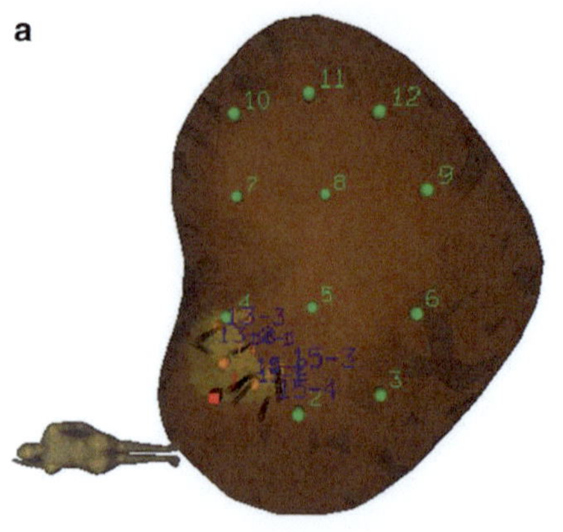

Fig. 7 Biopsy site planning and tracking (**a**) A *brown colored* three dimensional model of prostate created by fusion of MRI and US on Artemis and an automatically generated 12 core systematic biopsy plan is overlaid in addition to a region for targeted biopsy. (**b**) Recorded locations of targeted cores from two separate regions of interests are shown as *light brown cylinders*

also includes type of plan and other navigation data. This allows retrospective case review, with provision to enter PSA and pathology information.

Fusion-biopsy can be done in an outpatient setting, is less costly and less time consuming. However, this technique is still evolving and multicenter studies are needed to assess its accuracy.

Future Directions

In the past, increasing the magnetic field strength from 1.5 to 3 T has resulted in an increased intrinsic SNR and an increased spatial resolution. The utilization of 3 T multiparametric endorectal MRI has improved detection, localization, staging and risk stratification of prostate cancer. The wealth of information provided from multiparametric scans needs to be standardized for reporting and diagnosis. Using software to combine the information from different scans into a single comprehensive evaluation of prostate cancer is a possibility.

Ultra high field MR (7 T) is of immense interest for imaging and functional scans that are currently limited at strengths of 1.5 or 3 T, such as non-proton imaging and spectroscopy. In vivo safety and feasibility studies have been done at 7 T in healthy human volunteers to explore this avenue [64, 65]. However, extensive studies are required in normal and prostate cancer patients for characterization of prostate cancer.

Studies currently reporting MRI guided prostate biopsies demonstrate poor adherence to Standards for the Reporting of Diagnostic Accuracy (STARD) recommendations for the full and transparent reporting of diagnostic studies. To address this issue, it was recently proposed that reporting be done according to the Standards of reporting for MRI-targeted biopsies (START) checklist [66]. By following these guidelines, the quality of research published will be improved and pertinent questions regarding validity, importance and applicability of MRI-targeted biopsies will be more easily answered.

Disclosure Dr. Ashutosh Tewari discloses that he is the principal investigator on research grants from Intuitive Surgical, Inc. (Sunnyvale, California, USA) and Boston Scientific Corporation; he is a non-compensated director of Prostate Cancer Institute (Pune, India) and Global Prostate Cancer Research Foundation; he has received research funding from The LeFrak Family Foundation, Mr. and Mrs. Paul Kanavos, Craig Effron & Company, Charles Evans Foundation, and Christian and Heidi Lange Family Foundation.

References

1. Siegel R, Naishadham D, Jemal A. Cancer statistics, 2013. CA Cancer J Clin. 2013;63:11–30.
2. Malvezzi M, Bertuccio P, Levi F, La Vecchia C, Negri E. European cancer mortality predictions for the year 2013. Ann Oncol. 2013;24:792–800.
3. Jemal A, Ward E, Thun M. Declining death rates reflect progress against cancer. PLoS One. 2010;5: e9584.
4. Jang TL, Yossepowitch O, Bianco F, Scardino PT. Low risk prostate cancer in men under age 65: the case for definitive treatment. Urol Oncol. 2007;25:510.
5. Bonekamp D, Jacobs MA, El-Khouli R, Stoianovici D, Macura KJ. Advancements in MR imaging of the prostate: from diagnosis to interventions. Radiographics. 2011;31:677–703.
6. Merkle EM, Dale BM, Paulson EK. Abdominal MR imaging at 3 T. Magn Reson Imaging Clin N Am. 2006;14:17.
7. Barth MM, Smith MP, Pedrosa I, Lenkinski RE, Rofsky NM. Body MR imaging at 3.0 T: understanding the opportunities and challenges. Radiographics. 2007;27:1445–62.
8. Zaremba L. Guidance for industry and FDA staff: Criteria for Significant Risk Investigations of Magnetic Resonance Diagnostic Devices - Guidance for Industry and Food and Drug Administration Staff. 2003:14. Available at http://www.fda.gov/downloads/ MedicalDevices/DeviceRegulationandGuidance/ GuidanceDocuments/ucm072688.pdf. Accessed on 7 Oct 2014]
9. Sosna J, Pedrosa I, Dewolf WC, Mahallati H, Lenkinski RE, Rofsky NM. MR imaging of the prostate at 3 Tesla: comparison of an external phased-array coil to imaging with an endorectal coil at 1.5 Tesla. Acad Radiol. 2004;11:857.
10. Barentsz JO, Richenberg J, Clements R, et al. ESUR prostate MR guidelines 2012. Eur Radiol. 2012; 22:746–57.
11. Heijmink SW, Ftterer JJ, Hambrock T, et al. Prostate cancer: body-array versus endorectal coil MR imaging at 3 T—comparison of image quality, localization, and staging performance. Radiology. 2007;244:184–95.
12. Hricak H, White S, Vigneron D, et al. Carcinoma of the prostate gland: MR imaging with pelvic phased-array coils versus integrated endorectal–pelvic phased-array coils. Radiology. 1994;193:703–9.
13. Scheidler J, Hricak H, Vigneron DB, et al. Prostate cancer: localization with three-dimensional proton MR spectroscopic imaging—clinicopathologic study. Radiology. 1999;213:473–80.
14. Kim JK, Hong SS, Choi YJ, et al. Wash in rate on the basis of dynamic contrast enhanced MRI: usefulness for prostate cancer detection and localization. J Magn Reson Imaging. 2005;22:639–46.
15. Koh D-M, Collins DJ. Diffusion-weighted MRI in the body: applications and challenges in oncology. Am J Roentgenol. 2007;188:1622–35.
16. Morgan VA, Riches SF, Thomas K, et al. Diffusion-weighted magnetic resonance imaging for monitoring prostate cancer progression in patients managed by active surveillance. Br J Radiol. 2011;84:31–7.
17. Giannarini G, Petralia G, Thoeny HC. Potential and limitations of diffusion-weighted magnetic resonance imaging in kidney, prostate, and bladder cancer including pelvic lymph node staging: a critical analysis of the literature. Eur Urol. 2012;61(2):326–40.
18. Nicholson B, Theodorescu D. Angiogenesis and prostate cancer tumor growth. J Cell Biochem. 2004; 91:125–50.
19. Bigler SA, Deering RE, Brawer MK. Comparison of microscopic vascularity in benign and malignant prostate tissue. Hum Pathol. 1993;24:220–6.
20. Siegal JA, Yu E, Brawer MK. Topography of neovascularity in human prostate carcinoma. Cancer. 1995;75:2545–51.
21. Tofts PS, Wicks D, Barker GJ. The MRI measurement of NMR and physiological parameters in tissue to study disease process. Prog Clin Biol Res. 1991; 363:313.
22. Brix G, Semmler W, Port R, Schad LR, Layer G, Lorenz WJ. Pharmacokinetic parameters in CNS Gd-DTPA enhanced MR imaging. J Comput Assist Tomogr. 1991;15:621–8.
23. Ren J, Huan Y, Wang H, et al. Dynamic contrast-enhanced MRI of benign prostatic hyperplasia and prostatic carcinoma: correlation with angiogenesis. Clin Radiol. 2008;63:153–9.
24. Costello L, Franklin R. The intermediary metabolism of the prostate: a key to understanding the pathogenesis and progression of prostate malignancy. Oncology. 2000;59:269–82.
25. Costello LC, Franklin RB. The clinical relevance of the metabolism of prostate cancer; zinc and tumor suppression: connecting the dots. Mol Cancer. 2006; 5:17.
26. Costello LC, Liu Y, Franklin RB, Kennedy MC. Zinc inhibition of mitochondrial aconitase and its importance in citrate metabolism of prostate epithelial cells. J Biol Chem. 1997;272:28875–81.
27. Glunde K, Ackerstaff E, Mori N, Jacobs MA, Bhujwalla ZM. Choline phospholipid metabolism in cancer: consequences for molecular pharmaceutical interventions. Mol Pharm. 2006;3:496–506.
28. Scheenen TW, Ftterer J, Weiland E, et al. Discriminating cancer from noncancer tissue in the prostate by 3-dimensional proton magnetic resonance spectroscopic imaging: a prospective multicenter validation study. Invest Radiol. 2011;46:25–33.
29. Kurhanewicz J, Vigneron DB, Hricak H, Narayan P, Carroll P, Nelson SJ. Three-dimensional H-1 MR spectroscopic imaging of the in situ human prostate with high (0.24-0.7-cm^3) spatial resolution. Radiology. 1996;198:795–805.
30. Riches SF, Payne GS, Morgan VA, et al. MRI in the detection of prostate cancer: combined apparent diffusion coefficient, metabolite ratio, and vascular parameters. Am J Roentgenol. 2009;193:1583–91.

31. Turkbey B, Mani H, Shah V, et al. Multiparametric 3 T prostate magnetic resonance imaging to detect cancer: histopathological correlation using prostatectomy specimens processed in customized magnetic resonance imaging based molds. J Urol. 2011;186:1818–24.

32. Langer DL, van der Kwast TH, Evans AJ, et al. Intermixed normal tissue within prostate cancer: Effect on MR imaging measurements of apparent diffusion coefficient and T2—sparse versus dense cancers. Radiology. 2008;249:900–8.

33. Akin O, Sala E, Moskowitz CS, et al. Transition zone prostate cancers: features, detection, localization, and staging at endorectal MR imaging. Radiology. 2006;239:784–92.

34. Delongchamps NB, Beuvon F, Eiss D, et al. Multiparametric MRI is helpful to predict tumor focality, stage, and size in patients diagnosed with unilateral low-risk prostate cancer. Prostate Cancer Prostatic Dis. 2011;14:232–7.

35. Ikonen S, Kivisaari L, Vehmas T, et al. Optimal timing of post biopsy MR imaging of the prostate. Acta Radiol. 2001;42:70–3.

36. Qayyum A, Coakley FV, Lu Y, et al. Organ-confined prostate cancer: effect of prior transrectal biopsy on endorectal MRI and MR spectroscopic imaging. Am J Roentgenol. 2004;183:1079–83.

37. White S, Hricak H, Forstner R, et al. Prostate cancer: effect of postbiopsy hemorrhage on interpretation of MR images. Radiology. 1995;195:385–90.

38. Janssen M, Huijgensz P, Bourman A, Oe P, Donker A, Van Der Meulen J. Citrate versus heparin anticoagulation in chronic haernodialysis patients. Nephrol Dial Transplant. 1993;8:1228–33.

39. Peng Y, Jiang Y, Yang C, et al. Quantitative analysis of multiparametric prostate MR images: differentiation between prostate cancer and normal tissue and correlation with Gleason score—a computer-aided diagnosis development study. Radiology. 2013;267:787–96.

40. Zakian KL, Sircar K, Hricak H, et al. Correlation of proton MR spectroscopic imaging with Gleason score based on step-section pathologic analysis after radical prostatectomy. Radiology. 2005;234:804–14.

41. Hodge K, McNeal J, Terris M, Stamey T. Random systematic versus directed ultrasound guided transrectal core biopsies of the prostate. J Urol. 1989;142:71–4. discussion 4–5.

42. Raja J, Ramachandran N, Munneke G, Patel U. Current status of transrectal ultrasound-guided prostate biopsy in the diagnosis of prostate cancer. Clin Radiol. 2006;61:142–53.

43. Durkan G, Sheikh N, Johnson P, Hildreth A, Greene D. Improving prostate cancer detection with an extended core transrectal ultrasonography guided prostate biopsy protocol. BJU Int. 2002;89:33–9.

44. Bazinet M, Karakiewicz PI, Aprikian AG, et al. Value of systematic transition zone biopsies in the early detection of prostate cancer. J Urol. 1996;155:605–6.

45. Liu IJ, Macy M, Lai Y-H, Terris MK. Critical evaluation of the current indications for transition zone biopsies. Urology. 2001;57:1117–20.

46. Mitterberger M, Pinggera G, Horninger W, et al. Comparison of contrast enhanced color Doppler targeted biopsy to conventional systematic biopsy: impact on Gleason score. J Urol. 2007;178:464–8.

47. Trabulsi EJ, Sackett D, Gomella LG, Halpern EJ. Enhanced transrectal ultrasound modalities in the diagnosis of prostate cancer. Urology. 2010;76:1025–33.

48. Cantwell CP, Hahn PF, Gervais DA, Mueller PR. Prostate biopsy after ano-rectal resection: value of CT-guided trans-gluteal biopsy. Eur Radiol. 2008;18:738–42.

49. Shinohara K, Gulati M, Koppie TM, Terris MK. Transperineal prostate biopsy after abdominoperineal resection. J Urol. 2003;169:141–4.

50. Seaman EK, Sawczuk IS, Fatal M, Olsson CA, Shabsigh R. Transperineal prostate needle biopsy guided by transurethral ultrasound in patients without a rectum. Urology. 1996;47:353–5.

51. Thompson IM, Pauler DK, Goodman PJ, et al. Prevalence of prostate cancer among men with a prostate-specific antigen level 4.0 ng per milliliter. N Engl J Med. 2004;350:2239–46.

52. Pondman KM, Ftterer JJ, ten Haken B, et al. MR-guided biopsy of the prostate: an overview of techniques and a systematic review. Eur Urol. 2008;54:517–27.

53. Engelhard K, Hollenbach H, Kiefer B, Winkel A, Goeb K, Engehausen D. Prostate biopsy in the supine position in a standard 1.5-T scanner under real time MR-imaging control using a MR-compatible endorectal biopsy device. Eur Radiol. 2006;16:1237–43.

54. Hambrock T, Somford DM, Hoeks C, et al. Magnetic resonance imaging guided prostate biopsy in men with repeat negative biopsies and increased prostate specific antigen. J Urol. 2010;183:520–8.

55. Chun FK-H, Steuber T, Erbersdobler A, et al. Development and internal validation of a nomogram predicting the probability of prostate cancer Gleason sum upgrading between biopsy and radical prostatectomy pathology. Eur Urol. 2006;49:820–6.

56. Bott S, Young M, Kellett M, Parkinson M. Anterior prostate cancer: is it more difficult to diagnose? BJU Int. 2002;89:886–9.

57. Franiel T, Stephan C, Erbersdobler A, et al. Areas suspicious for prostate cancer: MR-guided biopsy in patients with at least one transrectal US-guided biopsy with a negative finding—multiparametric MR imaging for detection and biopsy planning. Radiology. 2011;259:162–72.

58. Vyas L, Acher P, Kinsella J, et al. Indications, results and safety profile of transperineal sector biopsies (TPSB) of the prostate: a single centre experience of 634 cases. BJU Int. 2014;114(1):32–7.

59. Seitz M, Shukla-Dave A, Bjartell A, et al. Functional magnetic resonance imaging in prostate cancer. Eur Urol. 2009;55:801–14.

60. Hata N, Jinzaki M, Kacher D, et al. MR imaging-guided prostate biopsy with surgical navigation software: device validation and feasibility. Radiology. 2001;220:263–8.

61. Beyersdorff D, Winkel A, Hamm B, Lenk S, Loening SA, Taupitz M. MR imaging-guided prostate biopsy with a closed MR unit at 1.5 T: initial results. Radiology. 2005;234:576–81.
62. Yakar D, Hambrock T, Hoeks C, Barentsz JO, Ftterer JJ. Magnetic resonance-guided biopsy of the prostate: feasibility, technique, and clinical applications. Top Magn Reson Imaging. 2008;19:291–5.
63. Zangos S, Herzog C, Eichler K, et al. MR-compatible assistance system for punction in a high-field system: device and feasibility of transgluteal biopsies of the prostate gland. Eur Radiol. 2007;17:1118–24.
64. Maas MC, Vos EK, Lagemaat MW, et al. Feasibility of T2 weighted turbo spin echo imaging of the human prostate at 7 tesla. Magn Reson Med. 2014;71(5):1711–9.
65. Kobus T, Bitz AK, van Uden MJ, et al. In vivo 31P MR spectroscopic imaging of the human prostate at 7 T: safety and feasibility. Magn Reson Med. 2012;68:1683–95.
66. Moore CM, Kasivisvanathan V, Eggener S, et al. Standards of reporting for MRI-targeted biopsy studies (START) of the prostate: recommendations from an International Working Group. Eur Urol. 2013;64:544–52.

Advanced Ultrasound Applications

Prostate Ultrasound Artifacts and How to Fix Them

Pat Fulgham

Introduction

Artifacts in ultrasound can be defined as depictions of structures or processes that do not accurately reflect the true underlying structure or process. That is, the ultrasound signal once transmitted is altered during transit inside the body in a manner that makes the returning signal and resultant image a distortion of the underlying reality. Thus, an artifact is not an error or mistake, just a logical misrepresentation based on the physics of ultrasound.

Once understood, artifacts may not only be corrected but used to gain additional clinical insight. The most effective way to approach artifacts is to (1) recognize and define them, (2) consider the possible physical and mechanical explanations for them, (3) make adjustments in technique and machine settings to correct or minimize them, if appropriate, and (4) derive any additional useful clinical information from them.

Examples of several types of artifacts are considered. Clinical images are presented to illustrate the pertinent points.

P. Fulgham, M.D., D.A.B.U., F.A.C.S. (✉)
Department of Urology, Texas Health
Presbyterian Dallas, 8230 Walnut Hill Lane,
Suite 014, Dallas, TX, USA
e-mail: pfulgham@airmail.net

Reverberation Artifact

Reverberation artifacts (often called multipath artifacts) are caused by sound waves bouncing back and forth between two or more reflectors (Fig. 1).

This type of artifact is quite common in transrectal scanning of the prostate and often arises from air trapping in the covering used to protect the probe (Fig. 2). It may also arise from gas in the rectum itself.

In scanning the prostate, the air bubble produces an artifact that may obscure distal anatomy (Fig. 3). This type of artifact can often be corrected by gently pressing the probe against the rectal wall to force the gas away from the crystal face. If that does not work, the probe should be removed and the condom cover re-prepared. Copious gel should be applied to help minimize air between the covering and the probe. Gas or stool in the rectum may also cause this artifact and does not usually respond to probe repositioning. In this circumstance, removing the probe and using a gloved finger to clear the gas and stool can be tried. Another type of reverberation artifact occurs when an ultrasound wave strikes gas and stool in the small intestine (Fig. 4).

Reverberation artifacts may also be seen when ultrasound waves strike any specular reflector. Examples of such reflectors in the prostate include needles, fiducial markers, and radioactive seeds (Fig. 5). This characteristic artifact is the

C.R. Porter and E.M. Wolff (eds.), *Prostate Ultrasound: Current Practice and Future Directions,*
DOI 10.1007/978-1-4939-1948-2_6, © Springer Science+Business Media New York 2015

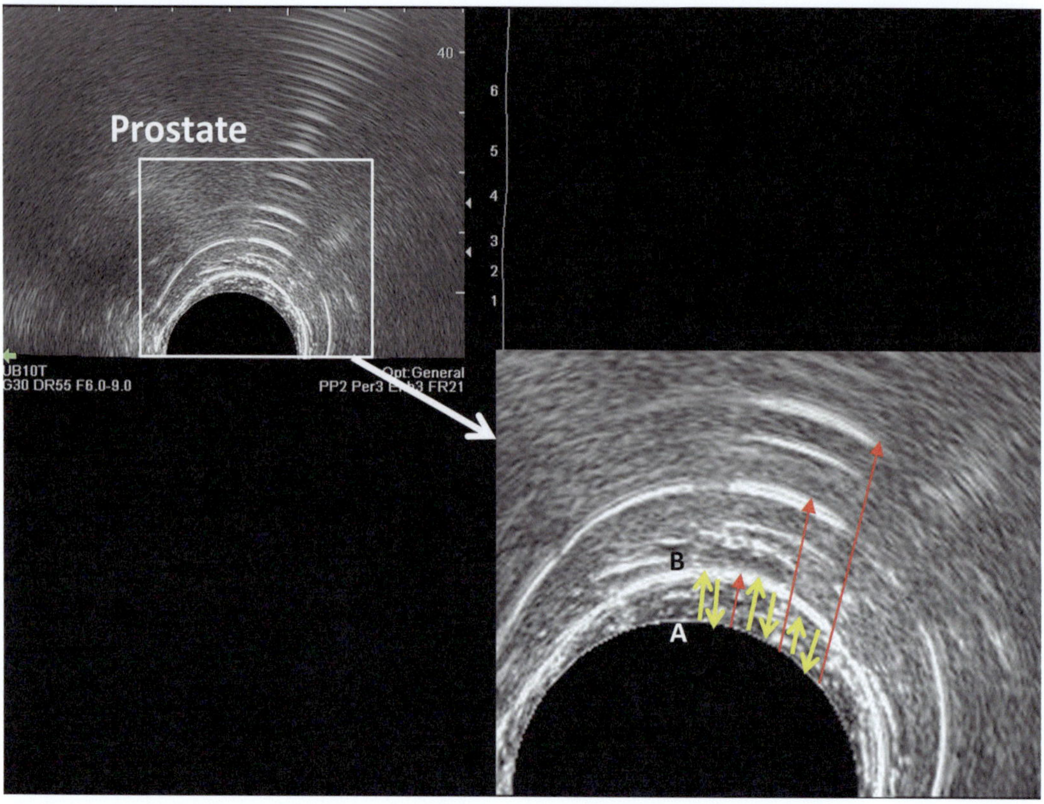

Fig. 1 As the incident wave bounces back and forth between surfaces A and B (*yellow arrows*), the returning waves are perceived by the probe as returning from reflectors progressively further from the probe face (*long red arrows*)

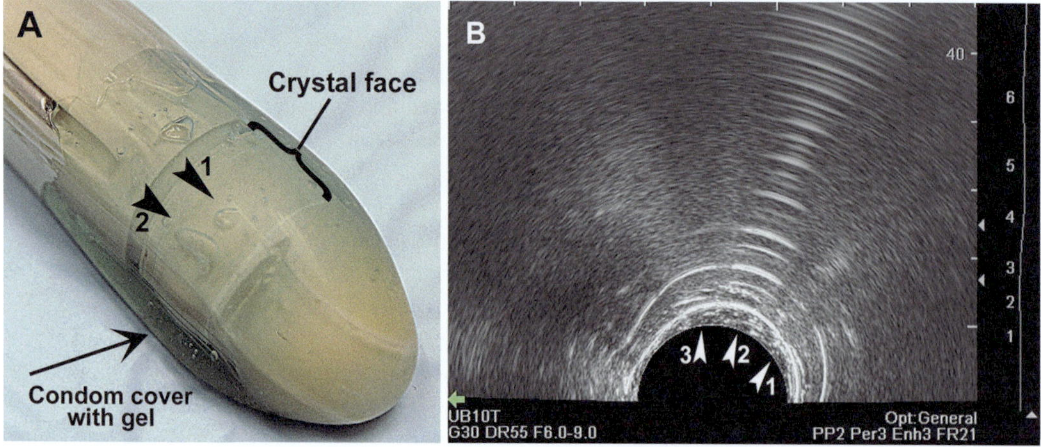

Fig. 2 A biplane probe with air bubbles overlying the transverse crystal (*arrowheads 1* and *2* in image **a**). *Arrowhead 1* in image (**a**) designates a bubble against the crystal surface. This produces a closely spaced reverberation artifact (*Arrowhead 1* in image **b**). *Arrowhead 2* in image (**a**) designates a bubble trapped beneath the probe cover. This produces a more hyperechoic and widely spaced reverberation artifact (*arrowhead 2* in image **b**). *Arrowhead 3* in image (**b**) represents the gel between the condom cover and the crystal face

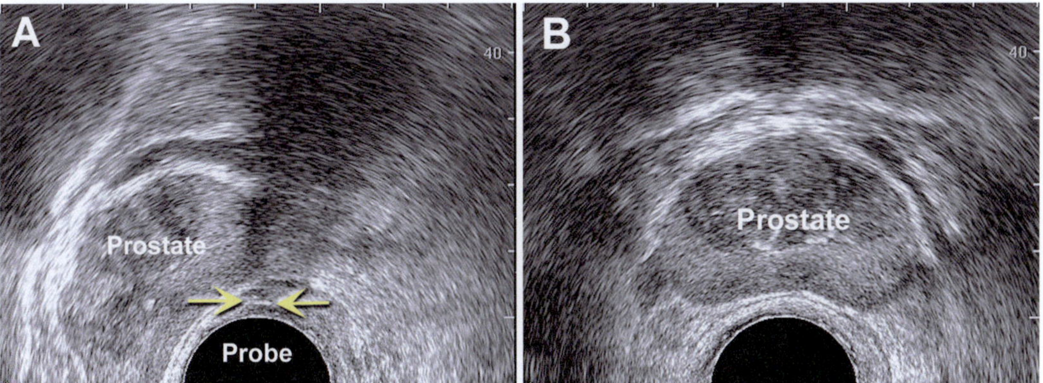

Fig. 3 (a) Reverberation artifact caused by air bubble trapped between probe crystal and probe cover resulting in a reverberation artifact (*yellow arrows*). If the probe is rotated within the rectum this artifact will remain. However, if air is trapped between the probe cover and the rectal wall the artifact will resolve with rotation or change in probe position. (**b**) Same prostate after the air bubble removed

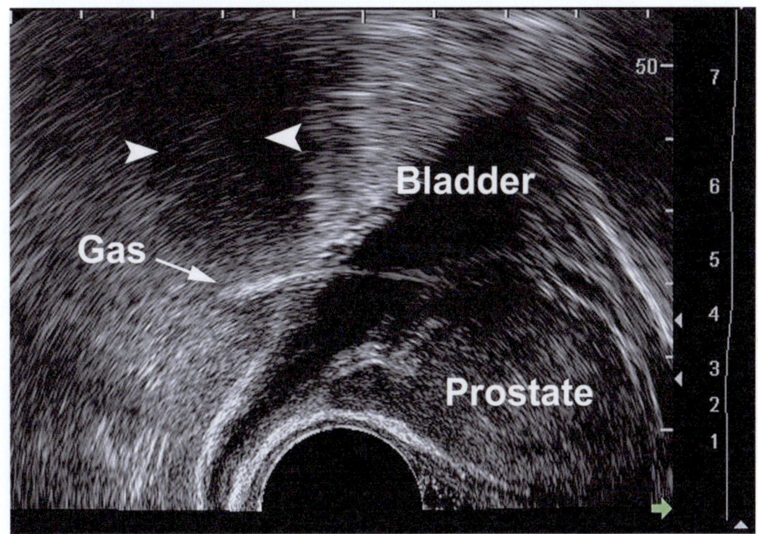

Fig. 4 Reverberation artifact caused by small intestine containing gas in the cul-de-sac posterior to the bladder on this sagittal view of the prostate causes acoustic shadowing (*arrowheads*) distally because of attenuation

result of reverberation of the waves between the leading and trailing edges of the structure. That is, for example, the wave strikes the front edge of a hollow needle and bounces back and forth between the front and back edge producing a distal artifact of diminishing echogenicity but equal distance from the needle (Fig. 5a, b). Similar patterns are seen for fiducial markers and seeds (Fig. 5c).

Compression Artifacts

Although compression does not technically produce an artifact (based on our original definition of artifact) it can cause distortions of anatomy and changes in echogenicity and blood flow. As such, compression may cause the sonographer to "misinterpret" the nature of the anatomic structure being interrogated. For

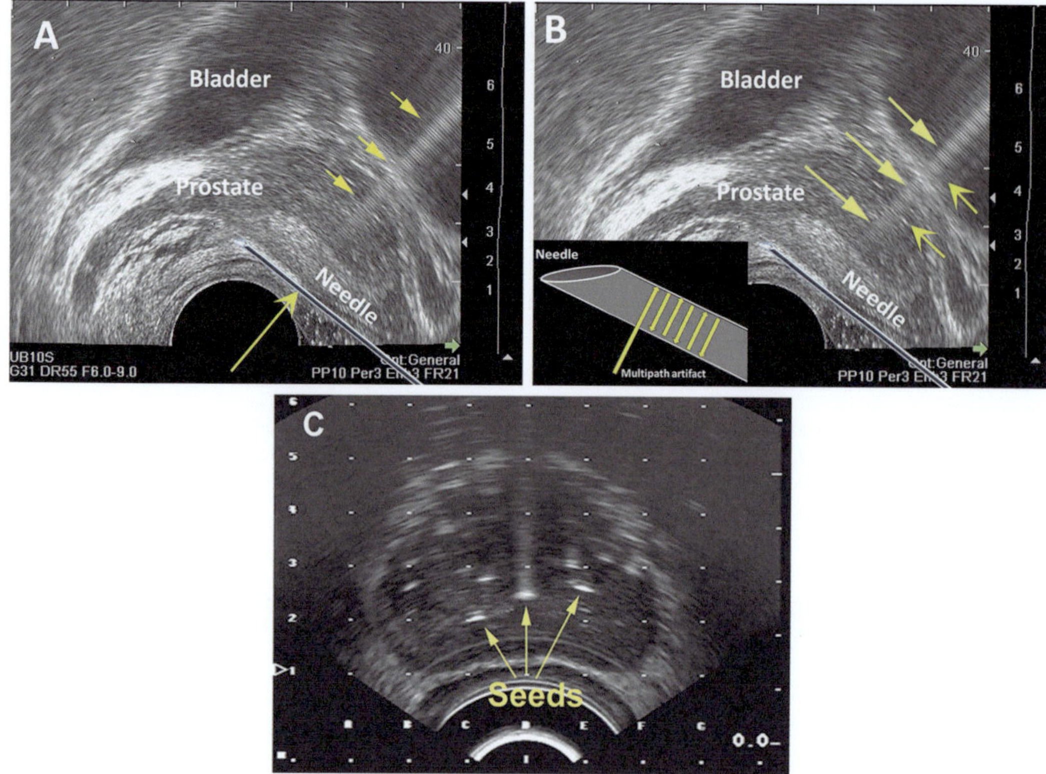

Fig. 5 Specular reflectors have a flat smooth surface. (**a**) Although sound waves strike the surface of the needle along its entire length, the reverberation artifact (*white arrows*) is most pronounced when the incident wave (*yellow arrows*) strikes perpendicular to the object. The *inset* in (**b**) shows the multipath artifact within the needle (*white arrows*). (**c**) Radioactive seeds also serve as specular reflectors in an ultrasound field. The reverberation artifact is most prominent when the incident wave strikes perpendicular to the reflector

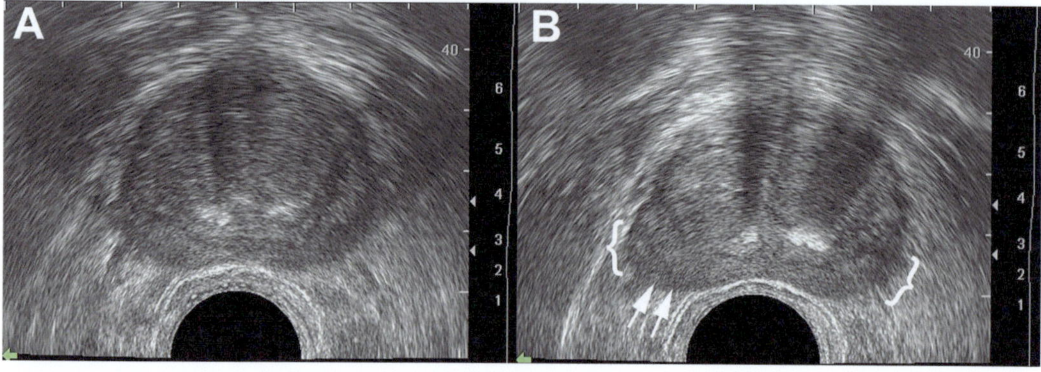

Fig. 6 A transverse ultrasound of the prostate with no compression (**a**). The same gland with compression of the rectal wall and prostate demonstrates capsular deformity (*arrows*) and induced hypoechogenicity (*brackets*) (**b**)

example, when the transrectal probe is pressed against the rectal wall it may deform the underlying prostate capsule and peripheral zone of the prostate, producing asymmetry and hypoechogenicity (Fig. 6).

Similarly, blood flow may be affected by the amount of force exerted against the rectal wall by the probe. Blood flow in the neurovascular bundle as well as the peripheral zone of the prostate may be diminished by probe pressure (Fig. 7).

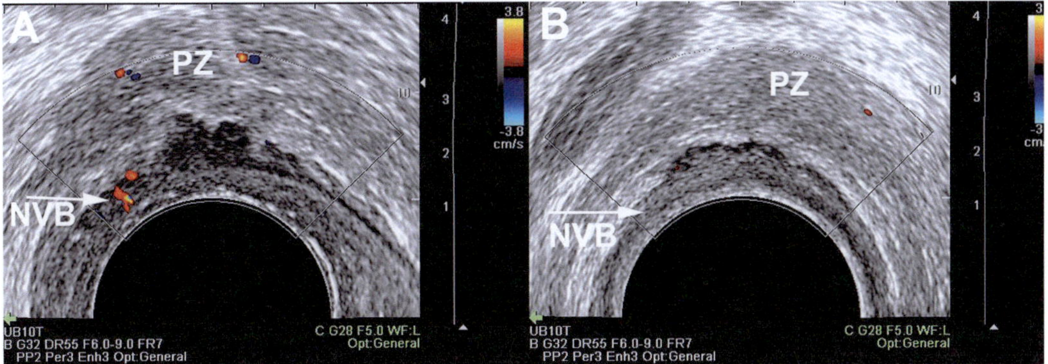

Fig. 7 (**a**) Normal blood flow on a transverse ultrasound of the prostate showing the expected flow in the peripheral zone (PZ) and the left neurovascular bundle (NVB). (**b**) Compression of the same prostate on the left side by a probe results in less demonstrated flow in the peripheral zone and left neurovascular bundle

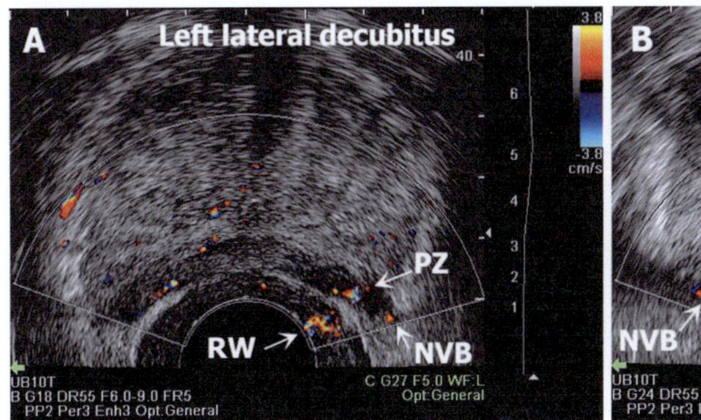
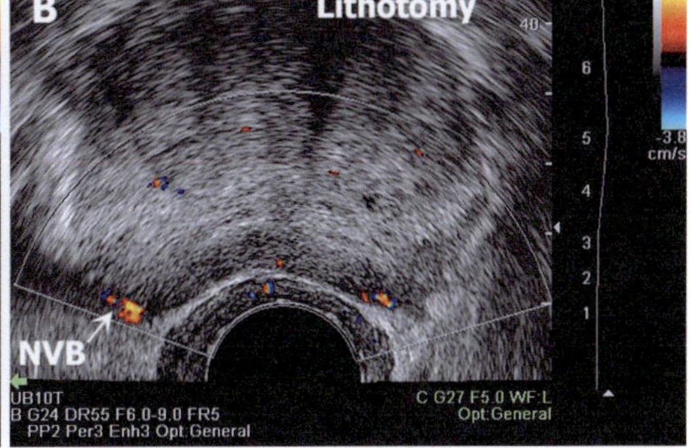

Fig. 8 (**a**) Color Doppler demonstrates increased flow in the peripheral zone (PZ) and neurovascular bundle (NVB) and rectal wall (RW) on the left side when the patient is in the left lateral decubitus position. (**b**) Same patient in the lithotomy position. The blood flow in the neurovascular bundles is more symmetric in this position

Artifacts of Patient Position

The interpretation of intra-prostatic blood flow has been used to identify areas of increased vascularity which could indicate underlying malignancy [1]. Some investigators have used the resistive index of intraprostatic vessels to predict the degree of bladder outlet obstruction [2]. Halpern et al. demonstrated that the position of the patient may affect the pattern of blood flow within the prostate [3]. Patients in the left lateral decubitus position will demonstrate increased blood flow in the left peripheral zone and neurovascular bundle, whereas blood flow will be symmetric from left to right when the same patient is evaluated in the supine position (Fig. 8). This phenomenon may be important if increased blood flow is being used as a marker for a possible isoechoic neoplasm.

Edging Artifacts

Edging artifacts occur when the angle of insonation is such that no sound waves are reflected back to the probe from a reflector. This is most obvious when a sound wave strikes a curved or rounded surface at the "critical angle" where their waves are neither reflected or refracted (Fig. 9).

In prostate ultrasound the two most common edging artifacts occur at the lateral margin of the peripheral zone [1] and at the lateral margin of the prostate [2] (Fig. 10). Edging artifact is also seen in the midline where the two rounded surfaces of the lateral lobes of the prostate come together (Fig. 11).

The edging artifact is frequently seen at the junction of the transition zone and peripheral zone on a transverse view of the prostate (Fig. 12).

If the edging artifact is obscuring information, this can be eliminated by changing the angle of insonation (Fig. 13).

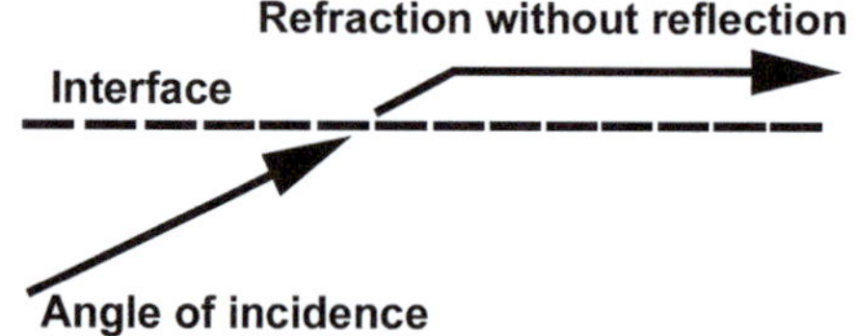

Fig. 9 When sound waves strike a surface or interface at a "critical angle," the wave is refracted without significant reflection

Acoustic Shadowing

Acoustic shadowing does not qualify, by our strict definition, as an artifact. Acoustic shadowing results from severe attenuation of a sound wave or reflection of a sound wave such that information about structures distal to the attenuator/reflector is lost or diminished. Thus acoustic shadowing is not a misrepresentation (as are artifacts) but a loss of information about reflectors in the sonofield.

In transrectal ultrasound of the prostate a common cause of acoustic shadowing is corpora amylacea. Corpora amylacea are proteinaceous deposits often in the junction between the transition zone and peripheral zone. Since there is a high impedance difference between the corpora amylacea and the surrounding prostatic parenchyma much of the sound wave energy is reflected and some is absorbed. As a consequence tissue and objects distal to the corpora amylacea are not seen and a hypoechoic or anechoic "shadow" is cast (Fig. 14).

Dystrophic calcification from previous infection or treatment for prostate cancer may create some acoustic shadowing (Fig. 15).

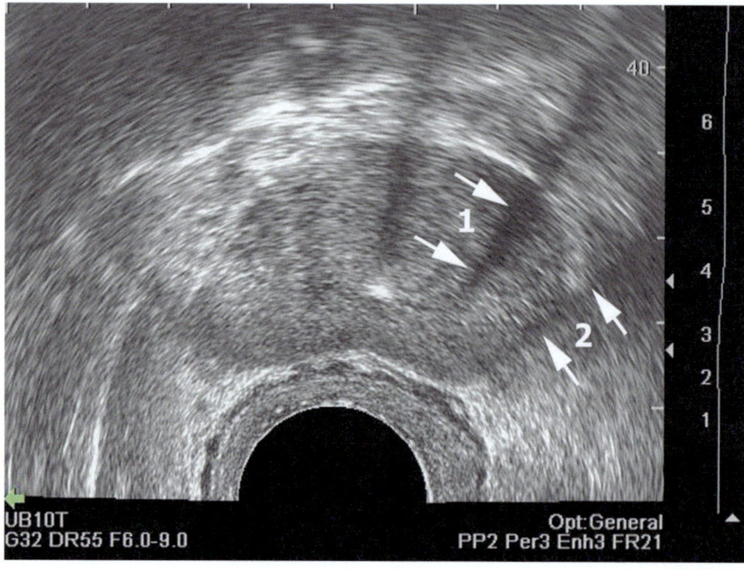

Fig. 10 Edging artifacts (*arrows*) seen at the lateral margins of the peripheral zone of the prostate (*1 arrows*) and at the lateral prostate capsule (*2 arrows*)

Acoustic shadowing may be distinguished from edging artifact since a change in the angle of insonation does not eliminate acoustic shadowing although it will change the direction of the resultant acoustic shadow (Fig. 16).

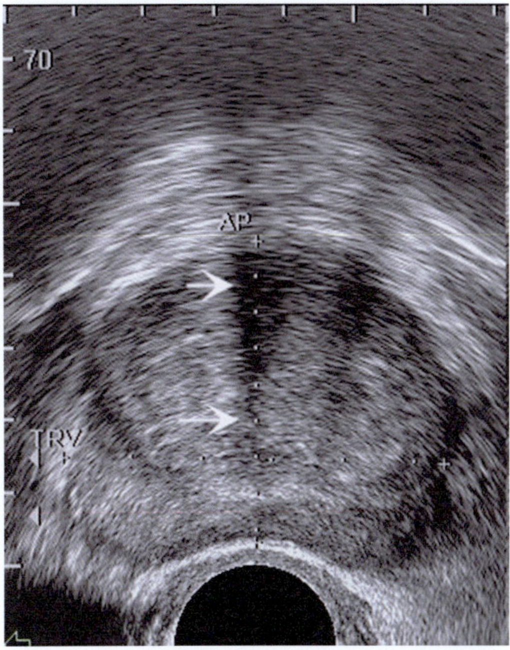

Fig. 11 Edging artifact (*arrows*) produced by transition zone and lobes meeting in the midline seen at the lateral margins of the peripheral zone of the prostate

Increased Thru Transmission

Increased thru transmission refers to the appearance of tissue distal to a structure or tissue that does not attenuate sound waves as much as the surrounding tissue. For example, fluid in a prostatic cyst does not attenuate sound waves as much as the surrounding prostatic tissue. The resulting sound waves are more energetic and when they strike the tissue distal to the cyst it appears hyperechoic compared to the surrounding tissue (Fig. 17).

Similar examples of increased thru transmission can be seen distal to utricular cysts and cysts in the seminal vesicles If imaging of tissue distal to a cystic structure is desired, it may be helpful to change the angle of insonation or decrease the sensitivity of the probe to that region of the sonographic field by adjusting the TGC curve.

Artifacts Associated with Doppler Imaging

Doppler imaging has been used in prostate ultrasound to identify areas of increased blood flow. Identification of areas of increased vascularity may improve the efficiency of detecting prostate

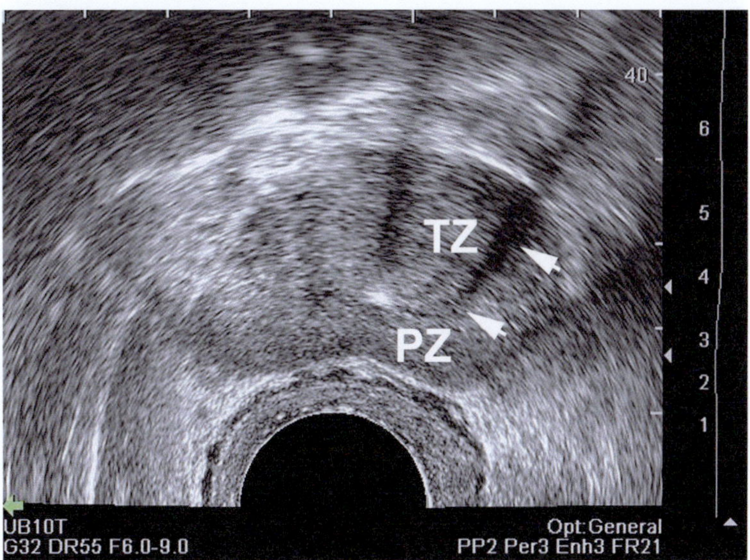

Fig. 12 Edging artifact (*arrows*) on transverse view of the prostate at the junction of the transition zone (TZ) and peripheral zone (PZ)

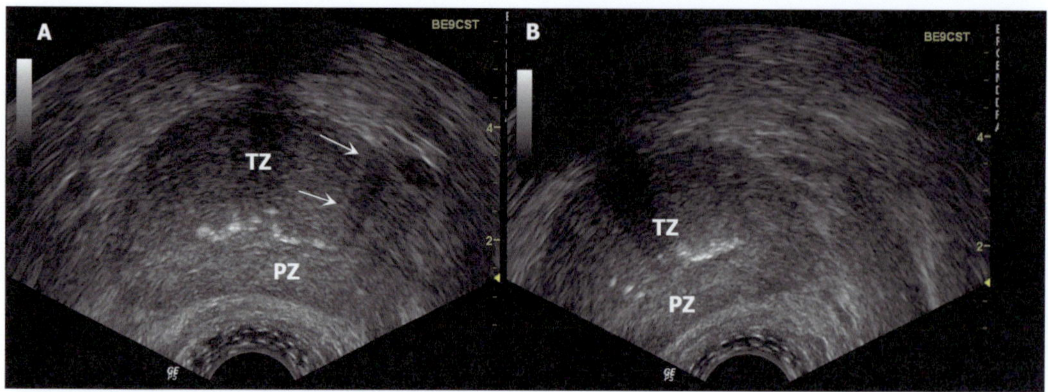

Fig. 13 (**a**) Edging artifact at junction of peripheral zone and transition zone can be eliminated (**b**) by moving the probe to change the angle of insonation

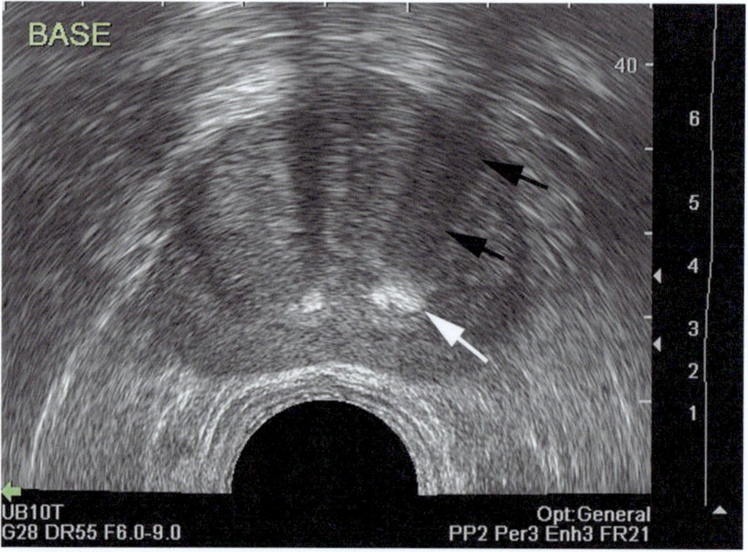

Fig. 14 In this transverse image of the prostate, an acoustic shadow (*black arrows*) is "cast" by highly reflective corpora amylacea (*white arrow*)

cancer [4]. It remains controversial whether unenhanced Doppler ultrasound significantly improves prostate cancer diagnosis.

Aliasing occurs when the Doppler frequency shift caused by flowing blood exceeds the sampling frequency by more than twofold (Nyquist Limit). Aliasing can misrepresent the velocity of blood flow (Fig. 18). Blood flow in prostatic capsular vessels is typically low, <0.2 m/s. Therefore, the frequency shift is typically low [2]. With appropriate velocity settings aliasing is infrequently encountered within the prostate.

The twinkle artifact occurs when sound waves strike a strong specular reflector. When color Doppler mapping is performed, a multicolored

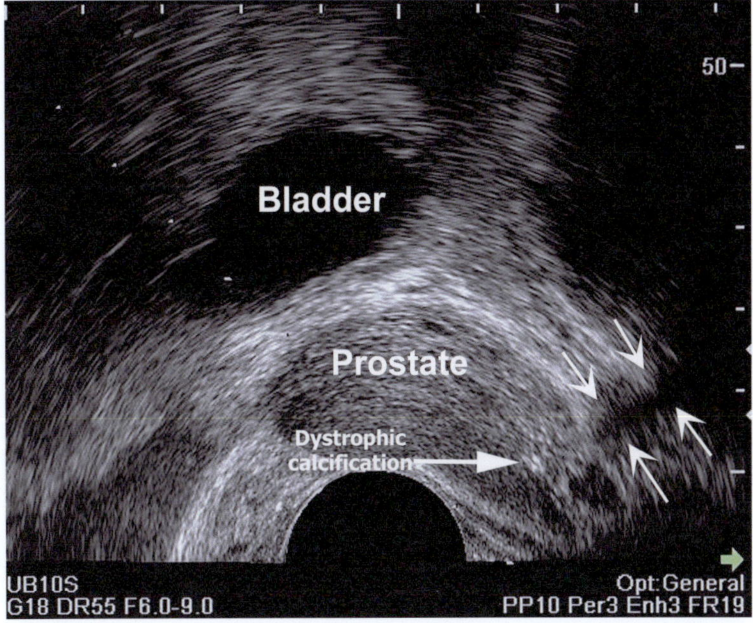

Fig. 15 Acoustic shadowing (*four white arrows*) caused by prostatitis with dystrophic calcification (dc) at the apex (*arrowhead*)

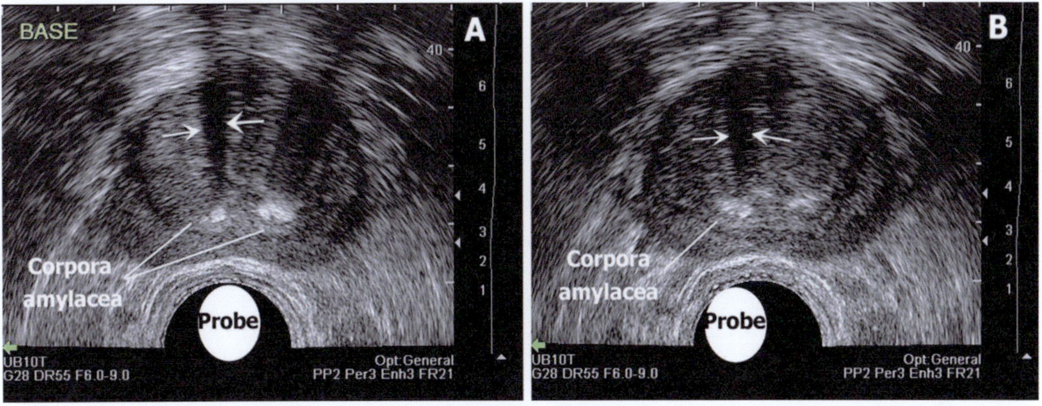

Fig. 16 Note that the acoustic shadowing in (**a**) is directly distal to probe (*arrows*). As the angle of insonation is changed in (**b**) the direction of the acoustic shadow changes (*arrows*)

shadow or trail is created distal to the reflector (Fig. 19).

This artifact simulates flow or motion when the object and tissue are stationary. Twinkle artifacts can be diminished by lowering the probe frequency or changing the angle of insonation.

Conclusions

Artifacts in prostate ultrasound scanning can usually be overcome by changing probe position or eliminating interfaces with large impedance differences (e.g., air–tissue or fluid–tissue interfaces).

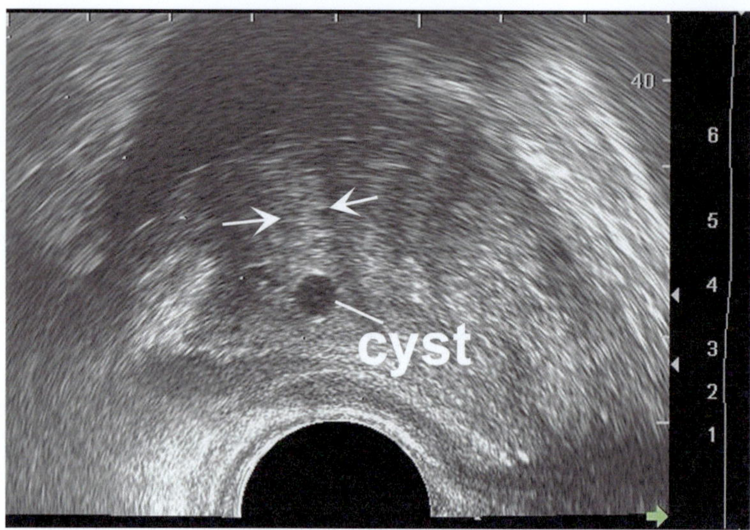

Fig. 17 Increased thru transmission causes tissue to appear hyperechoic compared to surrounding tissue (*arrows*) even though the tissues are histologically identical

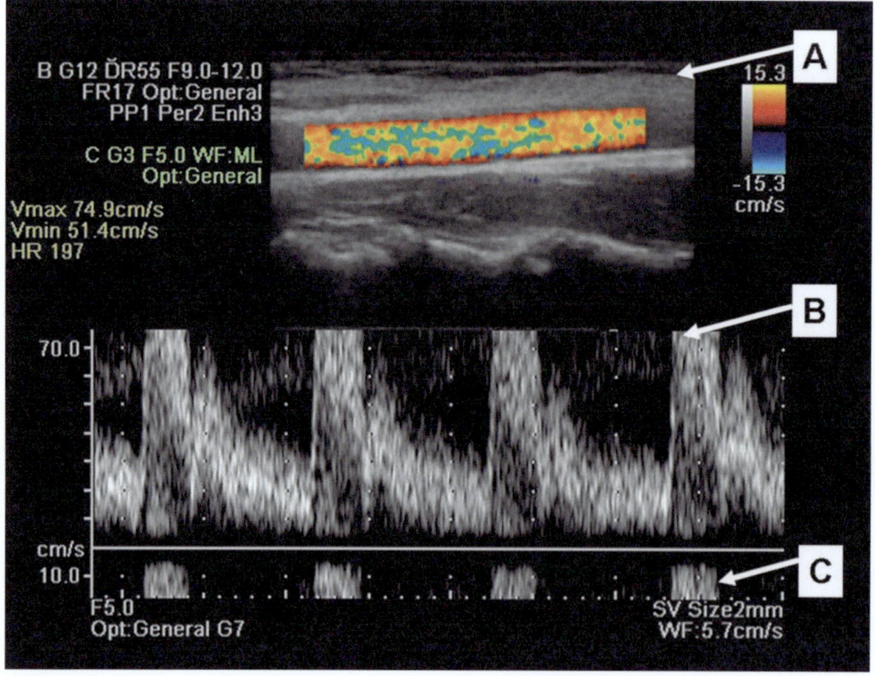

Fig. 18 Aliasing seen in this color Doppler image of the radial artery. (**a**) Shows apparently turbulent bidirectional flow. (**b**) Demonstrates "cropping" or wrapping of the velocity pattern on spectral Doppler. The truncated velocity peak is seen beneath the baseline (**c**)

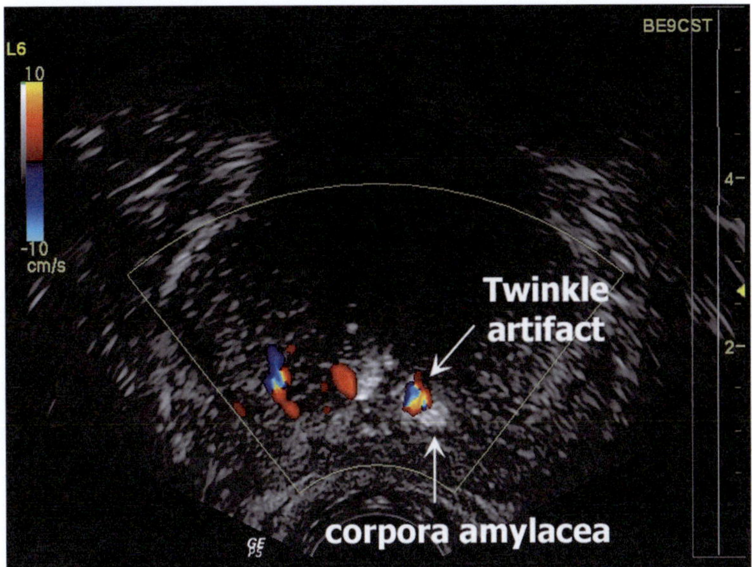

Fig. 19 Twinkle artifact (*arrow*) distal to a strong reflector, in this case corpora amylacea

A thorough understanding of the physics of artifacts is critical to producing good quality images that give a true understanding of the underlying structures of the prostate.

References

1. Trabulsi EJ, Sackett D, Gomella LG, Halpern EJ. Enhanced transrectal ultrasound modalities in the diagnosis of prostate cancer. Urology. 2010;76(5): 1025–33.

2. Zhang X, Gang L, Xuedong W, Xiaodong M, Linkun H, Yueqin Z, Hou J. Resistive index of prostate capsular arteries: a newly identified parameter to diagnose and assess bladder outlet obstruction in patients with benign prostatic hyperplasia. J Urol. 2012;188:881–7.

3. Halpern EJ, Frauscher F, Forsberg F, Strup SE, Nazarian LN, O'Kane P, Gomella LG. High-frequency Doppler ultrasound of the prostate: effect of patient position. Radiology. 2002;222:634–9.

4. Frauscher F, Klauser A, Volgger H, Halpern EJ, Pallwein L, Steiner H, Schuster A, Horninger W, Rogatsch H, Bartsch G. Comparison of contrast enhanced color Doppler targeted biopsy with conventional systematic biopsy: impact on prostate cancer detection. J Urol. 2002;167:1648–52.

Male Infertility and Prostate Ultrasound

Anna M. Lawrence and Thenu Chandrasekar

Introduction to Male Infertility

Infertility is a disease of increasing prevalence with approximately 15–20 % of couples that are attempting to become pregnant suffering from infertility [1]. It is estimated that in the developed world one in four couples will suffer from infertility and possibly 17–30 % in the developing world [2]. With the increase in the prevalence in infertility, the definitions, evaluation, and understanding of both male and female infertility has also increased. Consequently, the use of imaging, particularly ultrasound, to investigate causes of male infertility has increased. This chapter is focused on the use of ultrasound in the evaluation of male infertility.

Infertility as defined by the World Health Organization (WHO) [3] and the International Committee for Monitoring Assisted Reproductive Care [4] is "a disease of the reproductive system defined as the failure to achieve a clinical pregnancy after 12 months or more of regular unprotected sexual intercourse." The American Society of Reproductive Medicine [5] expands on this definition by stating that infertility is "defined by the failure to achieve a successful pregnancy after 12 months or more of appropriate, timed, unprotected intercourse or therapeutic donor insemination".

The increased understanding of infertility has made it apparent that female and male factors or a combination of both must be considered in the investigation of an infertile couple. Population studies completed as early as the 1980s, revealed that male factor infertility alone is responsible for up to 20 % of all infertile couples and an additional 30–40 % of couples have a component of male factor infertility. As such, up to 50–60 % of all infertile couples can be attributed in some part to the male partner [1].

In male factor infertility evaluation, the primary goal is to identify reversible etiologies of male infertility, which may increase the likelihood of conception through intercourse. Additionally, it is important to identify irreversible conditions in order to distinguish couples that may benefit from assisted reproductive techniques. Detection of etiologies that have no current available treatment is also important, as it allows couples to avoid the emotional and financial burden of attempting ineffective therapies.

A.M. Lawrence, M.Bc.H.B, F.R.A.C.S (✉)
Department of Urology, Auckland Hospital,
Auckland, New Zealand
e-mail: drannalawrence@gmail.com;
annamichele@hotmail.com

T. Chandrasekar, M.D.
Department of Urology, University of California
Davis Medical School, Lawrence Ellison Building,
4860 Y St., Suite 2200, Sacramento, CA, 95817, USA
e-mail: thenappan.chandrasekar@ucdmc.ucdavis.edu

C.R. Porter and E.M. Wolff (eds.), *Prostate Ultrasound: Current Practice and Future Directions*,
DOI 10.1007/978-1-4939-1948-2_7, © Springer Science+Business Media New York 2015

Classification of Male Infertility

There are numerous classifications of male factor infertility based on a variety of variables, including, (1) location of the abnormality causing infertility, (2) the abnormalities noted on semen parameters, (3) primary or secondary infertility, and (4) obstructive or non-obstructive abnormalities,

Location of Abnormalitiy

The location of the abnormality leading to male factor infertility is a valuable method of classification; by determining the location, the reversibility of the defect can be assessed. If it is reversible, then treatment options can be considered and prognosis of a successful pregnancy can be determined. The locations of the abnormalities causing male factor infertility are normally divided into pre-testicular, testicular, and post-testicular. The major etiologies within each category are listed in Table 1 [6].

Sperm Parameters

Semen analysis is a fundamental component of evaluating and defining the severity of male factor infertility [3, 6–8]. Semen analyses should always be conducted according to the WHO Laboratory Manual [3] in order to ensure standardization. The current standards for a normal semen analysis are defined in the fifth edition of the WHO Laboratory Manual, published in 2010, and can be reviewed in Table 2 [8, 9]. Classification based on semen analysis involves a wide variety of terminology, often misused in the public literature. A summary of the appropriate terminology is listed in Table 3 [6].

Primary and Secondary Infertility

Primary male factor infertility is defined as infertility in men who have never been able to conceive a child. In contrast, secondary male factor

Table 1 Etiologies of male factor infertility categorized by level of defect

Pre-testicular etiologies
Hypogonadotropic hypogonadism (congenital, acquired)
Coital Disorders (Erectile Dysfunction, Ejaculatory disorders) secondary to organic etiologies (diabetes mellitus, spinal injury, vascular/neurogenic, multiple sclerosis) and iatrogenic etiologies (RPLND, bladder neck surgery)
Primary testicular etiologies
Cryptorchidism (especially bilateral forms)
Infection or inflammation of the testes (Orchitis)
Testicular trauma
Testicular torsion
Varicocele
Gonadotoxic medications (including chemotherapy)
Radiation injury
Iatrogenic surgical injury (prior inguinal surgery)
Systemic diseases
Congenital etiologies
- Klinefelter's syndrome (47, XXY)
- Y-chromosome terminal deletions (Yq-)
- Structural autosomal abnormalities
Post-testicular etiologies
Obstructive/sub-obstructive lesions of the seminal tract (vasa deferentia, seminal vesicles, ejaculatory ducts)
Autoimmune infertility (autoimmunity against spermatozoa)
Infections and inflammation of the accessory glands (seminal vesicles, prostate, epididymis)
Congenital bilateral absence of the vasa deferentia

Table 2 WHO 2010 semen analysis parameters

Semen analysis component	Fifth percentile (95 % CI)
Semen Volume	1.5 mL (1.4–1.7)
Total Sperm Number	39 million (33–46)
Sperm Concentration	15 million/mL (12–16)
Vitality	58 % live (55–63)
Progressive Motility	32 % (31–34)
Total (Progressive + Nonprogressive Motility)	40 % (38–42)
Morphologically Normal Forms	4.0 % (3.0–4.0)

CI, confidence interval

infertility describes men who have previously conceived a child without assisted reproductive techniques but now is unable to achieve a successful pregnancy.

Table 3 Terminology based on semen analysis

Classification	Defining characteristics
Oligozoospermia	Sperm concentration $<15 \times 10^6$/mL, total sperm number $<39 \times 10^6$/mL
Asthenozoospermia	<32 % progressively motile spermatozoa
Teratozoospermia	<4 % morphologically normal spermatozoa
Oligo-astheno-teratozoospermia	Disturbance in all three parameters
Azoospermia	No spermatozoa in the ejaculate
Cryptozoospermia	Spermatazoa absent from fresh preparation, but observed in a centrifuged pellet
Aspermia	No ejaculate
Leucocytospermia	$> 1 \times 10^6$/mL leukocytes in the ejaculate

Obstructive and Non-obstructive

The importance of this classification lies in its prognostic value and the ability to then define the subsequent management for the patient. Obstructive etiologies frequently tend to have a good prognosis and, as described later, are often responsive to surgical interventions. Additionally, obstructive pathologies are *best-identified using ultrasound imaging*, and, as such, will be a major focus of the remainder of this chapter.

Evaluation of Male Infertility

Initial History

A complete and thorough history is the foundation of the evaluation for infertility. As there are a multitude of possible factors that may affect a patient's fertility and sexual function, a thorough medical, surgical, pharmaceutical (both legal and illicit), social and developmental history may help allude to these, and therefore focus further investigations. Key components of a sexual and fertility include enquiring about the length of time trying to conceive, frequency of sexual intercourse, previous

Table 4 Components of a thorough history in the evaluation of an infertile male

Reproductive/infertility history
Prior fertility/conceptions—current or previous partner, outcome
Prior fertility evaluation
Partner's fertility history and evaluation
Sexual history/Coital practices
Sexually transmitted diseases
Erectile function, lubrication
Frequency/timing of intercourse
Developmental history (onset of puberty, sexual characteristics)
Past medical history
Chronic illnesses
Genital trauma
Childhood history (cryptorchidism, torsion, midline defects)
Prior infections
Family history
Infertility history
Genetic conditions
Substance use or exposure
Prescription medication history
Drug abuses
Toxin exposure
Prior surgical history
Orchiopexy
Retroperitoneal/pelvic surgery
Herniorrhaphy
Vasectomy
Bladder neck/prostate surgery
Spinal surgery

fertility including any pregnancy or children, and any previous treatments for infertility

It is vital that this comprehensive history should encompass both long-term and short-term factors. Semen production has a 64-day cycle with 10–15 days for transit. During this period any disruption in spermatogenesis can cause an abnormal semen analysis, hence it is vital to expound any of these short term factors. At the same time long-term factors are also important to establish, as childhood chronic illness can cause long-term fertility changes [10]. The basis of a thorough history and factors/components to ask your patient when beginning their infertility evaluation are summarized in Table 4 [7, 11].

Table 5 Components of a thorough physical examination in the evaluation of an infertile male

General examination
Body habitus (height, weight, body dimensions)
Secondary sexual development (body hair, temporal balding)
Gynecomastia
Thyroid examination
Abdominal examination (Hepatomegaly)
Abdominal examination (Hepatomegaly)
Evidence of chronic illness (diabetes, hypertension, vasculitis, neuropathy)
Genitourinary examination
Phallus (chordee, hypospadias, Peyronie's)
Testes (size, masses, infection)
Epididymis (enlargement/induration, nodules, spermatoceles)
Spermatic cord (varicocele)
Vas deferens (presence or absence)
Inguinal region (hernia)
Prostate (nodules, infection, midline cysts)
Genitourinary infections

Physical Examination

Physical examination is another key component of the evaluation of the infertile male. Special attention should be given to the genitourinary examination; this portion of the exam may help identify testicular and post-testicular etiologies of infertility. The penis should be inspected for hypospadias, and the scrotum for testicular size, presence of bilateral spermatic cords, and other gross abnormalities of the scrotum such as the presence of a varicocele. The key components of the physical examination are found in Table 5 [7, 11].

Labwork

Laboratory tests in the evaluation of the infertile male can be extensive. The initial laboratory test should be the semen analysis (Tables 2 and 3). These findings, in addition to those from the comprehensive history and examination will help direct further tests as required for a patient's evaluation. In addition to the semen analysis, some key laboratory tests should include a complete blood cell count (to test for possible infection), renal and liver function studies, follicle stimulating hormone, luteinizing hormone and testosterone levels (to assess the hypothalamic–pituitary–gonadal axis), and a sexually transmitted infection evaluation. Additional laboratory test as may be ordered based on abnormal findings in the history, physical examination, and/or the initial laboratory test findings.

Imaging Modalities

While the ultrasound (transrectal, transperineal, and/or scrotal) remains the pillar of imaging for the infertile male, multiple imaging modalities are now available for the evaluation of an infertile male. Other modalities that may be utilized during the evaluation process include, but are not limited to, penile ultrasonography, abdominal ultrasonography, magnetic resonance imaging of the abdomen and pelvis, and PET scanning. A penile ultrasonography, using color Doppler, may be indicated if there is a history of Peyronie's disease, penile fractures, and erectile dysfunction. All of these may decrease the patient's sexual function, and henceforth cause decreased fertility [12, 13]. Abdominal ultrasound has a much more limited role in the evaluation process, as it is indicated to rule out associated renal abnormalities in patients with absent vasa deferentia. Occasionally, it may play a role in identifying renal or hepatic pathology as a contributor to infertility [12]. Magnetic Resonance Imaging has an emerging role in the evaluation of male infertility. It can provide a noninvasive alternative to traditional vasography, with or without endo-rectal coils, and is the gold standard for assessing the pituitary for possible adenomas causing hypothalamic–pituitary–gonadal axis. However it remains second line to ultrasonography for investigating possible causes of obstructive male infertility [12, 14]. As described in the remainder of this chapter, this imaging modality is an affordable, accessible, and versatile study that has an important role in a certain subset of infertile males.

Transrectal Ultrasound and Transperineal Ultrasound

Transrectal ultrasonography (TRUS) and transperineal ultrasound (TPUS) are important diagnostic tools in the field of male infertility. Historically diagnostic investigations of male infertility, such as vasography, were invasive, required general anesthetic, and had significant morbidity including iatrogenic stricture formation, vas obstruction, and radiation exposure. The vasograph has now given way to the ultrasound, and as the majority of the male reproductive system lies superficially, the ultrasound is an excellent non-morbid modality to evaluate the reproductive tract.

Transrectal ultrasonography is an imaging study that most urologists are familiar with due to its extensive use in the investigation of prostate cancer. It is most commonly performed in the outpatient setting and is both affordable and accessible. Transperineal ultrasonography is an alternative to the transrectal approach; however, it is not used as frequently and requires a general anesthetic.

Despite its low morbidity, ultrasonography is not recommended for all men undergoing evaluation for management of infertility, and as with all imaging it should only be completed when indicated. The indication for transrectal and transperineal ultrasonography in the evaluation of the infertile men is for the assessment of patients that present with possible obstructive infertility or infertility related to the absence or hypoplasia of the structures involved in ejaculation. These patients typically present with ejaculate volume of less than 1 cc. This ejaculate volume is by no means an accurate predictor of EDO [15, 16] and the absolute indications for transrectal ultrasonography are:

1. Low volume azoospermia in the absence of testicular atrophy and retrograde ejaculation.
2. Low-volume oligoasthenospermia or oligospermia, low volume ejaculate, and the absence of retrograde ejaculation.
3. Presence of midline cyst or asymmetry palpated on digital rectal exam.

4. Non-palpable vas deferens on physical exam [15–17].

Relative indications for obtaining a transrectal and/or transperineal ultrasound on an infertile male are more diverse and are not well established. These indications include:

1. Normal volume azoospermia or severe oligospermia.
2. Severe motility defects with normal physical examination.
3. Ejaculatory abnormality (by clinical history, including anejaculation, hematospermia, painful ejaculation, and explained retrograde ejaculation).
4. History suggestive of genital tract abnormality.

While not discussed in this chapter, it should be noted that scrotal ultrasound often accompanies prostate ultrasound in the evaluation of the infertile male.

Study Procedure

The procedure for transrectal ultrasonography for evaluation of male factor infertility is similar to the evaluation of the prostate for transrectal prostate biopsy. The patient is positioned in the left lateral decubitus position with the legs pulled up to the chest and the patient's perineum facing the examiner as demonstrated in Fig. 1. Digital rectal exam (DRE) should be the first step of the process with assessment for any palpable endorectal lesions; it may be possible to palpate the seminal vesicles for presence, and size. Since seminal vesicles are not usually palpable, this may be a sign of obstructive pathology. Following the DRE, a high-frequency (6.5–7.5 MHz) endorectal probe is inserted into the rectal vault using proper lubrication. Ideally, the probe should be placed with real time visualization of the rectal canal allowing safe and relatively pain free passage of the probe. Systematic ultrasonographic evaluation of the bladder, prostate, seminal vesicles, and ejaculatory ducts are completed in the axial and sagittal planes [12, 18].

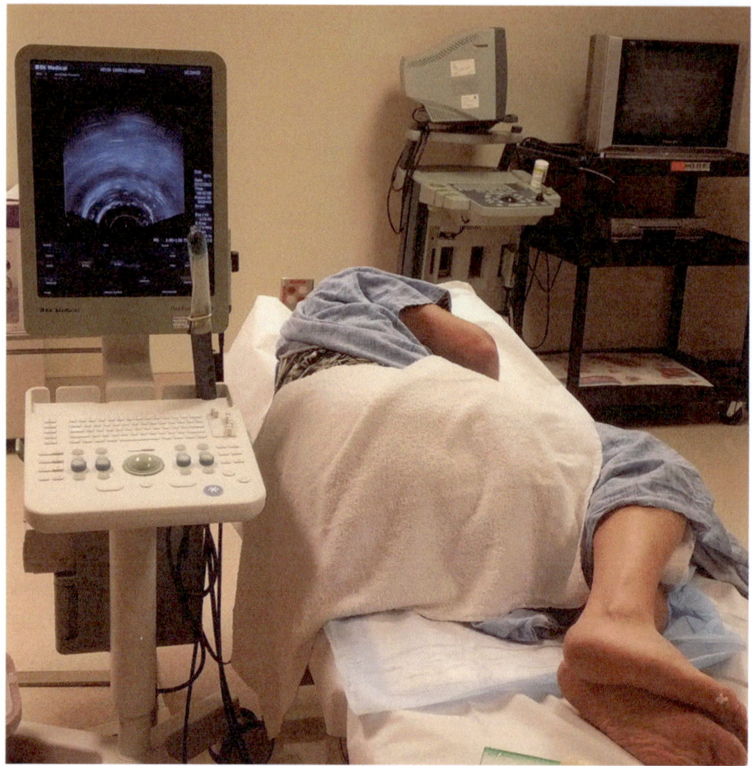

Fig. 1 Left lateral position for performing TRUS

Findings by Structures

Ejaculatory Ducts

The ejaculatory ducts are formed at the confluence of the seminal vesicles and the terminal portion of the vasa deferentia. They typically appear as small, hypoechoic-paired structures with a caliber of 2 mm and crossing the prostate gland obliquely to terminate in the urethra, lateral and proximal to the verumontanum.

Ejaculatory duct obstruction (EDO) is the diagnosis that is best identified using TRUS, and in the evaluation and management of male infertility is one of the few etiologies that has the potential to be reversible and can be managed surgically. EDO has both congenital and acquired causes, but the clinical presentations are very similar. Complete EDO occurs in less than one percent of infertile men, whereas incomplete

EDO is reportedly around 5 % [15]. Congenital etiologies of EDO include midline prostatic cystic lesions (described later), atresia or stenosis of the ejaculatory duct, and ejaculatory duct cysts. Acquired etiologies may be inflammatory or traumatic in origin, including calculus formation secondary to infection, stenosis following transurethral resection of the prostate, and cystic lesions from chronic obstruction (e.g., benign prostatic hypertrophy) [15].

Frequently patients with EDO may not have any antecedent history to delineate the etiology. Symptoms of EDO vary greatly, but reports have documented infertility, decreased force of ejaculate, pain on or after ejaculation, decreased ejaculate volume, hematospermia, perineal or testicular pain, history of prostatitis or epididymitis, low back pain, urinary obstruction, dysuria, or no symptoms [19]. The signs of EDO that warrant further investigation with TRUS include low ejaculate volume (<1 cc) and an otherwise normal physical

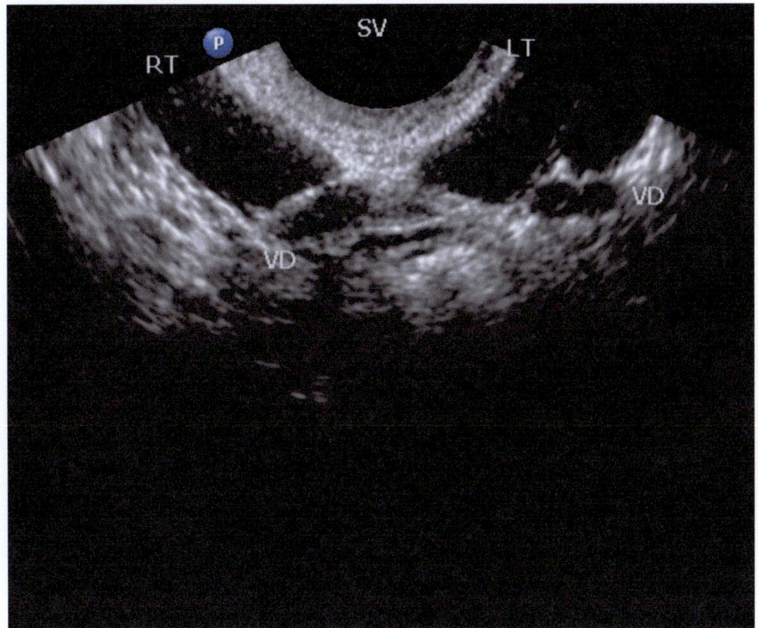

Fig. 2 Transrectal ultrasound in the transverse view demonstrating bilateral ejaculatory duct dilation

exam. Semen analysis, especially in the case of partial obstruction, may demonstrate a variety of abnormalities, including oligospermia or azoospermia, decreased motility, and decreased ejaculate volume [16, 17, 19]. TRUS findings suggestive of EDO (complete or partial) include midline cysts, dilated seminal vesicles, vasa ampulla or ejaculatory ducts, and/or hyperechoic regions suggestive of calcifications. However the presence of a dilated seminal vesicles, vasa ampulla, or ejaculatory duct is not seen in all cases of EDO, and conversely can be found to be dilated with no EDO [19, 20].

Dilation of the ejaculatory ducts is defined as a diameter greater than 2 mm. According to Kim et al. [16], the obstructed lumen of the ejaculatory duct (>2 mm diameter) is often best visualized in the sagittal images as a hypoechoic tubular structure entering the urethra at the level of the verumontanum as seen in Fig. 2. Even when visualized, concurrent seminal vesicle aspiration may be recommended prior to commencing any surgical treatment of EDO to confirm diagnosis.

Calcifications along the ejaculatory duct may be directly causing obstruction, but those in the prostate itself may be due to prior prostatic inflammation. The relationship between prostatic inflammation and EDO has not been clearly elucidated. Inflammatory involvement of the ducts themselves is thought to lead to stenosis or obstruction. In addition, changes in compliance of the ejaculatory duct walls may cause a functional obstruction. Whatever the underlying mechanism, the treatment remains the same [19]. EDO is treated via transurethral resection of the ejaculatory ducts (TURED), which was first described in 1973 by Farley and Barnes [21]. There have been several reports of successful treatment of infertility (i.e., successful pregnancy) following this technique, with success rates between 20 and 50 % [16, 22, 23]. Improved semen parameters and resolution of preoperative symptoms have also been demonstrated following TURED for symptomatic EDO and infertility [24].

Seminal Vesicles

The normal appearance of the seminal vesicles on TRUS are hypoechoic, paired elongated structures that lie cephalad to the prostate and

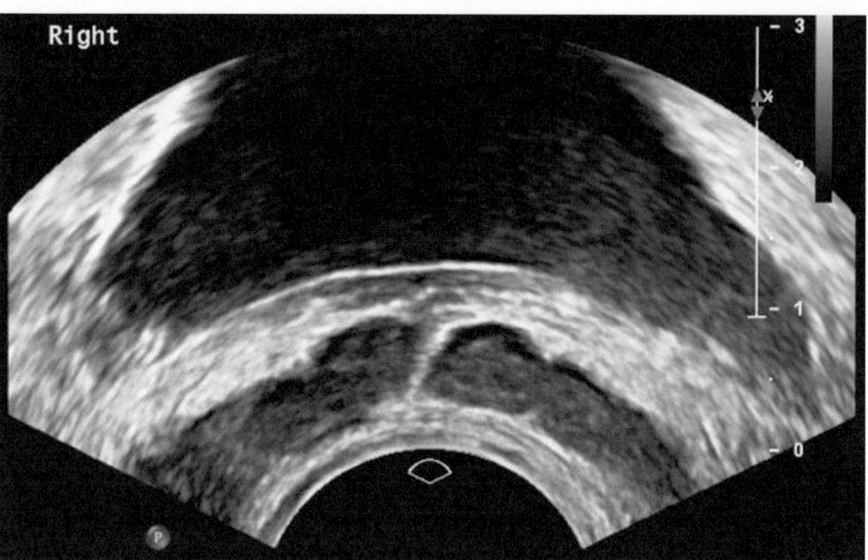

Fig. 3 Bilateral normal seminal vesicle

posterior to the urinary bladder, typically with a "bow-tie" configuration (Fig. 3). The seminal vesicles should be compared for symmetry and possible obstruction (Fig. 4). It is best to image the seminal vesicles in the longitudinal orientation and to follow their course by ultrasound to their insertion in the prostatic urethra. They can have fine internal echoes and a network of tubules with septations. According to most studies, they are typically less than 3 cm in length, 1.5 cm in width, and 1.5 cm in anteroposterior diameter, with a mean volume of approximately 14 mL [12].

The seminal vesicle is an important focus of the TRUS performed as part of the work-up of the infertile male, not only for diagnosis but also for intervention. There are a variety of pathologies that manifest as changes in the seminal vesicles and may account for male factor infertility. Seminal vesicle dilation is defined as diameter greater than 1.5 cm in transaxial imaging, as seen in Figs. 5 and 6 and this finding or asymmetry between the two seminal vesicles should raise suspicion for EDO [16]. However, it has become clear that seminal vesicle dilation is not a specific

finding to EDO alone and may not always identify patients with EDO [16, 19].

There have been various attempts to increase the specificity of TRUS findings for EDO in order to predict response to transurethral resection of ejaculatory ducts. The gold standard for investigatory imagery remains vasography, but the morbidity of this procedure is prohibitive. More recent developments include TRUS-guided seminal vesicle aspiration and TRUS-guided seminal vesiculography.

TRUS-guided seminal vesicle (SV) aspiration is a technique proposed by Jarow [25] in which the seminal vesicles are aspirated and the fluid is analyzed for evidence of an increased number of sperm compared to the patient's semen analysis. A finding of increased sperm in the SV aspirate (>3 sperm per high power field) confirms evidence of EDO due to reflux into the seminal vesicles and establishes intact spermatogenesis, which rules out more proximal obstruction and eliminates the need for testicular biopsy. This technique can also be employed for sperm retrieval in azoospermic patients. The morbidity of this procedure is low as contrast or dye mediums are

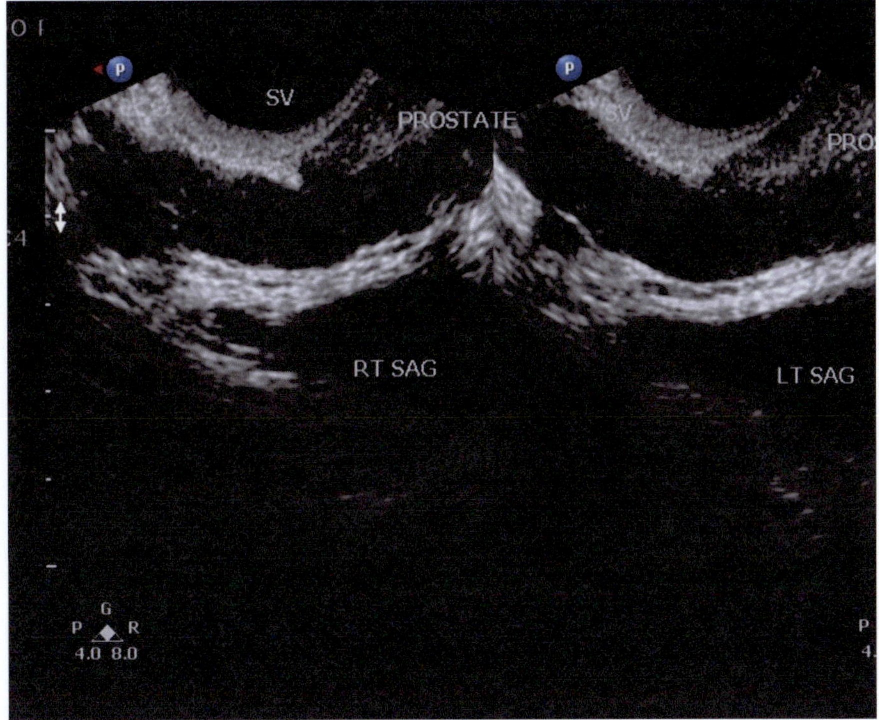

Fig. 4 Normal left and right seminal vesicles

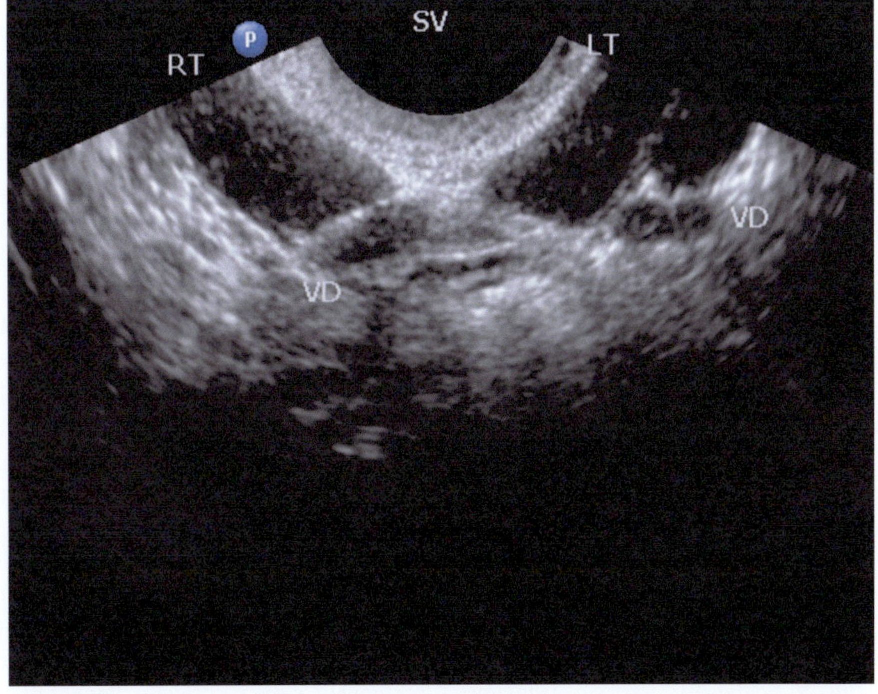

Fig. 5 Transrectal ultrasound in the sagittal view demonstrating dilation of bilateral seminal vesicles

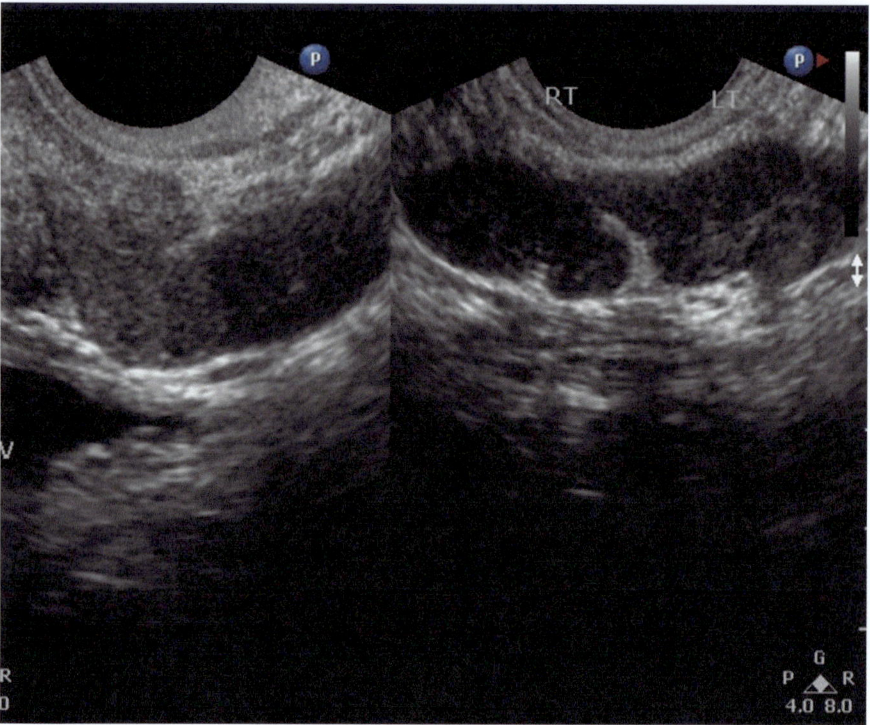

Fig. 6 Transrectal ultrasound in the sagittal view on the left side, and in transverse view on the right, demonstrating seminal vesicle dilation

avoided, and it can also be performed in an outpatient clinic setting. When Engin et al. [26] compared TRUS alone to TRUS-guided SV aspiration, they found that 15 % (2/13) of patients with normal TRUS had positive SV aspirates. Conversely, only 49 % of patients with TRUS findings suggestive of EDO had positive SV aspirates.

Seminal vesiculography is another technique that was developed as a potential part of the EDO evaluation algorithm. It provides a less invasive alternative to the traditional transscrotal vasography. In this technique, following the initial TRUS, a needle is used to access the seminal vesicles with fluoroscopic guidance. A contrast medium is injected into each seminal vesicle in an antegrade fashion while the bladder neck is occluded with a Foley catheter balloon. EDO is defined by the absence of contrast medium within the prostatic urethra. As a dynamic test of ejaculatory duct obstruction, Purohit [27] found that seminal

vesiculography was a more accurate predictor of response to transurethral resection of ejaculatory ducts. However, these results have to be balanced against the increased invasiveness of this procedure and the use of radiation and contrast compared to TRUS or TRUS-SV aspiration. As such, its role in the diagnostic evaluation of the infertile male has not yet been clearly defined. However, Purohit [27] has suggested that this dynamic study may yet warrant a more definite role.

Seminal vesicle dilation associated with adult polycystic kidney disease (APKD), referred to as megavesicles, is rarely associated with male infertility. Hendry et al. [28] described 6 patients with this finding and determined that the gross dilatation of the seminal vesicles seen on TRUS was not caused by obstruction but by atonicity. These ultrasonic appearances, when described previously, were incorrectly thought to be due to seminal vesicle cysts.

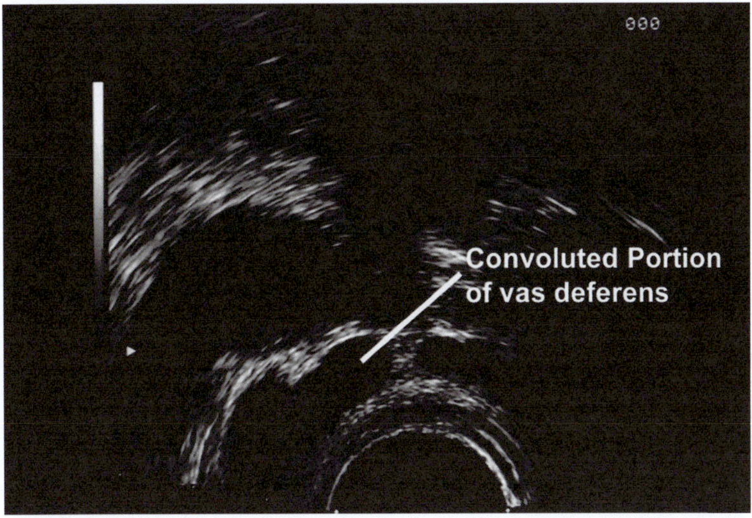

Fig. 7 Normal vasa deferentia

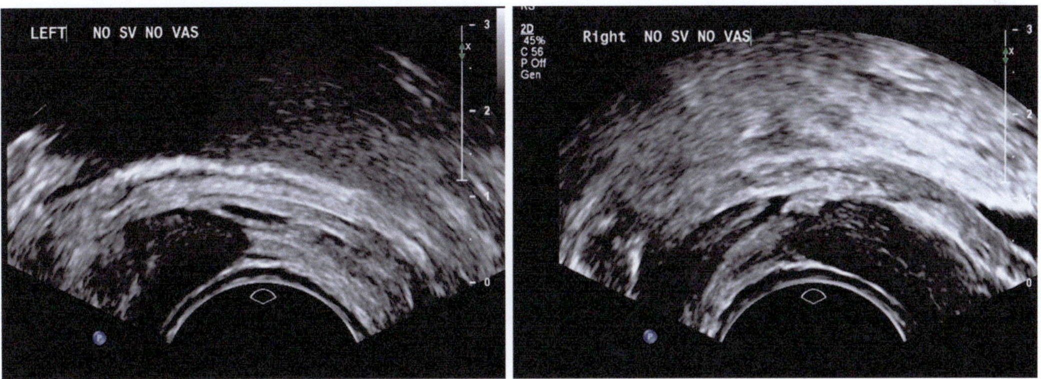

Fig. 8 Bilateral absence of seminal vesicle and vasa deferentia

Vasa Deferentia

On TRUS, the vasa deferentia are identified on axial imaging as a pair of oval, convoluted, tubular structures located medially to the seminal vesicles and cephalad to the prostate (Fig. 7). They have an echotexture similar to that of the seminal vesicles.

As previously mentioned, physical examination findings during the evaluation of an infertile male of non-palpable vas deferens, either unilaterally or bilaterally, or gaps in the vasa deferentia warrants a TRUS for further investigation.

A TRUS finding consistent with congenital bilateral absence of the vasa deferentia (CBAVD) is the absence of the ampulla of the vas deferens (Fig. 8) [12].

Unilateral non-palpable vas deferens is often associated with Wolffian duct abnormalities and potential renal abnormal development, warranting a renal ultrasound in addition to TRUS. Hall and Oates [29] demonstrated that a finding of unilateral absence of the vas deferens is often associated with abnormalities in the contralateral Müllerian duct system, including contralateral ejaculatory duct, epididymal or vasal obstruction, leading to infertility. Case reports have linked unilateral absence of the vas deferens with Klinefelter's Syndrome, the most common genetic condition associated with male infertility [30].

CBAVD is the most common cause of the congenital vas deferens obstruction. It is identified in approximately 2 % of patients being evaluated for infertility and accounts for 4–17 % of cases of obstructive azoospermia, except in patients with cystic fibrosis where CBAVD is identified in greater than 95 % of male suffers [7, 31]. It is important to note that up to 82 % of men with CBAVD have at least one mutation of the cystic fibrosis gene, and identification is therefore important for genetic counseling. Concurrent abnormalities of the Wolffian duct organs; epididymis, seminal vesicles, ejaculatory ducts; and kidneys (agenesis, ectopic kidneys) are also associated with CBAVD, with abnormalities of the seminal vesicle seen in 90 % of cases (complete absence noted 40 % of the time).

Prostate

TRUS for prostate pathology is a routine study familiar to most Urologists. It is a critical tool in the evaluation of prostate cancer and benign prostatic hypertrophy. However, in the evaluation of male infertility, the focus of TRUS is less commonly focused on the prostate. The typical ultrasonographic appearance of the prostate gland is a symmetric, triangular, and ellipsoid structure, with the base just inferior to the urinary bladder and seminal vesicles. The prostate should be imaged in two planes: longitudinal and transverse. The gland must be measured in 3 dimensions to obtain the appropriate data for gland volume. During the initial evaluation of the gland note must be made of any abnormal midline cystic structures, hypo-echoic masses, symmetry, and capsular integrity

The gland is typically hyperechoic, and the urethra is identified coursing through the midline. It often has a thin echogenic capsule. In a young male, it typically measures 20–25 mL in volume and 20 g in weight. It is approximately 4 cm in transverse diameter, 3 cm in the anteroposterior plane, and 4 cm in the craniocaudal direction [12].

When examining the prostate on TRUS for male factor infertility evaluation, midline cysts are important to identify. They are classified into two general categories: sperm containing and non-sperm-containing. Sperm-containing cysts are further separated into prostatic utricle cysts and Müllerian duct cysts. The difference between these two cysts is their embryologic origin, location and association with intersex disorders. Utricle cysts are endodermal in embryologic origin and are located near the verumontanum, while Müllerian duct cysts arise from the mesoderm and will lie near the prostatic base. Utricle cysts are associated with intersex disorders [16, 19].

Non-sperm-containing cysts are referred to as Wolffian duct cysts or ejaculatory duct cysts, and are much less common than sperm-containing cysts [16, 19]. Regardless of their origin, these cystic lesions can cause EDO by deviating the ejaculatory ducts medially or laterally or by causing external compression. Their role in EDO has been confirmed in multiple studies, with incidence much higher in infertile men than in fertile [32]. As with seminal vesicle dilation, presence of these cystic lesions is not pathognomonic for EDO. The finding of a midline cyst is an indication for further evaluation of these structures as a possible cause of EDO and male factor infertility.

If EDO is confirmed, treatment for all these midline cysts is a transurethral resection of the ejaculatory ducts. Studies on transurethral resection of the ejaculatory ducts have demonstrated that the response to this procedure is improved in patients with identifiable anatomic abnormality. TRUS at the time of transurethral resection of ejaculatory ducts may be useful to help identify the level or location of the cystic lesion that is to be resected. Resection requires excision through the cyst until the ejaculatory duct is in direct drainage into the prostatic urethra to ensure the resolution of obstruction of the ejaculatory ducts at this level.

Conclusion

Prostate (transrectal and transperineal) ultrasound has revolutionized the evaluation and investigation of male infertility, and its role will continue to expand in the future.

References

1. Thonneau P, Marchard S, Tallec A, Ferial M, Ducot B, Lansac J, Lopes P, Tabaste J, Spira A. Incidence and main causes of infertility in a resident population (1,850,000) of three french regions (1988–1989). Hum Reprod. 1991;6(6):811–6.
2. Boiven J, Bunting L, Collins JA, Nygren KG. International estimates of infertility prevalence and treatment-seeking: potential need and demand for infertility medical care. Hum Reprod. 2007;22(6):1506–12.
3. World Health Organization. WHO laboratory manual for the examination and processing of human semen. 5th ed. Geneva: World Health Organization; 2010.
4. Zegers-Hochschild F, Adamson GD, de Mouzon J, Ishihara O, Mansour R, Nygren K, Sullivan E, van der Poel S. The international committee for monitoring assisted reproductive care (ICMART) and the world health organization (WHO) revised glossary on ART technology, 2009. Hum Reprod. 2009;24(11):2683–7.
5. Practice Committee of the American Society for Reproductive Medicine. Definitions of infertility and recurrent pregnancy loss: a committee opinion. Fertil Steril. 2013;99(1):63.
6. Krausz C. Male infertility: pathogenesis and clinical diagnosis. Best Pract Res Clin Endocrinol Metab. 2011;25:271–85.
7. Sabanegh E, Agarwal A. Chapter 21:male infertility. In: Wein AJ, Kavoussi LR, Partin AW, Peters CA, editors. Campbell–Walsh urology. 10th ed. Philadelphia: WB Saunders Co; 2011.
8. Patel ZP, Niederberger CS. Male factor assessment in infertility. Med Clin N Am. 2011;95:223–34.
9. Cooper TG, Noonan E, von Eckardstein S, Auger J, Baker HW, Behre HM, Haugen TB, Kruger T, Wang C, Mbizvo MT, Vogelsong KM. World health organization reference values for human semen characteristics. Hum Reprod Update. 2010;16(3):231–45.
10. Kenney LB, Cohen LE, Schnorhavorian M, Metzger ML, Lockart B, Hijaya N, Duffey-Lind E, Constine L, Green D, Meacham L. Male reproductive health after childhood, adolescent, and young adult cancers: a report from the Children's oncology group. J Clin Oncol. 2012;30(27):3408–16.
11. Jose-Miller AB, Boyden JW, Frey KA. Infertility. Am Fam Physician. 2007;75(6):849–56.
12. Raza SA, Jhaveri KS. Imaging in male infertility. Radiol Clin N Am. 2012;50:1183–200.
13. Futterer JJ, Heijmink SW, Spermon JR. Imaging the male reproductive tract: current trends and future directions. Radiol Clin N Am. 2008;46:133–47.
14. Simpson WL, Rausch DR. Imaging of male infertility: pictorial review. Am J Radiol. 2009;192:98–107.
15. Donkol RH. Imaging in male-factor obstructive infertility. World J Radiol. 2010;2(5):172–9.
16. Kim ED, Lipshultz LI. Role of ultrasound in the assessment of male infertility. J Clin Ultrasound. 1996;24:437–53.
17. American Urological Association Education and Research, Inc. The optimal evaluation of the infertile male: AUA best practice statement. Linthicum (MD): American Urological Association Education and Research, Inc.; 2010 38 p
18. Edey AJ, Sidhu PS. Male infertility: role of imaging in the diagnosis and management. Imaging. 2008;20:139–46.
19. Fisch H, Lambert SM, Goluboff ET. Management of ejaculatory duct obstruction: etiology, diagnosis, and treatment. World J Urol. 2006;24:604–10.
20. Wessels EC, Ohori M, Grantmyre JE, et al. The prevalence of cystic dilatation of the ejaculatory ducts detected by transrectal ultrasound (TRUS) in a self-referred (screening) group of men (abstract 973). J Urol. 1992;147:456A.
21. Farley S, Barnes R. Stenosis of ejaculatory ducts treated by endoscopic resection. J Urol. 1973;109:664–6.
22. Shroeder-Printzen I, Ludwig M, Kohn F, Weidner W. Surgical therapy in infertile Men with ejaculatory duct obstruction: technique and outcome of a standardized surgical approach. Hum Reprod. 2000;15(6):1364–8.
23. Yurdaku T, Gokce G, Kilic O, Piskin MM. Transurethral resection of ejaculatory ducts in the treatment of complete ejaculatory duct obstruction. Int Urol Nephrol. 2008;40(2):369–72.
24. Turek PJ, Magana JO, Lipshultz LI. Semen parameters before and after transurethral surgery for ejaculatory duct obstruction. J Urol. 1996;155:1291–3.
25. Jarow JP. Seminal vesicle aspiration of fertile Men. J Urol. 1995;156:1005.
26. Engin G, Celtik M, Sanli O, Aytac O, Muradov Z, Kadioglu A. Comparison of transrectal ultrasonography and transrectal ultrasonography-guided seminal vesicle aspiration in the diagnosis of the ejaculatory duct obstruction. Fertil Steril. 2009;92(3):964–70.
27. Purohit RS, Wu DS, Shinohara K, Turek PJ. A propsective comparison of 3 diagnostic methods to evaluate ejaculatory duct obstruction. J Urol. 2004;171:232–6.

28. Hendry WF, Rickards D, Pryor JP, Baker LR. Seminal megavesicles with adult polycystic kidney disease. Hum Reprod. 1998;13(6):1567–9.
29. Hall S, Oates RD. Unilateral absence of the scrotal vas deferens associated with contralateral mesonephric duct anomalies resulting in infertility: laboratory, physical and radiographic findings, and therapeutic alternatives. J Urol. 1993;150(4):1161–4.
30. Baydilli N, Gokce A, Karabulut SY, Ekmekcioglu O. Klinefelter's syndrome with unilateral absence of Vas deferens. Fertil Steril. 2010;94(4):1529.
31. Stahl PJ, Stember DS, Goldstein M. Contemporary management of male infertility. Annu Rev Med. 2012;63:525–40.
32. Jarow JP. Transrectal ultrasonography of infertile Men. Fertil Steril. 1993;60:1035–9.

Application of Prostate Ultrasound for Benign Prostatic Hyperplasia and Male Urinary Stress Incontinence

Kasra Saeb-Parsy and Nikesh Thiruchelvam

Introduction

Benign prostatic hyperplasia (BPH) is a histo-pathological change that is seen in many men over the age of 40. Benign prostatic hyperplasia, although contributory, is not the sole cause of lower urinary tract symptoms (LUTS) in the aging male. Not all men with BPH will have lower urinary tract symptoms or indeed benign prostatic enlargement. There is a significant overlap among many different components, including benign prostatic enlargement (BPE), bladder outlet obstruction (BOO), lower urinary tract symptoms (LUTS), and BPH. This complex interaction was first described by Hald in 1989 [1] and is well demonstrated by Roehrborn [2] (Fig. 1).

Given this complex interaction it is very important to correctly identify men in the clinical setting in order to determine who will benefit from medical or surgical management.

BOO is a urodynamic diagnosis based on observation of increased detrusor pressure and reduced urinary flow rate during voiding [3]. Although urodynamic diagnosis, with use of pressure transducers, is the gold standard, it is an invasive and time-consuming investigation. There is a constant drive to diagnose BOO in the clinical setting with the aid of simple and less invasive methods of investigation. Over the years ultrasonography has become a useful tool in the armament of the urologist to help in the diagnosis of this common problem. Assessment of many components of the prostate and bladder using transabdominal and transrectal approaches may help in the diagnosis of BOO and this is discussed in detail.

Male stress incontinence is often iatrogenic and can occur following surgery on the prostate for benign disease (e.g., by holmium enucleation of the prostate or transurethral resection of the prostate, TURP) or following radical surgery on the prostate for prostate cancer (radical prostatectomy, RP). The latter can be performed by open surgery, laparoscopically assisted, or robotically assisted. Regardless of modality, each is associated with a degree of stress incontinence with rates varying based on definition, surgical expertise, and volume.

Prostate Volume

Although the most accurate means of assessing prostate volume (PV) is via the transrectal approach, with measurement of the height, width, and length of the prostate, most modern US machines can measure PV in the transverse view using the preset ellipsoid formula [4]. Yuen et al. studied the correlation between transrectal and

K. Saeb-Parsy, B.Sc., M.B.B.S., F.R.C.S. Urol (✉)
N. Thiruchelvam, M.B.B.S. B.Sc., M.R.C.S., M.D., F.R.C.S. Urol, F.E.B.U.
Department of Urology, Addenbrookes Hospital, Cambridge University Hospitals NHS Foundation Trust, Cambridge, UK
e-mail: kasra@doctors.org.uk;
Nikesh.thiruchelvam@addenbrookes.nhs.uk

C.R. Porter and E.M. Wolff (eds.), *Prostate Ultrasound: Current Practice and Future Directions*,
DOI 10.1007/978-1-4939-1948-2_8, © Springer Science+Business Media New York 2015

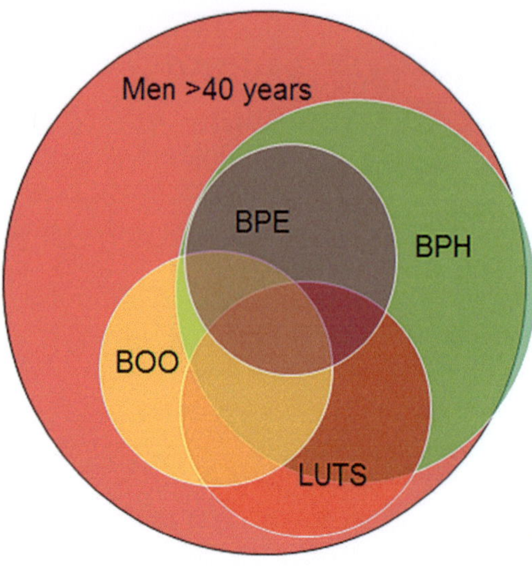

Fig. 1 Interaction between different components and their overlap. The size of the circles is not an indication of the proportion but merely to high light the complex overlap

transabdominal measurement of prostate volume in 22 patients under general anesthesia prior to TURP. They showed that the transabdominal ultrasound measurement of PV correlated well with the transrectal measurement of the same parameter when the bladder volume is less than 400 ml [5]. Although PV is also a useful index in the evaluation of BOO, it alone is not sufficiently accurate to diagnose BOO. Indeed, as described earlier, LUTS and BOO can exist in the absence of BPE. There is some evidence to suggest that the size of the prostate may be related to the severity of obstruction and progression of BPE. A study of f 2,115 men with lower urinary tract symptoms between the ages of 40 and 79 years with a 4 year follow-up revealed that men with PV of more than 30 g were threefold more likely to develop urinary retention [6]. A videourodynamics study (VUDS) of 324 consecutive men with LUTS by Kuo revealed that 65 % of men had evidence of BOO, and PV of 40 ml or more was associated with BOO with a sensitivity of approximately 95 % [7]. Conversely, Hirayama et al. found that in a study of 36 men with PV less than 20 ml, 60 % had evidence of obstruction on pressure flow studies [8]. Presence of median lobe or bladder neck stricture (despite a small prostate volume) may in part account for

the presence of BOO in this group of patients. In summary, prostate volume alone is not sufficiently accurate to exclude presence of BOO, however larger prostates are more likely to be associated with BOO.

Intravesical Prostatic Protrusions

Another parameter that can help with diagnosis of BOO is intravesical prostatic protrusions (IPP), as measured by the length of the prostate extending into the bladder in the sagittal plane. Volume of urine in the bladder will have a significant impact on the IPP. Yuen et al. have shown that the optimal bladder volume for the measurement of IPP is approximately 100–200 ml. Overdistension of the bladder (volume greater than 400 ml) leads to retraction of the prostate behind the symphysis pubis and inaccurate assessment of IPP. In contrast, under filling of the bladder (volume less than 100 ml) leads to over-estimation of IPP [5]. IPP can be graded as follows: Grade 1, 5 mm or less protrusion; grade 2, 5–10 mm protrusion; and grade 3, more than 10 mm protrusion as shown in Fig. 2 [4, 9]. In a prospective study of men over the age of 50, Chia et al. assessed the correlation between IP and BOO. In all, 125 patients had significant BOO, defined as a BOO index of >40. Of these men, 94 had grade 3 and 30 had grade 1–2 IPP, with a positive predictive value of 94 % and a negative predictive value of 79 % in Grade 3 IPP [9].

Similarly, Kegin et al. in a review of 206 patients with BPE found patients with grade 3 IPP had a statistically lower peak flow rate (Qmax), and a significantly higher maximum detrusor pressure (Pdet.max) and BOO index (BOOI) when compared to patients with grade 1–2 IPP ($p<0.05$ during urodynamic testing). The correlation coefficient (Spearman's rho) between IPP and Qmax, Pdet. max, and BOOI was −0.284, 0.252, and 0.456, respectively. They therefore concluded that IPP is a useful predictor in the assessment of patients with BOO. Patients with grade 3 IPP had more severe BOO and impaired detrusor function [10].

Lim et al. also showed that PV and IPP have a positive predictive value of 65 % and 72 %,

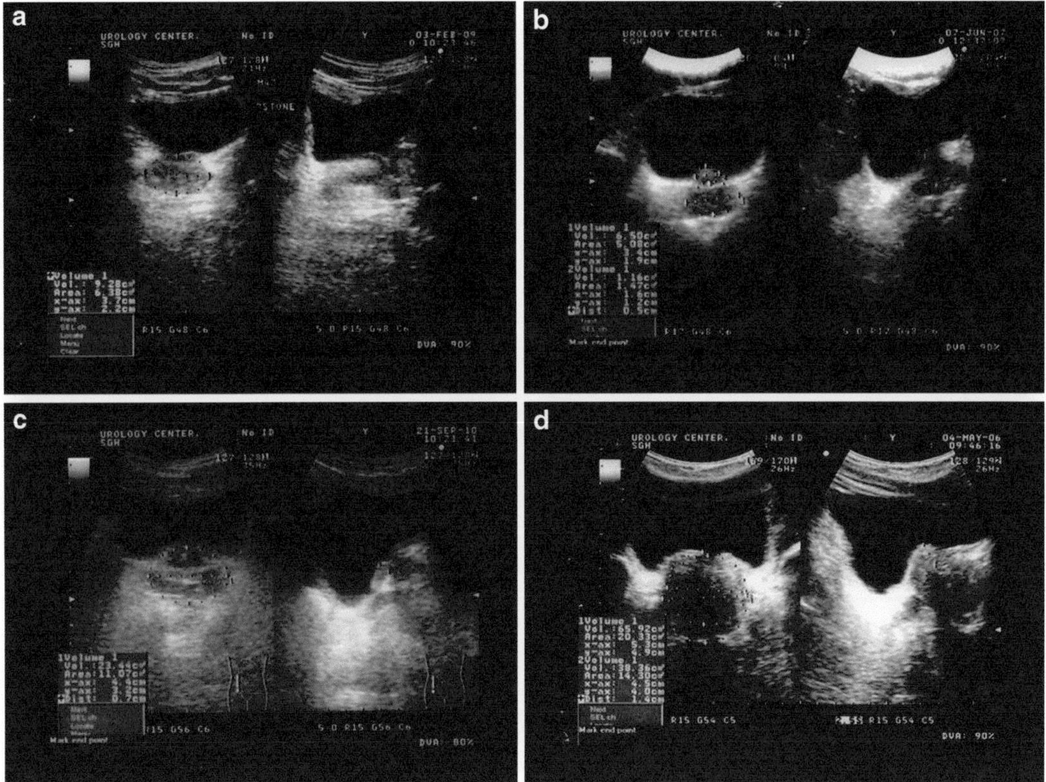

Fig. 2 (**a**) Normal prostate. (**b**) Intravesical prostatic protrusion (IPP) grade 1 prostate. (**c**) IPP grade 2 prostate. (**d**) IPP grade 3 prostate

respectively, for BOO. The Spearman rho correlation coefficients were 0.314 and 0.507 with the area under the receiver-operator characteristic curves of 0.637 and 0.772, for PV and IPP, respectively. Using a nominal regression analysis they concluded that IPP was a better indicator for BOO compared to PV [11].

Lee et al. showed that men with Grade 3 IPP who are on medical management are sevenfold more likely to progress over a mean follow-up period of 32 months [12].

Given the ease of IPP measurement it can be used as a surrogate marker in the initial assessment of men with LUTS as well risk stratification with regards to patients on conservative management with confirmed diagnosis of BOO. However, to date, this remains an experimental tool that has not entered widespread clinical practice. In a study of 111 patients with confirmed BPE, Aganovic et al. showed that grade 3 IPP was a superior indicator

for BOO, as compared to ultrasound measurement of bladder wall thickness (BWT) [13]. The authors also found that flow rate and age were useful predictors of BOO.

Transition Zone Index

Current generation US machines provide far superior image quality and allow a clear distinction between different zones of the prostate (Fig. 3, 4). As BPH arises in the transition zone tissue, some researchers advocate use of transition zone (TZ) index as an indicator for BOO. Transition zone index is calculated using a TRUS probe with the following formula: TZ volume/ total prostatic volume (TZV/TPV).

Greene et al. demonstrated that TZ volume is significantly increased in the clinical BPH group. They found the mean size of the transition zone

Fig. 3 (**a**) Sagittal (*top panel*) and (**b**) coronal (*bottom panel*) section of the prostate showing peripheral zone, transition zone, central zone, the verumontanum, the proximal urethral segment, as well as preprostatic sphincter, bladder neck, and ejaculatory duct

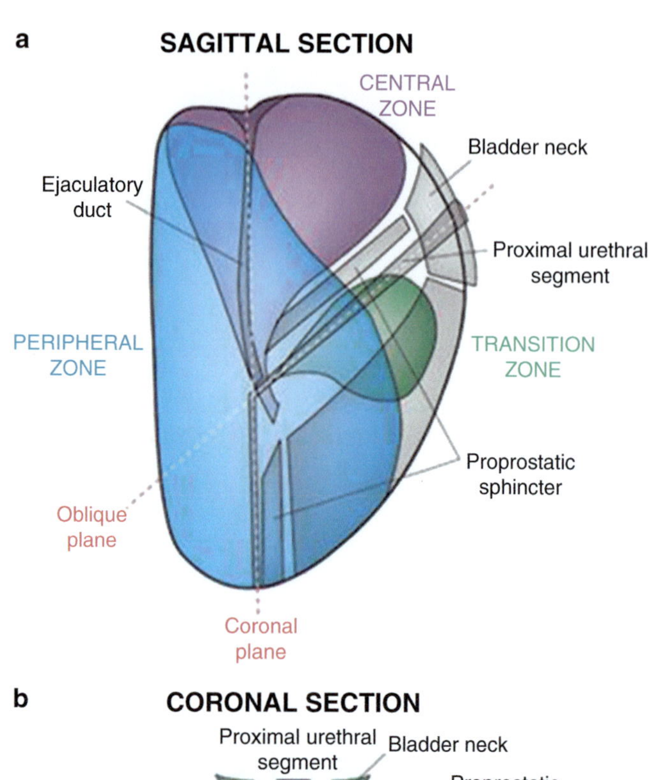

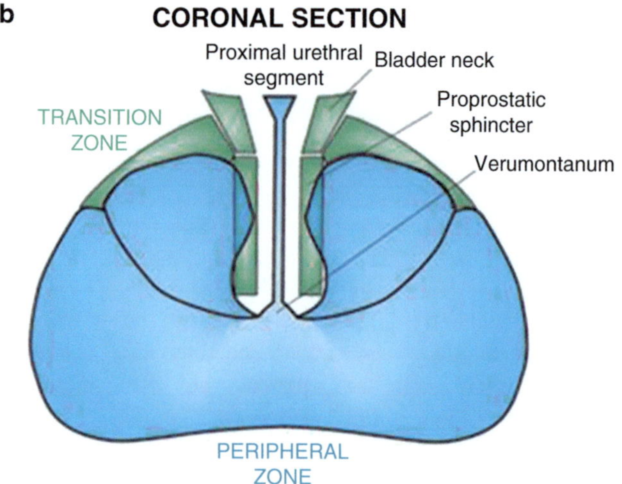

was 6.14±3.2 g in the normal group (as defined as no US features of BPH) and 24.81±14.4 g in the BPH group. The size of the transition zone increased significantly in relation to increased age of the patient [14]. Others have also demonstrated that application of TZ index can accurately identify patients with significant BOO.

Kaplan et al. conducted a prospective evaluation of 61 men with symptomatic BPH. They concluded that TZ Index demonstrated a significant correlation with American Urological Association symptom score (AUASS) ($r=0.75$; $p<0.001$) and peak flow rate ($r=0.71$; $p<0.001$). They concluded that TZ index may be valuable in the assessment of BOO [15].

Witjes et al. conducted a comprehensive study of 150 patients to establish the correlation between prostate volume, transition zone volume, transition zone index, and clinical and urodynamic investigations in patients with lower urinary tract symptoms. They concluded that there were very small differences between the correlations of total

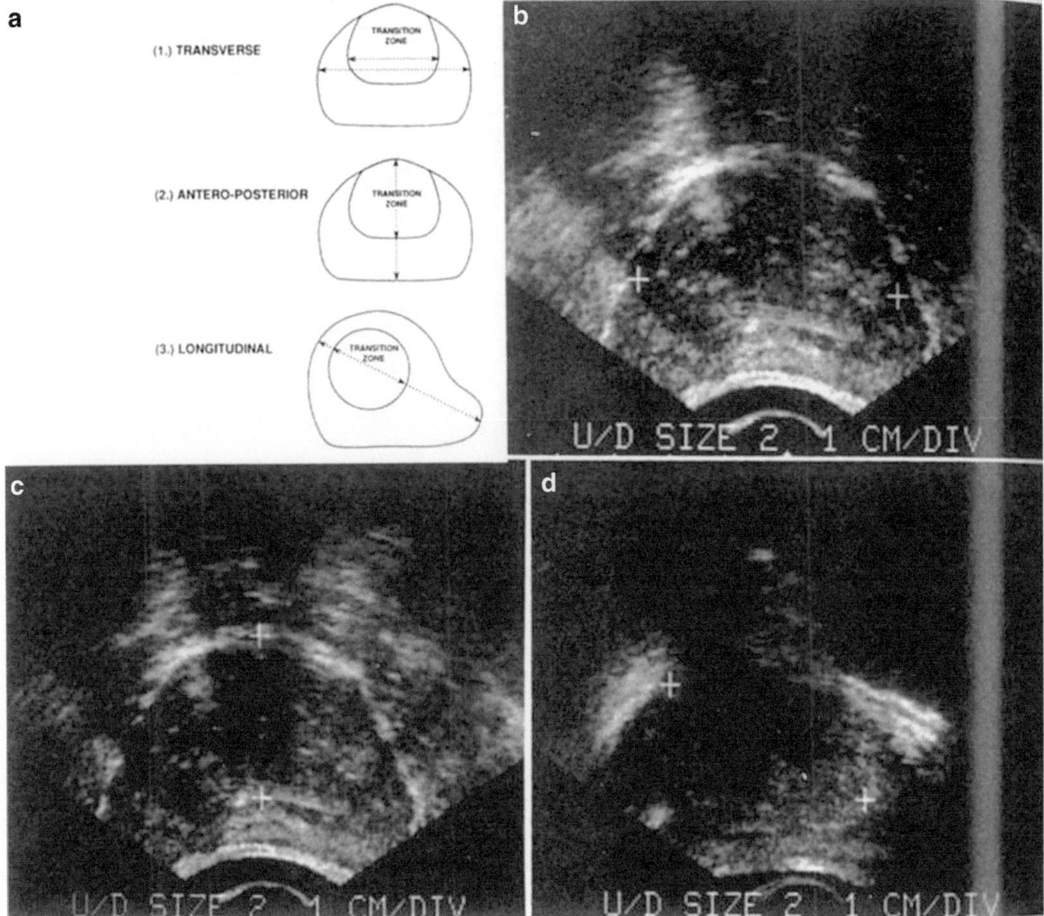

Fig. 4 (**a**) Measurements made of whole prostate gland and transition zone in each illustrated dimension: (**b**) transverse, (**c**) AP, and (**d**) longitudinal sonograms of prostate showing measurements in real time

prostate volume, TZ volume, and TZ index, and clinical and urodynamics variables. The addition of TZ index was of little value in the diagnosis and management of a patient with BOO. They also concluded that TZ index and other similar parameters should not be used in isolation to guide appropriate management [16].

Resistive Index

Resistive index (RI) can be employed to assess blood flow through a target organ. Modern generation US machines are able to utilize power Doppler transrectal ultrasound (TRUS) to cal-culate the RI in the prostate. Power Doppler uses the amplitude of the signal to calculate the density of red blood cells irrespective of velocity or flow direction. In order to measure RI the patient is placed in the standard left lateral position, and a 5.0–8.0 MHz end-fire TRUS probe is used. Pulsed-wave spectral Doppler images are obtained with the patient in the left lateral decubitus position. On the transverse view of the prostate, pulsatile waveforms of blood flow are obtained from the capsular artery and subjected to spectral waveform analysis. The pulsatile waveforms are then stabilized for a given Doppler spectrum, and the RI is measured using on-board software (Fig. 5) [17].

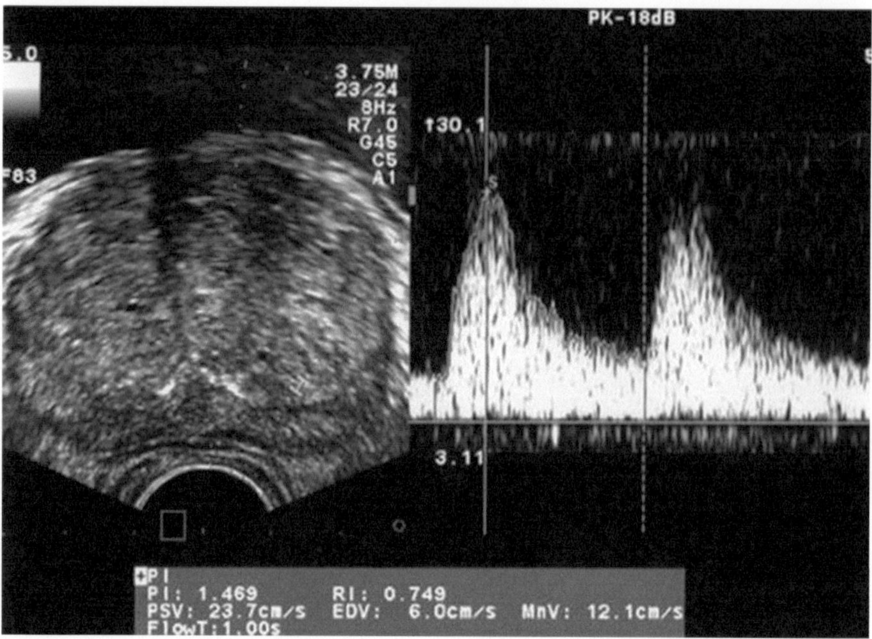

Fig. 5 Sample Doppler waveforms of blood flow at the capsular artery of the prostate. Systolic velocity and diastolic velocity are measured, and the RI is calculated using on-board software. PSV peak systolic velocity; EDV end diastolic velocity; PI pulsatility index; MnV mean velocity; FlowT flow time; RI resistive index

Tsuru et al. studied a total of 214 men aged between 48 and 86 years old with lower urinary tract symptoms. They found a significant correlation between the RI of capsular arteries and the International Prostatic Symptom Score (IPSS) ($r=0.389$; $p<0.0001$) and peak flow rate of uroflowmetry ($r=-0.393$; $p<0.0001$) [18].

Kojima et al. evaluated the utility of RI in 140 patients with symptoms suggestive of BOO. Their study showed that RI was also higher in patients with infravesical obstruction than those without (0.74 ± 0.06 vs. 0.70 ± 0.05, $p<0.005$). In their study, RI was significantly correlated with urodynamic parameters. They found that RI of 0.7 or more correctly identified 28 patients out of 33 (85 %) with obstruction, while 11 out of 24 patients (46 %) without obstruction had an RI less than 0.7 [19]. RI may not only be able to identify patients with BOO, but it may also help predict the patients who are likely to benefit from TURP. Haung et al. showed that RI accurately predicts the outcome of TURP. RI was more accurate in predicting effective outcome after TURP than bladder wall thickness. By combining measurements, the authors found that resistive index, detrusor wall thickness, and ultrasonic estimation of bladder weight had a combined positive predictive value of 96.3 % for successful surgical outcome [20].

It is postulated that the increase in RI noted in BOO is the result of lateral prostatic lobe enlargement compressing the prostatic capsule, with a resultant increase in RI of the capsular arteries. However, in patients with only enlargement of the median lobe as the cause of BOO, RI wound not be elevated. In addition, many conditions such as hypertension, atherosclerosis, and diabetes mellitus can lead to a decrease in tissue and vascular compliance and hence alter RI. Other limitations include the effects of drugs such as α-blockers, 5-α-reductase inhibitors, antihypertensives, and nonsteroidal antiphlogistics, which modulate the function of the capsular artery and tissue in the prostate and therefore will alter the RI. In summary, although RI can be useful in the diagnosis and prediction of surgical outcome in patients with BOO, there are many factors that can modulate the RI. As such, it is not accurate enough to replace the gold standard of urodynamics investigation of bladder function and confirmed BOO.

Bladder Wall Thickness and Bladder Weight

It is postulated that the increased work load of the bladder in the setting of BOO leads to an increase in bladder wall thickness (BWT). This has been confirmed both in animal models as well as in patients, where BOO leads to bladder smooth muscle hypertrophy and deposition of connective tissue [21, 22].

Oelke et al. conducted a study of 55 healthy adult patients to determine a normal range for BWT. They showed that BWT decreases rapidly until the bladder is filled up to 250 ml and, thereafter, remains almost stable until maximal bladder capacity. They concluded that BWT is best measured at the anterior bladder wall with a comfortably full bladder, with a minimal bladder volume of 250 ml (Fig. 6).

After enlargement of the digital ultrasound image (9.8×), the structures of the anterior bladder wall can be further analyzed. Mucosa and adventitia appear hyperechogenic, and the detrusor appears hypoechogenic (Fig. 7). The distance between the two hyperechogenic lines represents the detrusor wall thickness (DWT) that can be measured with the integrated measuring function of the ultrasound device (in this example 1.4 and 1.5 mm). Images and legend taken from Oelke et al., 2006.

They demonstrated that BWT was 1.4 mm in healthy men and 1.2 mm in healthy women. They also found that the age and BMI of the patient had no impact on BWT [23].

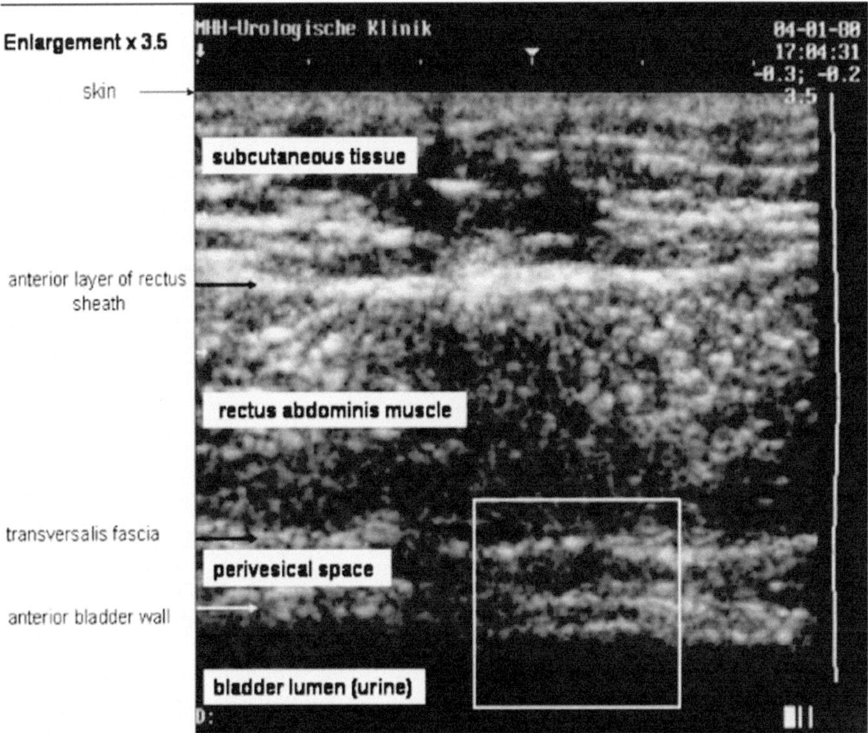

Fig. 6 Ultrasound image of the anterior abdominal wall and anterior bladder wall with a 7.5 MHz linear array positioned suprapubically. At low magnification of the ultrasound picture (3.5×), the anterior bladder wall can be identified

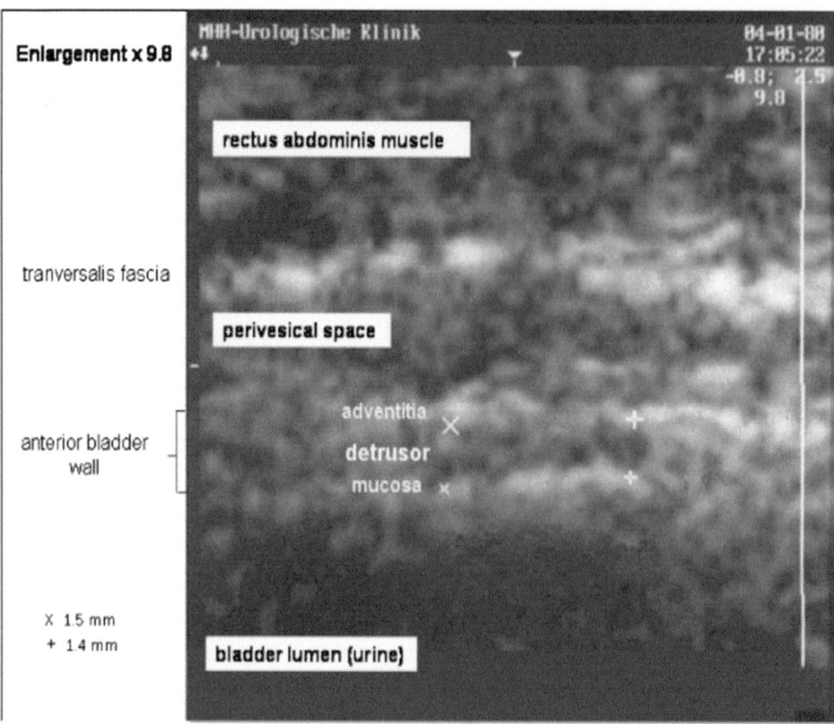

Fig. 7 After enlargement of the digital ultrasound image (9.8×), the structures of the anterior bladder wall can be further analyzed. Mucosa and adventitia appear hyperechogenic, while the detrusor appears hypoechogenic. The distance between the two hyperechogenic lines represents the detrusor wall thickness (DWT) that can be measured with the integrated measuring function of the ultrasound device (in this example 1.4 and 1.5 mm)

Kojima et al. assessed the accuracy of ultrasonic estimation of bladder weight (UEBW) as a maker for BOO. Assuming a spherical bladder UEBW was calculated on the basis of thickness of the bladder wall and the intravesical volume using transabdominal US. They concluded that UEBW did not alter with bladder filling and correlated well with actual bladder weight in cadavers. They demonstrated that UEBW in the obstructed group (49.7 ± 19.5 g) was significantly greater than that in the normal control group (25.6 ± 5.7 g; $p < 0.001$) or the non-obstructed group (28.4 ± 4.2 g; $p < 0.001$). They also showed that 94 % (45/48) of patients in the obstructed group had a UEBW greater than 35.0 g. They concluded that a cutoff value of 35 g for the UEBW has a diagnostic accuracy of 86.2 % in patients with BOO. They also showed that treatment of BOO lead to reduction of UEBW to a normal level after 3 months of treatment [24].

Manieri et al. evaluated BWT in patients with urodynamics-proven BOO. They found a statistically significant correlation between BWT and diagnosis of BOO on urodynamics. They showed that a cut off of 5 mm for BWT would identify 87.5 % with BOO, while BWT was less than 5 mm in 63.3 % of patients no evidence of BOO on pressure flow studies [25].

In a study of men with confirmed BOO on urodynamics, Oelke et al. demonstrated that BWT of 2 mm had a positive predictive value of 94 % and specificity of 95 %. Their results suggested a 89 % agreement between the results of BWT measurement and pressure–flow studies [26].

Blatt et al. assessed BWT in patients suspected of BOO or detrusor overactivity and correlated their data with urodynamics findings. They concluded that BWT does not change significantly in patients with non-neurogenic voiding dysfunction and hence cannot reliably predict bladder outlet obstruction or detrusor overactivity [27].

BWT and UEBW have been investigated in the community in healthy men. There is a weak correlation between BWT and body mass index and a similarly weak correlation between BWT or UEBW and the patient's weight (Bright et al. 2012). Bladder filling volume appeared to have a greater effect on BWT than on UEBW. There was large inter-observer and intra-observer variability when measuring BWT and UEBW. Disappointingly, the same investigators were unable to find a difference in UEBW among three groups of men with LUTS with varying flow rates [28, 29].

Measurement of UEBW and BWT is highly operator dependent. In addition, adequate bladder filling is often required, which can be challenging in many patients. In summary, UEBW and BWT, although noninvasive, currently lacks the necessary diagnostic accuracy in all patients to replace urodynamic study.

Prostatic Urethral Angle

It is commonly accepted that a high bladder neck can play a role in BOO and symptoms of LUTS; however, the effects of prostatic urethral angle are not clear. Cho et al. have demonstrated that prostatic urethral angle (PUA) can be calculated in the mid-sagittal plane of the prostate and recorded from 0 to 90° as shown in Fig. 8. They

also demonstrated that PUA is inversely related to maximal flow rate [30]. Park et al. evaluated the correlation between PUA and IPSS. They concluded that PUA had no statistically significant correlation with IPSS or IPSS storage symptoms. However, PUA had a significant correlation with IPSS voiding symptoms such as straining, which are surrogate markers of BOO ($p=0.047$). Patients with PUA 34° or more had a higher IPSS ($p=0.001$) [31]. It is important to bear in mind that patients with prostate size greater than 40 g were excluded from this study. Further studies are required to evaluate the effectiveness of PUA in diagnosis of patients with BOO.

Ultrasound, the Male Pelvic Floor, and Incontinence

Ultrasound is an evolving technique to investigate the male pelvic floor. Nahon et al. were able to demonstrate that transabdominal ultrasound was feasible and showed good correlation between pelvic floor contraction observed on ultrasound and by digital rectal examination. In those men who had undergone prostate cancer treatment, post-treatment continent men were also observed to have a greater movement of the bladder wall than incontinent men. Perineal ultrasound has also been used to assess male pelvic floor contraction and urethral and bladder neck

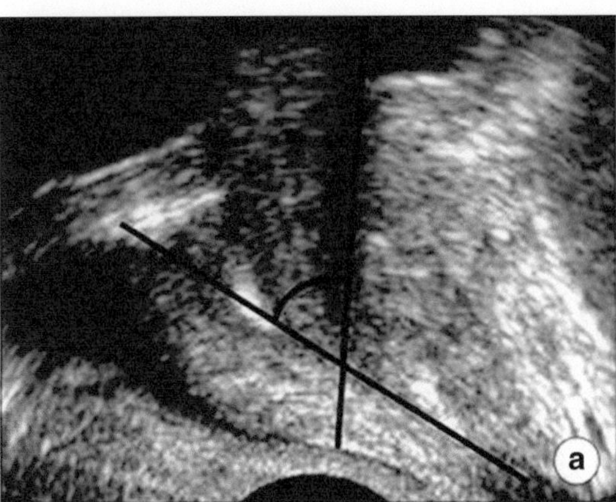
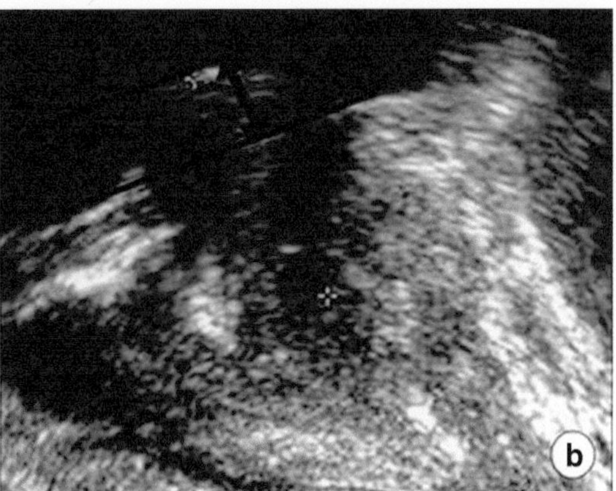

Fig. 8 (**a**) Prostatic urethral angle measured by TRUS shows 56°. (**b**) Intravesical prostatic protrusion measured by TRUS shows 53 mm

anatomy. Kirschner-Hermanns et al. revealed hypermobility of the proximal urethra, funneling of the bladder neck, voluntary pelvic floor contraction, and urethral and paraurethral fibrosis in post radical prostatectomy patients. They suggested that men with incontinence had differences in proximal urethal mobility and bladder neck opening. The same group reported high levels of reproducibility in male pelvic floor landmarks by perineal ultrasound (Najjari et al.). Displacement of male pelvic floor anatomical landmarks (including striated urethral sphincter, levator ani, and bulbocavernosus) by pelvic floor contraction has also been demonstrated and reproduced by Stafford et al.

The normal and abnormal male external sphincter is likely to play a role in male continence and incontinence post-prostate surgery. This structure is visible on MRI and recently has been described using transrectal ultrasound. By examining 52 men during transrectal ultrasound, Miano et al. described a hypoechoic area surrounding the urethra as the sphincter complex, with the proximal end defined as the area between the verumontanum and the prostate apex and the distal end defined by voluntary contraction of the external anal sphincter. These techniques are in their infancy in describing an important anatomical structure in the male pelvic floor [32–36].

Conclusions

Urodynamics study (pressure–flow measurements) remains the current gold standard in the diagnosis and management of BOO; however, it is an invasive procedure and time-consuming. There is a concerted drive to identify other parameters that can be measured more readily. With the advancement of US we are now able to accurately assess many aspects of the prostate and the bladder. Although many parameters such as IPP, PV, BWT, UEBWT, and PUA have been evaluated, they all lack the necessary sensitivity to replace the current gold standard. The majority of studies was conducted at single centers and reported small numbers of patients. In order to assess the usefulness of noninvasive US

parameters in the diagnosis of BOO and investigation of male stress urinary incontinence, further, large-scale multicenter studies are required. Currently noninvasive ultrasonic assessment of the prostate and bladder have not entered routine clinical practice to aid diagnosis of BOO or incontinence.

References

1. Hald T. Urodynamics in benign prostatic hyperplasia: a survey. Prostate. 1989;2:69–77.
2. Roehrborn CG. Pathology of benign prostatic hyperplasia. Int J Impot Res. 2008;20 Suppl 3:S11–8.
3. Abrams P, Cardozo L, Fall M, Griffiths D, Rosier P, Ulmsten U, et al. The standardisation of terminology of lower urinary tract function: report from the Standardisation Sub-committee of the International Continence Society. Neurourol Urodyn. 2002;21(2):167–78.
4. Foo KT. Decision making in the management of benign prostatic enlargement and the role of transabdominal ultrasound. Int J Urol. 2010;17(12):974–9.
5. Yuen JS, Ngiap JT, Cheng CW, Foo KT. Effects of bladder volume on transabdominal ultrasound measurements of intravesical prostatic protrusion and volume. Int J Urol. 2002;9(4):225–9.
6. Jacobsen SJ, Jacobson DJ, Girman CJ, Roberts RO, Rhodes T, Guess HA, et al. Natural history of prostatism: risk factors for acute urinary retention. J Urol. 1997;158(2):481–7.
7. Kuo HC. Clinical prostate score for diagnosis of bladder outlet obstruction by prostate measurements and uroflowmetry. Urology. 1999;54(1):90–6.
8. Hirayama A, Samma S, Fujimoto K, Yamaguchi A, Akiyama T, Fukui Y. Comparison of parameters to determine the cause of urinary disturbance in men with prostate volume less than 20 milliliters. Int J Urol. 2002;9(10):554–9. discussion 60.
9. Chia SJ, Heng CT, Chan SP, Foo KT. Correlation of intravesical prostatic protrusion with bladder outlet obstruction. BJU Int. 2003;91(4):371–4.
10. Keqin Z, Zhishun X, Jing Z, Haixin W, Dongqing Z, Benkang S. Clinical significance of intravesical prostatic protrusion in patients with benign prostatic enlargement. Urology. 2007;70(6):1096–9.
11. Lim KB, Ho H, Foo KT, Wong MY, Fook-Chong S. Comparison of intravesical prostatic protrusion, prostate volume and serum prostatic-specific antigen in the evaluation of bladder outlet obstruction. Int J Urol. 2006;13(12):1509–13.
12. Lee LS, Sim HG, Lim KB, Wang D, Foo KT. Intravesical prostatic protrusion predicts clinical progression of benign prostatic enlargement in patients receiving medical treatment. Int J Urol. 2010;17(1):69–74.

13. Aganovic D, Hasanbegovic M, Prcic A, Kulovac B, Hadziosmanovic O. Which is a better indicator of bladder outlet obstruction in patients with benign prostatic enlargemen-ntravesical protrusion of prostate or bladder wall thickness? Med Arh. 2012;66(5):324–8.

14. Greene DR, Egawa S, Hellerstein DK, Scardino PT. Sonographic measurements of transition zone of prostate in men with and without benign prostatic hyperplasia. Urology. 1990;36(4):293–9.

15. Kaplan SA, Te AE, Pressler LB, Olsson CA. Transition zone index as a method of assessing benign prostatic hyperplasia: correlation with symptoms, urine flow and detrusor pressure. J Urol. 1995;154(5):1764–9.

16. Witjes WP, Aarnink RG, Ezz-el-Din K, Wijkstra H, Debruyne EM, de la Rosette JJ. The correlation between prostate volume, transition zone volume, transition zone index and clinical and urodynamic investigations in patients with lower urinary tract symptoms. Br J Urol. 1997;80(1):84–90.

17. Shinbo H, Kurita Y, Nakanishi T, Imanishi T, Otsuka A, Furuse H, et al. Resistive index: a newly identified predictor of outcome of transurethral prostatectomy in patients with benign prostatic hyperplasia. Urology. 2010;75(1):143–7.

18. Tsuru N, Kurita Y, Masuda H, Suzuki K, Fujita K. Role of Doppler ultrasound and resistive index in benign prostatic hypertrophy. Int J Urol. 2002;9(8):427–30.

19. Kojima M, Ochiai A, Naya Y, Okihara K, Ukimura O, Miki T. Doppler resistive index in benign prostatic hyperplasia: correlation with ultrasonic appearance of the prostate and infravesical obstruction. Eur Urol. 2000;37(4):436–42.

20. Huang T, Qi J, Yu YJ, Xu D, Jiao Y, Kang J, et al. Predictive value of resistive index, detrusor wall thickness and ultrasound estimated bladder weight regarding the outcome after transurethral prostatectomy for patients with lower urinary tract symptoms suggestive of benign prostatic obstruction. Int J Urol. 2012;19(4):343–50.

21. Uvelius B, Persson L, Mattiasson A. Smooth muscle cell hypertrophy and hyperplasia in the rat detrusor after short-time infravesical outflow obstruction. J Urol. 1984;131(1):173–6.

22. Gilpin SA, Gosling JA, Barnard RJ. Morphological and morphometric studies of the human obstructed, trabeculated urinary bladder. Br J Urol. 1985;57(5):525–9.

23. Oelke M, Hofner K, Jonas U, Ubbink D, de la Rosette J, Wijkstra H. Ultrasound measurement of detrusor wall thickness in healthy adults. Neurourol Urodyn. 2006;25(4):308–17. discussion 18.

24. Kojima M, Inui E, Ochiai A, Naya Y, Ukimura O, Watanabe H. Ultrasonic estimation of bladder weight as a measure of bladder hypertrophy in men with infravesical obstruction: a preliminary report. Urology. 1996;47(6):942–7.

25. Manieri C, Carter SS, Romano G, Trucchi A, Valenti M, Tubaro A. The diagnosis of bladder outlet obstruction in men by ultrasound measurement of bladder wall thickness. J Urol. 1998;159(3):761–5.

26. Oelke M, Hofner K, Jonas U, de la Rosette JJ, Ubbink DT, Wijkstra H. Diagnostic accuracy of noninvasive tests to evaluate bladder outlet obstruction in men: detrusor wall thickness, uroflowmetry, postvoid residual urine, and prostate volume. Eur Urol. 2007;52(3):827–34.

27. Blatt AH, Titus J, Chan L. Ultrasound measurement of bladder wall thickness in the assessment of voiding dysfunction. J Urol. 2008;179(6):2275–8. discussion 8-9.

28. Bright E, Pearcy R, Abrams P. Automatic evaluation of ultrasonography-estimated bladder weight and bladder wall thickness in community-dwelling men with presumably normal bladder function. BJU Int. 2012;109(7):1044–9.

29. Bright E, Pearcy R, Abrams P. Ultrasound estimated bladder weight in men attending the uroflowmetry clinic. Neurourol Urodyn. 2011;30(4):583–6.

30. Cho KS, Kim JH, Kim DJ, Choi YD, Kim JH, Hong SJ. Relationship between prostatic urethral angle and urinary flow rate: its implication in benign prostatic hyperplasia pathogenesis. Urology. 2008;71(5):858–62.

31. Park YJ, Bae KH, Jin BS, Jung HJ, Park JS. Is increased prostatic urethral angle related to lower urinary tract symptoms in males with benign prostatic hyperplasia/lower urinary tract symptoms? Korean J Urol. 2012;53(6):410–3.

32. Kirschner-Hermanns R, Najjari L, Brehmer B, Blum R, Zeuch V, Maass N, et al. Two- and three-/four dimensional perineal ultrasonography in men with urinary incontinence after radical prostatectomy. BJU Int. 2012;109(1):46–51.

33. Miano R, Kim FJ, De Nunzio C, Mauriello A, Sansalone S, Vespasiani G, et al. Morphological evaluation of the male external urethral sphincter complex by transrectal ultrasound: feasibility study and potential clinical applications. Urol Int. 2012;89(3):275–82.

34. Nahon I, Waddington G, Adams R, Dorey G. Assessing muscle function of the male pelvic floor using real time ultrasound. Neurourol Urodyn. 2011;30(7):1329–32.

35. Najjari L, Hennemann J, Maass N, Kirschner-Hermanns RK. [Perineal ultrasound for diagnostics of male stress incontinence: comparative study on the application of urogynecological standards for men and women]. Urologe A. 2012;51(3):384–9.

36. Stafford RE, Ashton-Miller JA, Constantinou CE, Hodges PW. A new method to quantify male pelvic floor displacement from 2D transperineal ultrasound images. Urology. 2013;81(3):685–9.

Application of Prostate Ultrasound for Prostate Biopsy

Christopher R. Porter and Khanh N. Pham

Introduction

The evaluation of prostatic conditions prior to the advent of sonographic techniques relied on palpation of the gland and "blind" sampling techniques via needle aspiration and biopsy. With the development of B-mode ultrasound in the 1950s and probes capable of providing images to the clinician in real-time, gray-scale ultrasound became the standard method of prostate imaging for most prostate conditions. The position of the prostate in the pelvis, tucked beneath the pubis and anterior to the rectum, lends itself to the application of a transrectal approach. The transrectal approach to imaging the gland has become the standard of care for diagnostic evaluation of prostatic conditions, prostate biopsy and therapeutic approaches to prostate cancer.

The application of transrectal ultrasound is ubiquitous: virtually all urologists' offices, whether they are in a private small group setting or in the academic setting, have one or more ultrasound units with probes appropriate for transrectal imaging.

This chapter focuses on the application of transrectal ultrasound imaging to biopsy of the prostate. The chapter will encompass the initial evaluation of the gland, the techniques used to perform prostate biopsy, and references for documentation of the exam and patient safety.

History

Transrectal ultrasound (TRUS) guided prostate biopsy is the standard method for early detection of adenocarcinoma of the prostate. Prostate biopsy was first described in 1930 using a transperineal approach [1]. Seven years later Astraldi performed the first transrectal biopsy [2]. TRUS was first described in 1955 [3] and was widely used in practice by the 1970s [4]. In 1989 Hodge described the first systematic biopsy template (sextant) [5]. Further refinements have included an extended core biopsy scheme as well as modifications to pain control strategies.

Anatomy

Grossly the prostate is situated anterior to the rectum and beneath the pubic arch. The prostate is bordered laterally by the levator ani and superiorly by the bladder neck. Prostatic glandular anatomy is typically described in terms of zonal architecture (Fig. 1). The anterior fibromuscular stroma (AFS) is devoid of glandular tissue. The transition zone (TZ), which constitutes 5–10 % of normal prostate volume, gives rise to benign

C.R. Porter, M.D., F.A.C.S. (✉) • K.N. Pham, M.D.
Section of Urology and Renal Transplantation,
Virginia Mason, 1100 9th Ave, Mailstop C7-URO,
Seattle, WA 98101, USA
e-mail: Christopher.Porter@virginiamason.org

C.R. Porter and E.M. Wolff (eds.), *Prostate Ultrasound: Current Practice and Future Directions*,
DOI 10.1007/978-1-4939-1948-2_9, © Springer Science+Business Media New York 2015

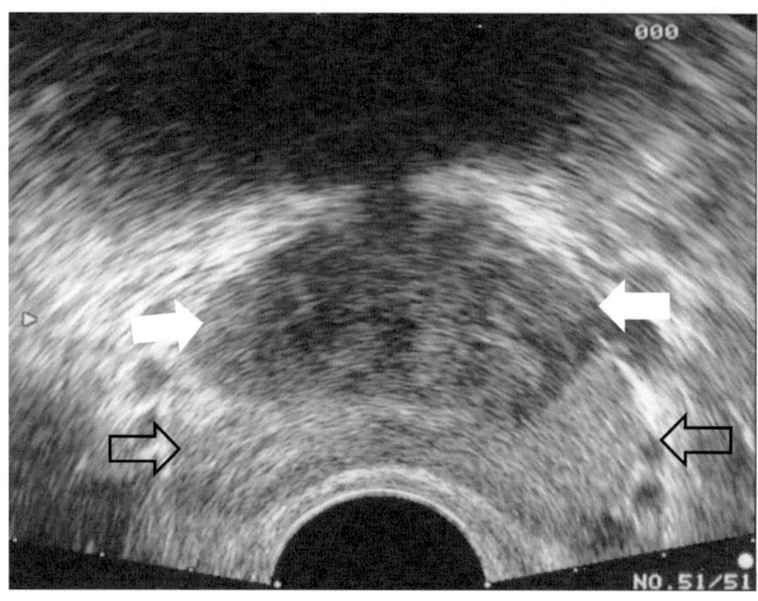

Fig. 1 Transrectal Ultrasound Image (7.5 MHz) of the prostate denoting the zonal anatomy. Hypoechoic region anteriorly corresponds to transition zone (*white arrows*). Peripheral zone (relatively more hyperechoic) lies posteriorly (*open arrows*)

prostatic hyperplasia (BPH) and is the zone or origin for 20 % of prostate cancers. The central zone (CZ) surrounds the ejaculatory ducts, makes up 20 % of the prostate volume, and gives rise to a minority of prostate tumors (5 %). Up to 75 % of the normal prostate volume is contained in the peripheral zone (PZ), which is the source of the majority of prostate cancers. These zonal distinctions are not always evident on ultrasound examination. However, in the presence of BPH, the PZ may be differentiated from the CZ. The paired seminal vesicles (SV), which are generally symmetrical in appearance, are located posteriorly.

Technique

Preparation

Patients undergoing a prostate needle biopsy should refrain from taking antiplatelet/anticoagulation medications (i.e., ASA/NSAIDs/clopidogrel/warfarin) 7 days prior to the procedure (Appendix Table A.1). Crawford et al. demonstrated that antibiotics taken 24 h prior to and continuing for 24 to 48 h post-procedure reduces bacterial septicemia [6]. While the septicemia rate following prophylaxis was reduced to less

than 1 %, this rate has risen over the last decade [7] This has been due in large part to an increased incidence of extended-spectrum beta-lactamase-producing (ESBL) *Escherichia coli* that tend to be resistant to ciprofloxacin, ceftriaxone, sulbactam/ampicillin, and cefazolin. Generally imipenem and piperacillin-tazobactam are effective agents against ESBL-producing *E. coli* [8, 9].

Recent literature from Taylor et al. has demonstrated a potential benefit in targeted antimicrobial prophylaxis based on rectal swab culture results [10]. Targeted antimicrobial prophylaxis was associated with a decrease in the incidence of infectious complications after biopsy caused by fluoroquinolone-resistant organisms as well as a decrease in the overall cost of care. Cost-effectiveness analysis revealed that targeted prophylaxis yielded a cost savings of $4,499 per TRUS-guided prostate biopsy infectious complication averted. Additionally, an enema may be given the night prior to and the morning of the procedure. Less rectal content increases visibility by reducing interference and decreases the rate of bacteremia [11]. Prophylactic antibiotic use may need to be modified based on local patterns of bacterial resistance. Shakil et al. evaluated the use of outpatient parenteral prophylaxis with ertapenem for multidrug-resistant *E. coli* rectal colonization identified on rectal swab cultures [12]. All patients received ertapenem one day prior to and on the day of biopsy with no infectious complications.

Special considerations should be made for patients at risk for infective endocarditis and patients with a history of total joint replacement. Prophylaxis against infective endocarditis, with appropriate antibiotics, such as gentamicin and ampicillin [13], is recommended by the American Heart Association. Patients at high risk for infective endocarditis include those with: (1) prosthetic cardiac valves or prosthetic material used for cardiac valve repair, (2) previous infective endocarditis, (3) congenital heart defects, and (4) cardiac transplant recipients with valve regurgitation [14]. The American Academy of Orthopedic Surgeons (AAOS) guidelines [15] state that clinicians should consider antibiotic prophylaxis for all total joint replacement patients prior to any invasive procedure that may cause bacteremia. For genitourinary procedures the AAOS recommends ciprofloxacin 60 min prior to the biopsy.

Anesthesia

It is accepted that TRUS guided prostate biopsy can be painful [16, 17]. Patient perception of this procedure is a major source of anxiety and a deterrent for undergoing biopsy. Nijs and associates demonstrated that 18 % of patients in a population based screening program refused biopsy due anticipated pain [18]. Li et al. investigated the effect of diazepam on pain perception during and after prostate biopsy in a prospective, randomized placebo-controlled trial and found no benefit in the treatment group based on patient questionnaires and the visual analog pain scale [19]. Nash and colleagues first conducted a randomized, double-blind study evaluating the effect of infiltration of 1% lidocaine in the vascular pedicles of 64 patients undergoing PNB [20]. The mean pain scores on the side injected with drug were significantly lower than the control side. Numerous investigators have demonstrated decreased pain with various pre-procedural periprostatic local anesthetic strategies (including a meta-analysis of 14 studies examining 994 procedures) [20–23]. Conversely, a small number of studies have shown no benefit [24–26].

There have been several different periprostatic injection techniques described. The most common strategy involves injection of local anesthetic between the base of the prostate and the seminal vesicles, causing a wheal between the corresponding seminal vesicle and the prostate gland from the rectal wall (Fig. 2) [27–29]. Other authors have described injecting the prostatic plexus in the area of the apex of the prostate [21, 30],

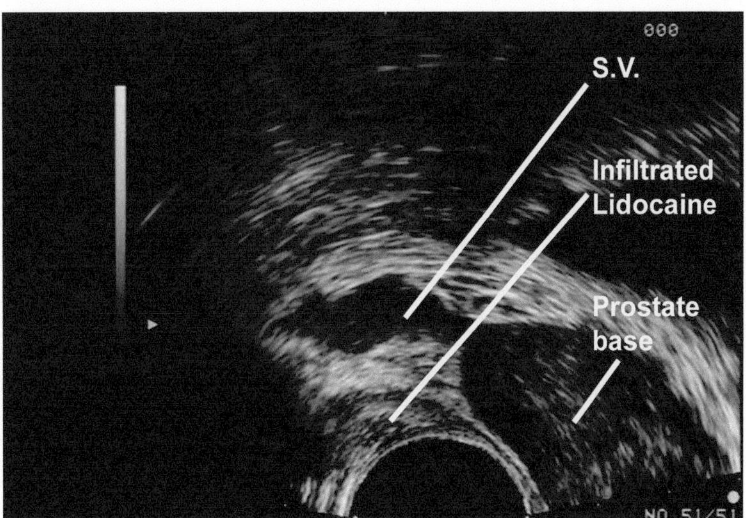

Fig. 2 Transrectal Ultrasound Image (7.5 MHz) of the Prostate—Sagittal view. Hypoechoic region posterior to the gland represents local anesthetic injection site

A majority of studies advocate bilateral injections [22, 27–29]. The administered anesthetic described varies from 1 to 2 % lidocaine [20, 21, 25, 28], with a meta-analysis showing a cumulative anesthetic dose varying from 2.5 to 20 ml [23].

Transrectal Biopsy

Patients are typically placed in the left lateral decubitus position. Digital rectal exam is performed and any palpable lesions are noted with respect to their location on the gland. A 7.5 MHz probe is typically used. The probe is activated and placed using the ultrasound image to guide the probe gently beyond the anal sphincter and adjacent to the prostate: it is recommended to perform this slowly and carefully to minimize patient discomfort. TRUS should be performed in the sagittal and the transverse planes using gray-scale ultrasound. The gland is then inspected using color and power Doppler in both planes for presence of lesions demonstrating increased flow with respect to other PZ areas of the gland. Abnormalities are recorded by image saving mechanisms (either paper hard copy or electronic). Localization of all lesions is performed in real time and documented. Following instillation of local anesthesia, prostate volume calculations should be carried out. These volumes can be calculated through a variety of formulas that assume the prostate to be that of a geometric shape.

(a) Ellipse: ($\pi/6 \times$ transverse diameter $\times$ AP diameter $\times$ longitudinal diameter)
(b) Sphere: ($\pi/6 \times$ transverse diameter^3)
(c) Prolate (egg shaped): ($\pi/6 \times$ transverse diameter$^2 \times$ AP diameter)

These formulas estimate weight as well as volume, as 1 cm^3 equals 1 g of prostatic tissue. The specific gravity of prostate tissue is approximately 1.02 g/cm.^{3}

Volume measurements of the TZ and bladder volume may be carried out and recorded depending on the preference of the physician. The integrity of the surrounding structures should be evaluated, including examination of the bladder wall, seminal vesicles, and anal canal up to the level of the prostate.

PSA Density (PSAD)

Calculating prostate volume allows the use of PSA density (PSAD) defined as the ratio of serum PSA-to-prostate volume. PSAD is thought to improve cancer detection (sensitivity) and reduce the number of unnecessary biopsies (specificity). Djavan and colleagues demonstrated PSAD and TZ PSA density were significantly higher in subjects diagnosed with prostate cancer on initial and repeat biopsies [31]. The authors routinely calculate PSAD and record it in real time; however, their data do not support basing the decision to perform prostate biopsy solely on this parameter.

Prostatic and Paraprostatic Cysts

As the prostate is examined, focal cystic areas can often be noted. These cysts can vary in size and when associated with BPH are due to cystic dilatation of TZ glands. Other common cysts include acquired prostatic retention cysts, which represent dilatation of glandular acini. Acquired prostatic retention cysts may occur in any zone and are not associated with BPH. Other cysts are less common, but have important associations or implications. Utricular and Müllerian duct cysts are congenital midline or paramedian cysts. Utricular cysts are intraprostatic in nature. Arising from a dilated utricle originating at the verumontanum, these communicate with the urethra and can be associated with cryptorchidism and hypospadias [32]. Müllerian duct cysts are located retrovesically and originate from Müllerian remnants. They have no communication to the urethra and can be associated with calculi and renal agenesis [33]. Ejaculatory cysts, arising from an obstructed ejaculatory duct, can be located in a midline or paramedian position. These can be associated with seminal vesicle obstruction and may contain calculi. Seminal vesicle cysts are found lateral to the prostate and are secondary to congenital hypoplasia of the ejaculatory duct [34]. Unilateral in nature, they may contain calculi and are associated with renal agenesis and epididymitis. Prostatic abscesses can be associated with surgery, prostatitis, or epididymitis [35].

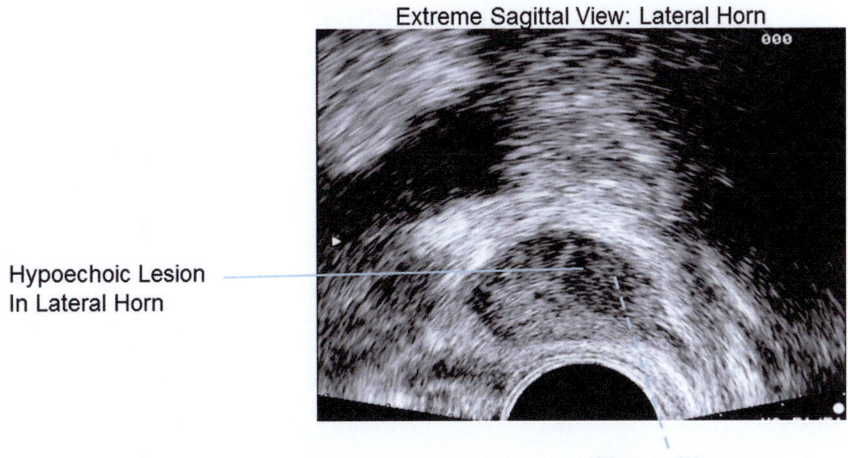

Fig. 3 Transrectal Ultrasound Image (7.5 MHz) of the Prostate—Extreme sagittal view. Hypoechoic lesion in the lateral horn represents an area of increased suspicion for malignancy

Hypoechoic Lesions

The gland should be examined for hypoechoic lesions. The classic appearance of prostate cancer is a round/oval hypoechoic lesion located in the PZ (Fig. 3). Contemporary series have noted the presence of these lesions is a less sensitive sign for prostate cancer than once thought, with hypoechoic lesions being malignant at a rate of 17–57 % [36]. However, a continued valuable asset of TRUS is directed biopsy of these lesions. Absence of hypoechoic lesions is not a contraindication to biopsy as 39 % and 1 % of prostate tumors are isoechoic and hyperechoic, respectively [37]. TRUS has a known poor specificity in regard to presence of a hypoechoic lesion. Entities that also have a hypoechoic appearance on TRUS include granulomatous prostatitis [38], prostatic infarction [39], lymphoma [40], and TZ BPH [41].

Color Doppler

Color Doppler (CD) is a tool that attempts to allow TRUS to differentiate benign from malignant tissue. CD measures the frequency shift in sound waves as a measurement of the velocity of blood flow (Fig. 4). This capitalizes on the hypervascular appearance of prostate cancer due to increased microvessel density secondary to increased angiogenesis versus benign tissue [42]. Cornud et al. noted that in patients with clinical T1c disease, high-risk pathologic features (extracapsular extension and seminal vesicle invasion) were present more often in tumors with a positive CD signal versus those with the absence of a positive CD signal [43]. Another study demonstrated a 2.6-fold increase in the rate of detection of prostate cancer versus conventional gray-scale ultrasound [36]. Halpern and Strup demonstrated CD sensitivity and specificity to diagnose prostate cancer at 27 % and 84 %, respectively [44]. This is an improvement in specificity with respect to gray-scale imaging (sensitivity 44 %, specificity 71 %). However, 45 % of cancers still went undetected by any ultrasound modality. Arger has suggested that pathologic groups, based on high, intermediate, and low Gleason grade scores, were not separable by vascular measurement [45]. While several studies [43, 46, 47] have demonstrated increased cancer detection using CD-targeted focal biopsy strategies, there remain enough questions to preclude replacement of a systematic biopsy approach [48].

Biopsy Strategies

The advent of the sextant biopsy technique, that is systematic biopsy of the apex, mid, and base of

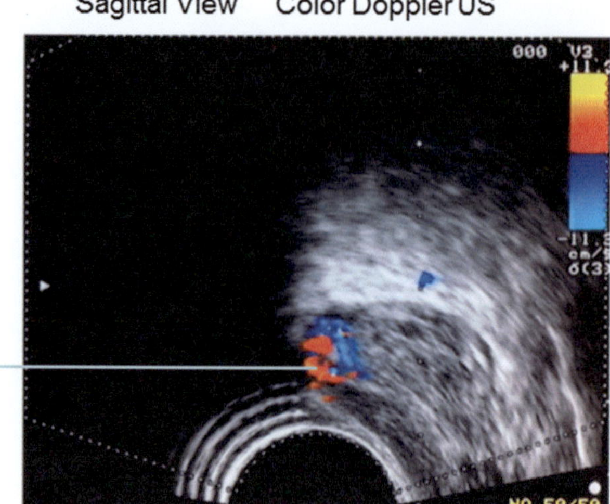

Fig. 4 Transrectal Ultrasound Image, Color Doppler, of the Prostate—Sagittal view. Colored area in the posterior lateral aspect of the gland represents an area of increased vascular flow relative to the surrounding parenchyma

Table 1 Prostate cancer detection rates with extended core biopsy

Study	Number of Cores/Biopsy	Prostate Cancer Detection %
Eskew [50]	6	26.1
	13	40.3
Babian [51]	6	20
	11	30
Presti [52]	6	33.5
	8	39.7
	10	40.2
Naughton [53]	6	26
	12	27

the prostate on each side of the gland, represented an improvement in prostate cancer detection over site-specific biopsies of hypoechoic lesions or palpable abnormalities [5]. With this limited template there is still concern for a high false negative rate. In a repeat biopsy series, Levine et al. demonstrated a false negative rate of 30 % in men with an abnormal digital rectal examination and/ or elevated serum PSA [49].

Refinements have focused on the importance of increased number of cores, as well as including laterally directed biopsies. Many groups have reported series (Table 1) in which improved cancer detection rates were achieved by including additional laterally directed cores and/or increasing the number cores taken from 6 to as many as 13

[49–53]. Investigators have demonstrated a lack of usefulness for TZ and SV sampling on initial biopsy with only 2.1 % and 3.7 % of biopsies being positive, respectively [54, 55]. The spatial distribution of cancer foci in patients with negative initial biopsies or with a prostate gland volume larger than 50 cc may vary compared to those with prostate carcinomas diagnosed on initial biopsy. In these cases, special emphasis on the apico-dorsal peripheral and transitional zones should be considered [56, 57]. Biopsy of the SV is not recommended unless a palpable abnormality is appreciated.

It is generally recommended that 10–12 biopsies of the gland be obtained with attention to the lateral horns. Technique is important in obtaining laterally directed biopsies (Fig. 5). It should be recalled that the Tru-Cut needle travels between 17 mm and 24 mm depending on the manufacture's standard. The user must appropriately guide the angle of the biopsy to maximize its position laterally on the gland, particularly when the lateral horns are approached.

Repeat Biopsy

For the patient who has had a previous negative biopsy but a persistent PSA elevation or abnormal DRE, an additional biopsy may be considered.

Fig. 5 Transrectal Ultrasound Image (7.5 MHz) of the Prostate—Sagittal view. Laterally directed TRUS biopsy

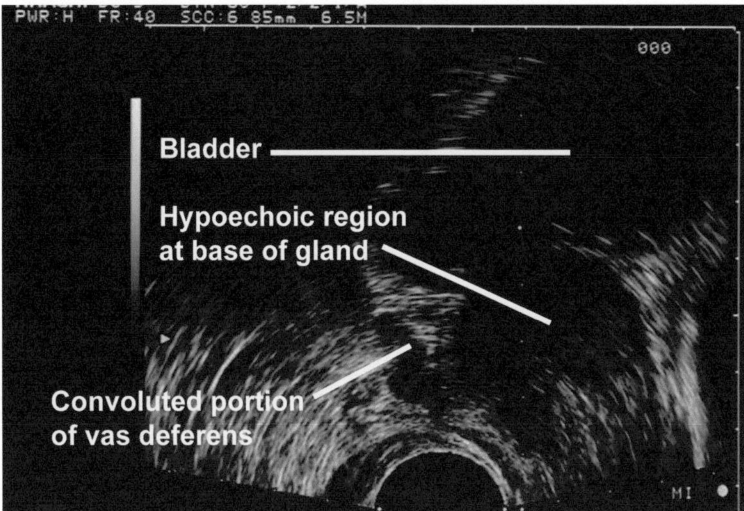

Sagital view: 7.5 MHz probe
Dotted line represents biopsy position

During repeat biopsy the standard extended core biopsy protocol should be carried out. Additionally any sites of ultrasound abnormality and any sites of high grade prostatic intraepithelial neoplasia (HGPIN) or atypical small acinar proliferation (ASAP) should be sampled [58]. The aforementioned strategy of apico-dorsal peripheral and TZ biopsies should be included. It is well established that as successive biopsies are obtained, a decreased rate of prostate cancer detection will be observed with each additional biopsy [59]. A large series of over 1,100 men undergoing biopsy as directed by PSA screening found an initial prostate cancer detection rate of 34 % [60]. This declined to 19, 8, and 7 % on biopsies 2 thru 4, respectively. This was echoed by Djavan in the European Prostate Cancer Detection Study, in which 1,051 men with a PSA value of 4–10 ng/ml had a detection rate of 22 % on primary biopsy [61]. This declined to 10, 5, and 4 %, respectively, on subsequent biopsies 2, 3, and 4. The use of free and total PSA, along with prostate cancer antigen 3 (PCA3) may allow risk stratification of patients for additional prostate biopsy. Catalona et al. proposed the use of the percentage of free PSA to reduce unnecessary biopsies in patients with a PSA values between 4.0 and 10.0 ng/ml and a palpably benign gland [62]. In this study Catalona suggested that patients with a free PSA of less than 25 % were significantly more likely to have a positive biopsy.

PCA3 encodes a prostate-specific messenger ribonucleic acid (mRNA) that serves as the target for a novel urinary molecular assay for prostate cancer detection [63]. It also has potential as an aid in identifying men with a high probability of a positive (repeat) biopsy. PCA3 mRNA concentration is measured in urine collected after digital rectal examination (DRE). Haese et al. compared PCA3 to percent free PSA and biopsy results in 463 men undergoing repeat biopsy [64]. The overall positive repeat biopsy rate was 28 %. The probability of a positive repeat biopsy increased with rising PCA3 scores. The PCA3 score (cut point of 35) was superior to percent free PSA (cut point of 25 %) for predicting repeat prostate biopsy outcomes.

Saturation Biopsy

Saturation biopsy has a role in maximizing prostate cancer detection rates in select patients at high risk for prostate cancer in the setting of a prior negative biopsy. Protocols have been described using both transrectal and transperineal approaches [65]. Various series have shown detection rates of 30–34 % [66–69]. One drawback to this procedure is the need for these biopsies to be performed under sedation in a hospital setting. However, there are circumstances that warrant more extensive gland sampling. These include: (1) a persistent rise in serum PSA, (2) new DRE abnormalities, and (3) low volume cancers for which a surveillance approach is being considered. The standard transrectal approach has a theoretical limitation due to its limited ability to obtain anterior prostatic tissue, particularly at the apex. The technique described below focuses on the transperineal approach with glandular mapping.

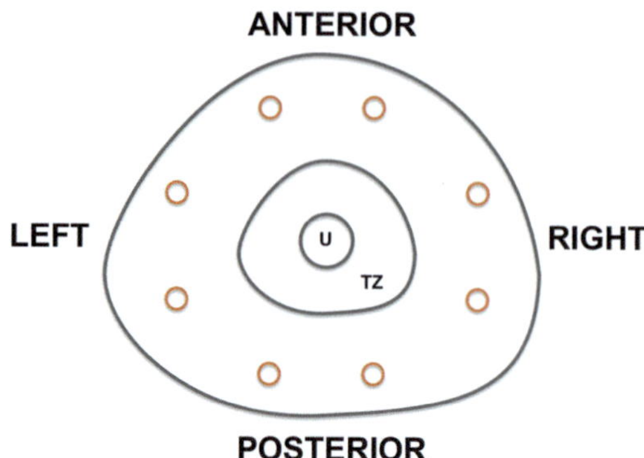

Fig. 6 Template for TRUS Biopsy

Transrectal Ultrasound-Guided Transperineal Prostate Biopsy using the Brachytherapy Template

Indications for transrectal ultrasound-guided transperineal prostate biopsy (TRUS/TPB) include: men with further worrisome serum PSA changes or DRE abnormalities after one or more negative standard biopsies or those considering active surveillance (AS) for prostate cancer. Gershman and colleagues evaluated 34 patients with prior negative prostate biopsies despite persistently elevated PSA and found prostate cancer in 17 (50 %) patients, with prostate cancer noted in the anterior prostate in 14 (82 %) [70]. Furthermore, with recent increasing use of AS to manage men with low-risk prostate cancer, proper staging is of utmost importance. Shapiro et al. previously reported that more than one-third of patients managed with AS are upgraded at the time of a repeat biopsy or RP [71]. In an analysis of 64 patients with clinically insignificant PCa as defined by Epstein criteria who were under consideration for active surveillance, Taira et al. showed that initial TRUS BX underestimates disease extent, with 46 (72 %) patients found to have clinically significant prostate cancer and 25 (45 %) patients with cancer had higher Gleason grade pathology following TP BX [72]. Katz and colleagues evaluated the accuracy of TPB compared to pathology specimens from 78 patients who underwent radical prostatectomy for

localized prostate cancer. In their cohort, they found the sensitivity and specificity of TPB for prostate cancer detection were 86 % and 83 %, respectively [73].

Stereotactic TPB is performed using a standard brachytherapy template and the ultrasound device together with a brachytherapy stepper device [74]. Patients are appropriately counseled on the risks and benefits of the procedure and surgical consent is obtained. Similar pre-biopsy precautions are taken as per those outlined above for the transrectal technique. Antibiotic considerations to cover for skin flora are made instead of for rectal flora.

Under a general anesthetic patients are placed in the lithotomy position. Intravenous antibiotics are administered, a DRE is again performed and any lesions noted. As in the case of transrectal biopsies, the prostate is scanned in gray-scale and color Doppler and any abnormalities are recorded. The transrectal probe is placed in the brachytherapy stepper device and synchronized with the ultrasound device. Prostate volumes are again obtained and recorded. The prostate is divided into 12 sections: 4 quadrants each at the base, mid gland, and apex. Tissue cores are harvested using a standard Tru-Cut needle biopsy instrument beginning at the apical quadrants. Twenty-four core samples are targeted in both the sagittal and axial views. A representation of the template that is obtained from the base, mid gland, and apex is shown in Fig. 6. Specimens are placed in individual jars and reported accordingly. Patients are discharged with oral antibiotics and analgesics.

TRUS after Definitive Treatment and Hormonal Ablative Therapy

External beam radiotherapy (EBRT) decreases the size of the prostate gland. Small areas of cancer that have moderate or severe radiation effects tend to appear isoechoic while large (greater than 4 mm) foci of cancer usually show little radiation effect, and these foci typically appear hypoechoic [75]. When the urologist and patient are seeking proof of local relapse, prostate needle biopsy is usually performed as described in the transrectal ultrasound-guided manner.

With the exception of the presence of well-distributed foreign bodies, long-term changes after brachytherapy resemble EBRT. [76] Biopsies of the gland are obtained in the same fashion as described above.

Whittington described the effects of luteinizing hormone-releasing hormone (LHRH) on prostate tissue [76]. The median decrease in prostate volume as a result of androgen deprivation was 33 %. The reduction in volume was greatest in men with the largest initial gland volume (59 %) and least in men with the smallest glands (10 %). It is rare that further biopsies will be required after hormonal ablation; however, if biopsies are required it is very important to notify the pathologist as to the presence of hormonal ablation given the histologic changes that usually occur in these situations.

After radical prostatectomy, presence of lesions (hyper or hypoechoic) interrupting the tapering of the bladder to the urethra, representing the anastomotic plane, is considered worrisome for recurrence [77]. One notable exception is nodules noted anterior to the anastomosis, which may represent the ligated dorsal venous complex. [78] Biopsies of the bladder neck/vesico-urethral anastomosis are possible. The target for biopsy is usually small and care is required to accurately map the anatomy prior to biopsy. The typical area to concentrate on is between the bladder neck and the external sphincter. The urologist is reminded to exhibit extreme caution around the sphincter.

Complications

Transrectal ultrasound-guided needle biopsy is safe for diagnosing prostate cancer. Complications do arise after a prostate needle biopsy, with few major but frequent minor self-limiting complications. Vagal response, secondary to pain/anxiety, occurs in 1.4–5.3 % of patients [69]. This is generally responsive to hydration and placing the patient in the Trendelenburg position. Hematuria is quite common immediately following biopsy (71 %), with 47 % of patients having limited hematuria resolving over 3–7 days [79]. Hematospermia is observed in 9–36 % of biopsies and may persist for several months [7, 78]. Rectal bleeding is seen after 2–8 % of biopsies [7, 79]. Frequently, the bleeding is mild, and can be controlled with digital pressure. More severe cases, or bleeding that is not controlled with conservative approaches, can be managed with rectal packing [80] using a tampon or gauze or can be addressed with endoscopic injection of vasoconstrictive agents or ligation of bleeding vessels during colonoscopy [81]. Acute urinary retention requiring catheter drainage occurs up to 0.4 % of the time [81]. Men with enlarged prostates or severe baseline lower urinary tract symptoms are at an increased risk [79, 82]. In the pre-prophylaxis era, Thompson demonstrated a bacteremia rate of 100 % with a bacteruria rate of 87 %. This decreased to 44 % and 16 %, respectively, with enema alone [83]. Crawford et al. administered 48 h of carbenicillin and noted bacteruria to decrease from 36 % to 9 % versus the control group [6]. The incidence of fever in the treatment group was 17 % compared to 48 % in the control group. Antibiotic prophylaxis is now standard of care. Berger demonstrated fever (>38.5 °C) in 0.8 % of 4,303 patients receiving a 5-day course of ciprofloxacin [7]. Similarly, a study administering 1 to 3 days of ciprofloxacin noted a fever incidence of 0.6 % [84]. Seeding of prostate cancer in the needle tract is rare, but is reported in the literature. It is seen more commonly in the form of perineal recurrences after transperineal biopsy [85, 86], but has been reported after TRUS biopsy [87]. Perineal recurrence has a poor prognosis [86], while rectal seeding has been shown to be responsive to hormonal therapy as well as EBRT. [88] Hara et al. demonstrated increased circulating PSA mRNA in men following positive biopsy [89]; however, the risk of developing metastatic disease is thought to be low [58].

A more thorough description of complications following prostate biopsy is detailed in the next chapter.

Findings

HGPIN & ASAP

High-grade intraepithelial neoplasia (HGPIN) is detected on needle biopsy in 1–25 % of patients [90]. HGPIN was thought to be a precursor lesion for adenocarcinoma, and historically, its presence prompted rebiopsy at 3–6 months in the absence of prostate cancer in the biopsy specimen [91–93]. Lefkowitz et al. noted that with the extended 12-core biopsy technique, the repeat biopsy cancer detection rate was 2.3 %. They recommended repeat biopsy was not indicated for HGPIN in the absence of any other findings [94]. Atypical small acinar proliferation (ASAP) demonstrates gland proliferation without atypia and has an incidence of 5 % of men undergoing biopsy [95, 96]. The association with prostate cancer is stronger than with HGPIN, with the cancer detection rates on subsequent biopsies ranging from 51 to 75 % [97–100]. Repeat systematic biopsy of the prostate is recommended for patients with pathology demonstrating ASAP.

Predicting Outcomes Following Local Treatment

The pathologic elements obtained during needle biopsy, including number of cores positive, percent/length of cancer in each core, and localization of cores, may contribute important prognostic information. Clinical under-staging by TRUS PNB occurs, but it is reduced in the era of extended core strategies [101, 102]. The number/percent of cores positive has been shown to be correlated with prostate cancer extracapsular extension (ECE), surgical margin status, tumor volume and stage, seminal vesicle involvement, and presence of lymph node metastasis [103–106]. Length of tumor tissue involved in each core can also be measured. Longer tumor lengths, or higher percentage of core positivity, have been strongly associated with the presence of ECE, SV involvement, and biochemical recurrence following treatment [107–110]. Biopsy site-specific percent core positivity is predictive of sextant site of extension, which can aid in identification of appropriate candidates for nerve sparing surgery [111].

Summary

Transrectal biopsy technique using prophylactic antibiotics, local analgesia, and an extended core technique is safe and allows detection of prostate cancer while providing important prognostic information.

Appendix: Pre-procedure Medication Review

Prior to surgery it is important to review **<u>all</u> <u>medications</u>** you are taking with your physician as some products may increase your risk of bleeding. These include prescription, over-the-counter (OTC), and herbal products. **Please notify your physician if you are taking any of the following medications.*** Medications are listed by their generic name, with the some common brand names in parenthesis.

Always consult your health care provider if you are unsure if you are taking a medication that may increase your bleeding risk.
[a]Includes pills, liquids, teas, etc.

Table A.1 List of medications to be avoided prior to biopsy

Prescription and OTC Medication:	Topical Medication (cream, gel, ointment, etc.):
Aminosalicylic acid (*Paser*)	Diclofenac (*Flector, Solaraze, Voltaren*)
Aspirin (numerous, e.g., *Bayer, Bufferin, Ecotrin, Fiorinal, Aspergum, Alka-Seltzer, Percodan, Anacin, Goody's, Zorprin*)	Trolamine (e.g., *Aspercreme, Mobisyl, Myoflex*)
Celecoxib (*Celebrex*)	Methyl salicylate (e.g., *SalonPas, Icy Hot*)
Choline magnesium trisalicylate	**Ophthalmic Medication:**
Clopidogrel (*Plavix*)	Bromfenac (*Xibrom*)
Cilostazol (*Pletal*)	Diclofenac (*Voltaren*)
Diclofenac (*Cataflam, Voltaren, Arthrotec*)	Flurbiprofen (*Ocufen*)
Diflunisal	Ketorolac (*Acular*)
Dipyridamole (*Aggrenox, Persantine*)	Nepafenac (*Nevanac*)
Etodolac (*Lodine*)	**Injectable Medication:**
Fenoprofen	Enoxaparin (*Lovenox*)
Flurbiprofen	Dalteparin (*Fragmin*)
Ibuprofen (e.g., *Advil, Midol, Motrin*)	Fondaparinux (*Arixtra*)
Indomethacin (*Indocin*)	Heparin (*HepFlush, Hep-Lock*)
Ketoprofen (*Orudis*)	Tinzaparin (*Innohep*)
Ketorolac (*Toradol*)	Ketorolac (*Toradol*)
Magnesium salicylate (e.g., *Doan's, Momentum*)	**Herbals/Natural Products[a]:**
Meclofenamate	Aloe
Mefenamic acid (*Ponstel*)	Bilberry
Meloxicam (*Mobic*)	Cayenne
Nabumetone (*Relafen*)	Dong Quai
Naproxen (e.g., *Aleve, Naprosyn, Pamprin, Treximet*)	Feverfew
Oxaprozin (*Daypro*)	Fish Oil
Piroxicam (*Feldene*)	Flaxseed Oil
Salicylamide (e.g., *BC Fast Pain Relief, Lobac*)	Garlic
Salsalate	Ginger
Sulindac (*Clinoril*)	Gingko Biloba
Ticlopidine (*Ticlid*)	Ginseng
Tolmetin	Glucosamine Chondroitin
Warfarin (*Coumadin, Jantoven*)	Golden Seal
- Many OTC headache, allergy, cough, and cold products also contain aspirin, ibuprofen, or naproxen.	**Supplement Oils:**
- Tylenol is okay. Take as instructed.	Vitamin E

References

1. Ferguson R. Prostatic neoplasms; their diagnosis by needle puncture and aspiration. Am J Surg. 1930;9:507.
2. Astraldi A. Diagnosis of cancer of the prostate; biopsy by rectal route. Urol Cutaneous Rev. 1937;41:421.
3. Wild J. Fourth annual conference in ultrasound therapy. Presented at the, 1955.
4. Wantanabe H, Kato H, Kato T. Diagnostic application of ultrasonotomography to the prostate. Nippon Hinyokika Gakkai Zasshi. 1968;59:273.
5. Hodge KK, McNeal JE, Terris MK, et al. Random systematic versus directed ultrasound guided transrectal core biopsies of the prostate. J Urol. 1989;142:71.
6. Crawford ED, Haynes Jr AL, Story MW, et al. Prevention of urinary tract infection and sepsis following transrectal prostatic biopsy. J Urol. 1982;127:449.
7. Berger AP, Gozzi C, Steiner H, et al. Complication rate of transrectal ultrasound guided prostate biopsy: a comparison among 3 protocols with 6, 10 and 15 cores. J Urol. 2004;171:1478.
8. Cannon Jr GM, Smaldone MC, Paterson DL. Extended-spectrum beta-lactamase gram-negative

sepsis following prostate biopsy: implications for use of fluoroquinolone prophylaxis. Can J Urol. 2007;14:3653.

9. Ozden E, Bostanci Y, Yakupoglu KY, et al. Incidence of Acute Prostatitis Caused by Extended-Spectrum beta-Lactamase-producing Escherichia coli After Transrectal Prostate Biopsy. Urology. 2009;74: 119–23.

10. Taylor AK, Zembower TR, Nadler RB, Scheetz MH, Cashy JP, Bowen D, Murphy AB, Dielubanza E, Schaeffer AJ. Targeted antimicrobial prophylaxis using rectal swab cultures in men undergoing transrectal ultrasound guided prostate biopsy is associated with reduced incidence of postoperative infectious complications and cost of care. J Urol. 2012;187(4):1275–9.

11. Lindert KA, Kabalin JN, Terris MK. Bacteremia and bacteriuria after transrectal ultrasound guided prostate biopsy. J Urol. 2000;164:76.

12. Shakil J, Piracha N, Prasad N, Kopacz J, Tarasuk A, Farrell R, Urban C, Mariano N, Wang G, Segal-Maurer S. Use of outpatient parenteral antimicrobial therapy for transrectal ultrasound-guided prostate biopsy prophylaxis in the setting of community-associated multidrug-resistant Escherichia coli rectal colonization. Urology. 2014;83(4):710–3.

13. Dajani AS, Taubert KA, Wilson W, et al. Prevention of bacterial endocarditis: recommendations by the American Heart Association. Clin Infect Dis. 1997; 25:1448.

14. Nishimura RA, Carabello BA, Faxon DP, et al. ACC/ AHA 2008 guideline update on valvular heart disease: focused update on infective endocarditis: a report of the American College of Cardiology/ American Heart Association Task Force on Practice Guidelines: endorsed by the Society of Cardiovascular Anesthesiologists, Society for Cardiovascular Angiography and Interventions, and Society of Thoracic Surgeons. Circulation. 2008;118:887.

15. Bratzler DW, Houck PM. Antimicrobial prophylaxis for surgery: an advisory statement from the National Surgical Infection Prevention Project. Clin Infect Dis. 2004;38:1706.

16. De Sio M, D'Armiento M, Di Lorenzo G, et al. The need to reduce patient discomfort during transrectal ultrasonography-guided prostate biopsy: what do we know? BJU Int. 2005;96:977.

17. Soloway MS. Do unto others–why I would want anesthesia for my prostate biopsy. Urology. 2003; 62:973.

18. Nijs HG, Essink-Bot ML, DeKoning HJ, et al. Why do men refuse or attend population-based screening for prostate cancer? J Public Health Med. 2000;22:312.

19. Li R, Ruckle HC, Creech JD, Culpepper DJ, Lightfoot MA, Alsyouf M, Nicolay L, Jellison F, Baldwin DD. A Prospective, Randomized, Controlled Trial Assessing Diazepam to Reduce Perception and Recall of Pain During Transrectal Ultrasonography-Guided Biopsy of the Prostate. J Endourol. 2014;28(7):881–6.

20. Nash PA, Bruce JE, Indudhara R, et al. Transrectal ultrasound guided prostatic nerve blockade eases systematic needle biopsy of the prostate. J Urol. 1996;155:607.

21. Schostak M, Christoph F, Muller M, et al. Optimizing local anesthesia during 10-core biopsy of the prostate. Urology. 2002;60:253.

22. Trucchi A, De Nunzio C, Mariani S, et al. Local anesthesia reduces pain associated with transrectal prostatic biopsy. A prospective randomized study. Urol Int. 2005;74:209.

23. Hergan L, Kashefi C, Parsons JK. Local anesthetic reduces pain associated with transrectal ultrasound-guided prostate biopsy: a meta-analysis. Urology. 2007;69:520.

24. Bozlu M, Atici S, Ulusoy E, et al. Periprostatic lidocaine infiltration and/or synthetic opioid (meperidine or tramadol) administration have no analgesic benefit during prostate biopsy. A prospective randomized double-blind placebo-controlled study comparing different methods. Urol Int. 2004;72:308.

25. Vanni AP, Schaal CH, Costa RP, et al. Is the periprostatic anesthetic blockade advantageous in ultrasound-guided prostate biopsy? Int Braz J Urol. 2004;30:114.

26. Walsh K, O'Brien T, Salemmi A, et al. A randomised trial of periprostatic local anaesthetic for transrectal biopsy. Prostate Cancer Prostatic Dis. 2003;6:242.

27. Adamakis I, Mitropoulos D, Haritopoulos K, et al. Pain during transrectal ultrasonography guided prostate biopsy: a randomized prospective trial comparing periprostatic infiltration with lidocaine with the intrarectal instillation of lidocaine-prilocain cream. World J Urol. 2004;22:281.

28. Obek C, Ozkan B, Tunc B, et al. Comparison of 3 different methods of anesthesia before transrectal prostate biopsy: a prospective randomized trial. J Urol. 2004;172:502.

29. Rabets JC, Jones JS, Patel AR, et al. Bupivacaine provides rapid, effective periprostatic anesthesia for transrectal prostate biopsy. BJU Int. 2004;93:1216.

30. Nambirajan T, Woolsey S, Mahendra V, et al. Efficacy and safety peri-prostatic local anesthetic injection in trans-rectal biopsy of the prostrate: a prospective randomized study. Surgeon. 2004;2:221.

31. Djavan B, Zlotta A, Remzi M, et al. Optimal predictors of prostate cancer on repeat prostate biopsy: a prospective study of 1,051 men. J Urol. 2000; 163:1144.

32. Gregg DC, Sty JR. Sonographic diagnosis of enlarged prostatic utricle. J Ultrasound Med. 1989; 8:51.

33. McDermott V, Orr JD, Wild SR. Duplicated mullerian duct remnants associated with unilateral renal agenesis. Abdom Imaging. 1993;18:193.

34. King BF, Hattery RR, Lieber MM, et al. Congenital cystic disease of the seminal vesicle. Radiology. 1991;178:207.

35. Zagoria RJ. Genitourinary Radiology. In: Thrall JH, editor. The Requisites. 2nd ed. Philadelphia: Mosby; 2004. p. 335–8.

36. Frauscher F, Klauser A, Volgger H, et al. Comparison of contrast enhanced color Doppler targeted biopsy with conventional systematic biopsy: impact on prostate cancer detection. J Urol. 2002;167:1648.

37. Shinohara K, Scardino PT, Carter SS, et al. Pathologic basis of the sonographic appearance of the normal and malignant prostate. Urol Clin North Am. 1989;16:675.

38. Terris MK, Macy M, Freiha FS. Transrectal ultrasound appearance of prostatic granulomas secondary to bacillus Calmette-Guerin instillation. J Urol. 1997;158:126.

39. Purohit RS, Shinohara K, Meng MV, et al. Imaging clinically localized prostate cancer. Urol Clin North Am. 2003;30:279.

40. Varghese SL, Grossfeld GD. The prostatic gland: malignancies other than adenocarcinomas. Radiol Clin North Am. 2000;38:179.

41. Ramey JR, H. EJ, Gomella LG. Ultrasonography and Biopsy of the Prostate. In: Wein AJ, editor. Campbell-Walsh Urology. Ninthth ed. Philadelphia: Saunders; 2007. p. 2883–95. vol. 3.

42. Bigler SA, Deering RE, Brawer MK. Comparison of microscopic vascularity in benign and malignant prostate tissue. Hum Pathol. 1993;24:220.

43. Cornud F, Hamida K, Flam T, et al. Endorectal color Doppler sonography and endorectal MR imaging features of nonpalpable prostate cancer: correlation with radical prostatectomy findings. AJR Am J Roentgenol. 2000;175:1161.

44. Halpern EJ, Strup SE. Using gray-scale and color and power Doppler sonography to detect prostatic cancer. AJR Am J Roentgenol. 2000;174:623.

45. Arger PH, Malkowicz SB, VanArsdalen KN, et al. Color and power Doppler sonography in the diagnosis of prostate cancer: comparison between vascular density and total vascularity. J Ultrasound Med. 2004;23:623.

46. Okihara K, Kojima M, Nakanouchi T, et al. Transrectal power Doppler imaging in the detection of prostate cancer. BJU Int. 2000;85:1053.

47. Kelly IM, Lees WR, Rickards D. Prostate cancer and the role of color Doppler US. Radiology. 1993;189:153.

48. Halpern EJ, Frauscher F, Strup SE, et al. Prostate: high-frequency Doppler US imaging for cancer detection. Radiology. 2002;225:71.

49. Levine MA, Ittman M, Melamed J, et al. Two consecutive sets of transrectal ultrasound guided sextant biopsies of the prostate for the detection of prostate cancer. J Urol. 1998;159:471.

50. Eskew LA, Bare RL, McCullough DL. Systematic 5 region prostate biopsy is superior to sextant method for diagnosing carcinoma of the prostate. J Urol. 1997;157:199.

51. Babaian RJ, Toi A, Kamoi K, et al. A comparative analysis of sextant and an extended 11-core multisite directed biopsy strategy. J Urol. 2000;163:152.

52. Presti Jr JC, Chang JJ, Bhargava V, et al. The optimal systematic prostate biopsy scheme should include 8 rather than 6 biopsies: results of a prospective clinical trial. J Urol. 2000;163:163.

53. Naughton CK, Miller DC, Mager DE, et al. A prospective randomized trial comparing 6 versus 12 prostate biopsy cores: impact on cancer detection. J Urol. 2000;164:388.

54. Terris MK, Pham TQ, Issa MM, et al. Routine transition zone and seminal vesicle biopsies in all patients undergoing transrectal ultrasound guided prostate biopsies are not indicated. J Urol. 1997;157:204.

55. Epstein JI, Walsh PC, Sauvageot J, et al. Use of repeat sextant and transition zone biopsies for assessing extent of prostate cancer. J Urol. 1997;158:1886.

56. Mazal PR, Haitel A, Windischberger C, et al. Spatial distribution of prostate cancers undetected on initial needle biopsies. Eur Urol. 2001;39:662.

57. Chang JJ, Shinohara K, Hovey RM, et al. Prospective evaluation of systematic sextant transition zone biopsies in large prostates for cancer detection. Urology. 1998;52:89.

58. Katsuto Shinohara VM, Chi T, Carroll P. Prostate Needle Biopsy Techniques and Interpretation. In: Voegelzang NJ, Debruyne FMJ, Shipley WU, Linehan WM, editors. Genitourinary Oncology. 3rd ed. Philadelphia: Lippincott; 2006. p. 111–9.

59. Djavan B, Remzi M, Marberger M. When to biopsy and when to stop biopsying. Urol Clin North Am. 2003;30:253.

60. Keetch DW, Catalona WJ, Smith DS. Serial prostatic biopsies in men with persistently elevated serum prostate specific antigen values. J Urol. 1994;151:1571.

61. Djavan B, Ravery V, Zlotta A, et al. Prospective evaluation of prostate cancer detected on biopsies 1, 2, 3 and 4: when should we stop? J Urol. 2001;166:1679.

62. Catalona WJ, Partin AW, Slawin KM, et al. Use of the percentage of free prostate-specific antigen to enhance differentiation of prostate cancer from benign prostatic disease: a prospective multicenter clinical trial. JAMA. 1998;279:1542.

63. Wang R, Chinnaiyan AM, Dunn RL, et al. Rational approach to implementation of prostate cancer antigen 3 into clinical care. Cancer. 2009;115:3879–86.

64. Haese A, de la Taille A, van Poppel H, et al. Clinical utility of the PCA3 urine assay in European men scheduled for repeat biopsy. Eur Urol. 2008;54:1081.

65. Bott SR, Henderson A, McLarty E, et al. A brachytherapy template approach to standardize saturation prostatic biopsy. BJU Int. 2004;93:629.

66. Lane BR, Zippe CD, Abouassaly R, et al. Saturation technique does not decrease cancer detection during follow up after initial prostate biopsy. J Urol. 2008;179:1746.

67. Borboroglu PG, Comer SW, Riffenburgh RH, et al. Extensive repeat transrectal ultrasound guided prostate biopsy in patients with previous benign sextant biopsies. J Urol. 2000;163:158.

68. Stewart CS, Leibovich BC, Weaver AL, et al. Prostate cancer diagnosis using a saturation needle biopsy technique after previous negative sextant biopsies. J Urol. 2001;166:86.

69. Fleshner N, Klotz L. Role of "saturation biopsy" in the detection of prostate cancer among difficult diagnostic cases. Urology. 2002;60:93.

70. Gershman B, Zietman AL, Feldman AS, McDougal WS. Transperineal template-guided prostate biopsy for patients with persistently elevated PSA and multiple prior negative biopsies. Urol Oncol. 2013;31(7):1093–7.

71. Shapiro RH, Johnstone P. Risk of Gleason Grade Inaccuracies in Prostate Cancer Patients Eligible for Active Surveillance. Urology. 2012;80:661–6.

72. Taira AV, Merrick GS, Bennett A, Andreini H, Taubenslag W, Galbreath RW, Butler WM, Bittner N, Adamovich E. Transperineal template-guided mapping biopsy as a staging procedure to select patients best suited for active surveillance. Am J Clin Oncol. 2013;36(2):116–20.

73. Katz DJ, Pinochet R, Richards KA, Godoy G, Udo K, Nogueria L, Cronin AM, Fine SW, Scardino PT, Coleman JA. Comparison of transperineal mapping biopsy results with whole-mount radical prostatectomy pathology in patients with localized prostate cancer. Prostate Cancer. 2014;2014:781438.

74. Moran BJ, et al. Re-biopsy of the Prostate With Stereotactic Transperineal Technique. J Urol. 2006;176:1376–81.

75. Egawa S, Wheeler TM, Scardino PT. The sonographic appearance of irradiated prostate cancer. Br J Urol. 1991;68:172.

76. Whittington R, Broderick GA, Arger P, et al. The effect of androgen deprivation on the early changes in prostate volume following transperineal ultrasound guided interstitial therapy for localized carcinoma of the prostate. Int J Radiat Oncol Biol Phys. 1999;44:1107.

77. Kapoor DA, Wasserman NF, Zhang G, et al. Value of transrectal ultrasound in identifying local disease after radical prostatectomy. Urology. 1993;41:594.

78. Goldenberg SL, Carter M, Dashefsky S, et al. Sonographic characteristics of the urethrovesical anastomosis in the early post-radical prostatectomy patient. J Urol. 1992;147:1307.

79. Rodriguez LV, Terris MK. Risks and complications of transrectal ultrasound guided prostate needle biopsy: a prospective study and review of the literature. J Urol. 1998;160:2115.

80. Maatman TJ, Bigham D, Stirling B. Simplified management of post-prostate biopsy rectal bleeding. Urology. 2002;60:508.

81. Brullet E, Guevara MC, Campo R, et al. Massive rectal bleeding following transrectal ultrasound-guided prostate biopsy. Endoscopy. 2000;32:792.

82. Raaijmakers R, Kirkels WJ, Roobol MJ, et al. Complication rates and risk factors of 5802 transrectal ultrasound-guided sextant biopsies of the prostate within a population-based screening program. Urology. 2002;60:826.

83. Thompson PM, Pryor JP, Williams JP, et al. The problem of infection after prostatic biopsy: the case for the transperineal approach. Br J Urol. 1982;54:736.

84. Desmond PM, Clark J, Thompson IM, et al. Morbidity with contemporary prostate biopsy. J Urol. 1993;150:1425.

85. Moul JW, Bauer JJ, Srivastava S, et al. Perineal seeding of prostate cancer as the only evidence of clinical recurrence 14 years after needle biopsy and radical prostatectomy: molecular correlation. Urology. 1998;51:158.

86. Moul JW, Miles BJ, Skoog SJ, et al. Risk factors for perineal seeding of prostate cancer after needle biopsy. J Urol. 1989;142:86.

87. Bastacky SS, Walsh PC, Epstein JI. Needle biopsy associated tumor tracking of adenocarcinoma of the prostate. J Urol. 1991;145:1003.

88. Koppie TM, Grady BP, Shinohara K. Rectal wall recurrence of prostatic adenocarcinoma. J Urol. 2002;168:2120.

89. Hara N, Kasahara T, Kawasaki T, et al. Frequency of PSA-mRNA-bearing cells in the peripheral blood of patients after prostate biopsy. Br J Cancer. 2001;85:557.

90. Meng MV, Shinohara K, Grossfeld GD. Significance of high-grade prostatic intraepithelial neoplasia on prostate biopsy. Urol Oncol. 2003;21:145.

91. Oyasu R, Bahnson RR, Nowels K, et al. Cytological atypia in the prostate gland: frequency, distribution and possible relevance to carcinoma. J Urol. 1986;135:959.

92. Prange W, Erbersdobler A, Hammerer P, et al. Significance of high-grade prostatic intraepithelial neoplasia in needle biopsy specimens. Urology. 2001;57:486.

93. Davidson D, Bostwick DG, Qian J, et al. Prostatic intraepithelial neoplasia is a risk factor for adenocarcinoma: predictive accuracy in needle biopsies. J Urol. 1995;154:1295.

94. Lefkowitz GK, Sidhu GS, Torre P, et al. Is repeat prostate biopsy for high-grade prostatic intraepithelial neoplasia necessary after routine 12-core sampling? Urology. 2001;58:999.

95. Helpap BG, Bostwick DG, Montironi R. The significance of atypical adenomatous hyperplasia and prostatic intraepithelial neoplasia for the development of prostate carcinoma. An update. Virchows Arch. 1995;426:425.

96. Helpap B, Bonkhoff H, Cockett A, et al. Relationship between atypical adenomatous hyperplasia (AAH), prostatic intraepithelial neoplasia (PIN) and prostatic adenocarcinoma. Pathologica. 1997;89:288.

97. Iczkowski KA, Chen HM, Yang XJ, et al. Prostate cancer diagnosed after initial biopsy with atypical small acinar proliferation suspicious for malignancy is similar to cancer found on initial biopsy. Urology. 2002;60:851.

98. Iczkowski KA, MacLennan GT, Bostwick DG. Atypical small acinar proliferation suspicious for malignancy in prostate needle biopsies: clinical significance in 33 cases. Am J Surg Pathol. 1997;21:1489.

99. Alsikafi NF, Brendler CB, Gerber GS, et al. High-grade prostatic intraepithelial neoplasia with adjacent atypia is associated with a higher incidence of cancer on subsequent needle biopsy than high-grade prostatic intraepithelial neoplasia alone. Urology. 2001;57:296.

100. Park S, Shinohara K, Grossfeld GD, et al. Prostate cancer detection in men with prior high grade prostatic intraepithelial neoplasia or atypical prostate biopsy. J Urol. 2001;165:1409.

101. Javidan J, Wood DP. Clinical interpretation of the prostate biopsy. Urol Oncol. 2003;21:141.

102. Makhlouf AA, Krupski TL, Kunkle D, et al. The effect of sampling more cores on the predictive accuracy of pathological grade and tumour distribution in the prostate biopsy. BJU Int. 2004;93:271.

103. Wills ML, Sauvageot J, Partin AW, et al. Ability of sextant biopsies to predict radical prostatectomy stage. Urology. 1998;51:759.

104. Ravery V, Boccon-Gibod LA, Dauge-Geffroy MC, et al. Systematic biopsies accurately predict extracapsular extension of prostate cancer and persistent/recurrent detectable PSA after radical prostatectomy. Urology. 1994;44:371.

105. Badalament RA, Miller MC, Peller PA, et al. An algorithm for predicting nonorgan confined prostate cancer using the results obtained from sextant core biopsies with prostate specific antigen level. J Urol. 1996;156:1375.

106. D'Amico AV, Whittington R, Malkowicz SB, et al. Clinical utility of percent-positive prostate biopsies in predicting biochemical outcome after radical prostatectomy or external-beam radiation therapy for patients with clinically localized prostate cancer. Mol Urol. 2000;4:171.

107. Naya Y, Slaton JW, Troncoso P, et al. Tumor length and location of cancer on biopsy predict for side specific extraprostatic cancer extension. J Urol. 2004;171:1093.

108. Freedland SJ, Aronson WJ, Terris MK, et al. Percent of prostate needle biopsy cores with cancer is significant independent predictor of prostate specific antigen recurrence following radical prostatectomy: results from SEARCH database. J Urol. 2003;169:2136.

109. Freedland SJ, Csathy GS, Dorey F, et al. Percent prostate needle biopsy tissue with cancer is more predictive of biochemical failure or adverse pathology after radical prostatectomy than prostate specific antigen or Gleason score. J Urol. 2002;167:516.

110. Freedland SJ, Csathy GS, Dorey F, et al. Clinical utility of percent prostate needle biopsy tissue with cancer cutpoints to risk stratify patients before radical prostatectomy. Urology. 2002;60:84.

111. Elliott SP, Shinohara K, Logan SL, et al. Sextant prostate biopsies predict side and sextant site of extracapsular extension of prostate cancer. J Urol. 2002;168:105.

Prostate Ultrasound Complications and Patient Safety

Frederick A. Gulmi and Miguel Pineda

Abbreviations

STAI	State-Trait Anxiety Inventory
TRUS	Transrectal ultrasound
NSAID	Nonsteroidal anti-inflammatory drug
TURP	Transurethral resection of prostate
MIC	Minimum inhibitory concentration
SEER	Surveillance Epidemiology and End Results
UTI	Urinary tract infection
IIEF	International Index of Erectile Function
SHIM	Sexual Health Inventory for Men
IPSS	International Prostate Symptom Score
QOL	Quality of life

Introduction

Between 800,000 to 1 million transrectal ultrasound (TRUS)-guided prostate biopsies are performed in the United States each year [1]. Despite the potential benefit of undergoing TRUS biopsy (i.e., diagnosing prostate cancer at an early, treatable stage), the procedure is associated with a wide variety of minor and major complications.

Prior to the actual procedure patients can suffer from anxiety and the anxiety may persist for weeks afterwards [2]. The source of the anxiety ranges from worrying about the discomfort of the procedure to the fear of being diagnosed with cancer. The physical consequences from a biopsy procedure include anal pain and discomfort from the insertion of the rectal sonogram probe, as well as pain from the needle punctures for both the anesthetic injection and tissue sampling [3]. Some of the more common complications are relatively mild, usually requiring nothing more than observation and reassurance, and mostly consist of blood in the semen, urine, or per rectum [4–7]. Other, less common, minor complications include irritative voiding symptoms such as dysuria and frequency [8]. Erectile dysfunction has also been documented, sometimes afflicting patients before the procedure, but also occurring after the biopsy and lasting for weeks in some cases [2, 9].

Major complications requiring admission to the hospital are rare. The majority are infectious in nature and a result of rectal bacteria entering the bloodstream and prostate tissue through the needle puncture sites. Rates of hospital admissions for these major complications vary from 0.8 to 3.5 % [10–13]. These rates have been increasing in recent years and, as a result, more research into the etiology, prevention, and treatment of these infections has been conducted. These new efforts will undoubtedly reverse this trend of increasing infectious complications and hospital admissions in the coming years.

F.A. Gulmi, M.D. (✉) • M. Pineda, M.D.
Department of Urology,
Brookdale University Hospital and Medical Center,
1 Brookdale Plaza, Brooklyn, NY 11212, USA
e-mail: fgulmi@brookdale.edu;
Miguel.a.pineda@gmail.com

C.R. Porter and E.M. Wolff (eds.), *Prostate Ultrasound: Current Practice and Future Directions*,
DOI 10.1007/978-1-4939-1948-2_10, © Springer Science+Business Media New York 2015

Anxiety

There are many possible reasons for a man to be anxious while awaiting a prostate biopsy. The fear of being diagnosed with having cancer, the method of obtaining the biopsy via a trans rectal approach, the anticipated pain and bleeding, as well as the mere fact that a sexual organ is being disturbed can all form the basis of the stress [14]. Baseline levels of anxiety in the general population of older men are generally low at about 15 % [15], but went as high as two thirds in a study of patients awaiting prostate biopsy, with 19 % reporting anxiety of severe grade (4–4.5 on a scale of 5) [2]. Anxiety-associated complaints such as loss of work days due to anxiety and erectile dysfunction while awaiting biopsy were also reported. Predictors for worse anxiety included younger age, patients with more than two relatives who had a history of prostate cancer, and men with high anxiety levels according to the State-Trait Anxiety Inventory (STAI), a validated scale for measuring anxiety [16]. Patients who had higher levels of anxiety before the biopsy were found to complain of more pain from the procedure [2, 17]. For 6 % of patients, anxiety was treated with anxiolytics before biopsy, and these patients in general reported less pain during biopsy than those who did not take medication [2]. The highest levels of anxiety occurred 7 days after the biopsy, just before the pathology report was given to the patient. Gustafsson et al. also found that anxiety, as measured by serum cortisol levels, was highest just before patients were informed of their biopsy results and subsequently decreased by 2 weeks following biopsy regardless of the pathological findings [18]. Patients that were diagnosed with prostate cancer were significantly more likely to report sustained levels of anxiety 30 days following biopsy compared to those patients who were found to have no cancer (75 % vs. 14 %, respectively, $p=0.01$). Based on their results, the authors of this study stressed the importance of expediently informing patients of their results, since this improves anxiety levels in all patients, especially those who have a negative pathology result.

Pain

The physical pain that comes from a TRUS biopsy is multifactorial. The passage of the probe via penetration results in the initial transient period of discomfort and may last for the entirety of the procedure. The shifting of the probe to reach the different areas of the prostate may also add to the discomfort of this phase. The more significant pain is due to the actual needle penetration of the prostate capsule, usually by the biopsy needle. The penetration of the needle through the rectal mucosa is not thought to be a significant contributor to pain because the punctures are performed above the dentate line into a region of the rectal wall where fewer nerve fibers reside [14].

Number of Cores and Patterns

According to the American Urologic Association (AUA) White Paper on Optimal Techniques of Prostate Biopsy and Specimen Handling (2013), the use of 10–12-core extended-sampling protocols increases cancer detection rates compared to traditional sextant sampling while also decreasing the rate of repeat biopsies due to the higher negative predictive value than traditional sextant biopsies [19]. The complications of the traditional technique involving six biopsies without anesthesia were studied by Raaijmaker et al. in 2002. They found that out of 5,676 questionnaires that were filled out, 286 (7.5 %) patients reported pain after the biopsy, with 18 (0.3 %) reporting use of analgesics [11]. More generally, they found that previous prostatitis as well as younger age was associated with more pain after biopsy. Rodriguez and Terris found that 30 % of patients experienced moderate to severe discomfort in their prospective series of complications associated with the standard sextant biopsy protocol [3]. They found that the amount of discomfort was not associated with the number or location of biopsies. However, this study was not based on a visual analogue scale but instead executed via telephone interview.

Peyromaure et al. used a 10 core biopsy approach, adding 4 peripheral biopsies to the original sextant technique, and found that 47 % of their 275 patients reported the experience to be painful, with the majority of these classifying the pain as slight (67 %) [17]. Naughton et al. performed a prospectively randomized study where they directly compared pain and morbidity between patients undergoing 6 versus 12 biopsies and found that there was no difference in pain with more biopsy cores [20]. On the other hand, Berger et al. recommended that when the number of biopsy specimens is increased, more analgesia might be required because of the increasing subjective sensation of pain during the procedure [24].

Types of Anesthesia

Local: Periprostatic

Local analgesia for prostate biopsy was not initially standard practice. In the early 2000s, Soloway outlined the benefits of periprostatic anesthesia, strongly touting the decreased pain and discomfort that can be achieved with a rather quick, easy, and well-tolerated step [21]. Aside from the anal discomfort, pain from a prostate biopsy is due to the violation of the prostatic capsule or stroma by needles. Innervation to the prostate is from the spinal roots of S2 to S5 as well as the sympathetic chain through the presacral and hypogastric plexus [22]. These nerves are found in the posterolateral prostate and are thus easily reached via a transrectal probe. Several techniques for accessing these nerves have been devised over the years.

The initial periprostatic analgesic injection technique was described by Nash in 1996 and consisted of an injection at the junction of the base of the prostate and seminal vesicles. In his study, Nash injected either 5 ml of 1 % lidocaine or placebo on one side of the prostate and did not inject anything in the opposite side. Pain scores were then compared and it was found that patients had significantly less pain on the side where lidocaine was used [23]. Berger et al. also injected in this same prostate-seminal vesicle junction and decided to stop recruiting for the study after 100 patients because of the significantly lower pain

recorded by the patients who received lidocaine [24]. Soloway's group injected at two different locations on each side of the prostate—one between the rectal wall and base of the seminal vesicles and the other at the lateral aspect of the prostate. Injection at both of these sites resulted in significantly reduced pain levels compared to placebo [21, 25].

In two different studies, Seymour and Rodriguez injected local anesthetic in the opposite end of the prostate, the bilateral apex [26, 27]. Both groups found that this approach was sufficient at numbing the entire gland, suggesting that the injected bolus was able to spread from the apex, under Denonvilliers fascia, all the way to the angle of the prostate and seminal vesicle, thereby reaching and achieving the desired effect on the nerves at the lateral borders.

Taverna et al. took a minimalistic approach and advocated a single 10 ml dose of lidocaine given at the prostatic midline between Denonvilliers fascia and prostatic fascia. This approach resulted in 93 % of patients who received the analgesic reporting only a slight discomfort with biopsy and 7 % requiring an additional 1 cc of lidocaine [28].

In order to determine the most appropriate dose of 1 % lidocaine injection as well as the best location for its administration, Özden et al. designed a study that consisted of seven groups of 25 patients each. Group 1 received 5 cc of saline, and groups 2–7 received 2.5, 5, or 10 cc of 1 % lidocaine injected as local anesthesia at basal or basal plus apical locations. The only group that was not significantly different than the control was the group with 2.5 cc of lidocaine bilaterally injected at the base. The most effective pain control was reported in the groups that received 10 ml injections. Patients who received the combination of basal and apical injections had a lower mean pain score than those receiving only basal injections, although this did not achieve statistical significance [29].

Lee-Elliot et al. studied the effects of longer acting analgesics on patients undergoing prostate biopsies [30]. Their goal was to determine whether relieving pain not only during the biopsy, but also immediately and in the days following the biopsy would lead to patients being more willing to undergo a repeat biopsy in the future if needed. They found that when a combination of lidocaine and bupivacaine was injected, patients had the same pain score during biopsy, but significantly lower pain scores 1 h after biopsy, as well as every day until day 7, when compared to lidocaine injection alone. Despite the improvement in intensity of pain when the combination of lidocaine and bupivacaine was employed, the patients were equally unwilling to undergo a repeat biopsy if needed, compared to patients who received only the lidocaine treatment.

Local: Intraprostatic

The concept of injection of analgesic directly into the prostatic stroma was introduced by Mutaguchi et al. [31]. In their study, lidocaine was infiltrated directly into the prostate at two or three sites on the right and left sides from the base to apex. They compared this to the more traditional injection at the junction between the seminal vesicles and prostate and found significantly lower pain scores during biopsy in patients given the intraprostatic injection. Other indexes, including pain after biopsy, duration and location of pain, and post-procedure use of analgesics taken for late pain, were not significantly different between the two groups. This approach is based on the fact that traditional injection at the junction of the prostate and seminal vesicles reaches the posterior nerves of the prostate but not the fibers of the pelvic plexus that travel on the lateral prostatic surface to join the anterior surface [32]. Analgesic injected directly into the prostate exerts its effects on all of the abovementioned nerves.

Lee et al. went one step further and looked at the combination of periprostatic in combination with intraprostatic analgesia and found that this combination was better at controlling pain during the biopsy than the periprostatic injection alone or the intraprostatic injection alone [33]. However, none of the three techniques were better than the rest in reducing the anal pain from the probe insertion. The superiority of the combination of intraprostatic and periprostatic injection of analgesic compared to periprostatic alone was confirmed by Cam et al. in the following year

[34]. This study consisted of two groups, the first received periprostatic and intraprostatic lidocaine and the second received periprostatic lidocaine and intraprostatic 0.95 % NaCl. The patients in the first group were significantly more likely to report no pain during and after the biopsy (64 % and 62 %, respectively) compared with those in the second group (27 % and 25 %, respectively).

Suppositories

Minimally invasive approaches for pain control for prostate biopsy, which mitigate the need for an injection of anesthetic, have been studied. When Issa et al. compared the effects of 10 cc of 2 % lidocaine gel administered transrectally 10 min before biopsy to control, the median pain score during transrectal prostate biopsy was significantly lower at 2 (range 1–5) vs. 5 (range 1–7) ($p=0.00001$) [35]. In contrast, Duc et al. found that 15 ml of 2 % lidocaine gel administered 15 min before biopsy had no significant effect on the perception of pain compared to regular sono gel in a prospective randomized study [36], and Chang et al. and Chevik et al. came to similar conclusions [37, 38]. In one randomized study, Rodriguez et al. reported that bilateral periprostatic nerve block at the apex resulted in less pain compared to lidocaine gel, even though the mean number of core biopsies taken was greater in the group receiving the periprostatic block [27]. However, when a combination of lidocaine gel along with periprostatic lidocaine injection was studied, it proved to be better at pain control than either method alone [39]. The questionable effect of transrectal administration of lidocaine gel for pain control during prostate biopsy may be due to poor local absorption directly into the prostate via the rectal wall.

Ragavan et al. examined the effects of diclofenac, a nonsteroidal anti-inflammatory (NSAID) suppository on prostate biopsy pain in a nonblinded manner. Patients were randomized into one of three groups: diclofenac suppository alone, periprostatic injection alone, and a combination of the two. Pain during the procedure was lower in the injection alone and combination groups, highlighting the importance of the injection for immediate pain. Conversely, pain on the evening of the procedure was lowest for the diclofenac and combination group, revealing the long-term pain relief of diclofenac [40]. This study showed the importance of administration of analgesics not just at the time of the procedure itself but also for post-procedure pain as well, be it by pre-op NSAID suppositories or more traditional post-op oral pain medications.

Pelvic Plexus Block

Injection of analgesic into the pelvic plexus was first studied by Wu et al. In their double-blind study, patients received bilateral injections of 5 ml of either 1 % lidocaine or sterile normal saline under ultrasound guidance lateral to the seminal vesicles prior to their prostate biopsy [41]. When compared to the placebo, there was no significant change in pain perception. In contrast, when Akpinar et al. compared pelvis plexus block to the more traditional periprostatic nerve block they found that patients had significantly less pain during the anesthetic injection and the actual prostate biopsy with the plexus block [42]. The differing findings from these two studies may be due to the fact that Akpinar et al. used Doppler guidance to locate the pelvic plexus, injected a smaller amount of analgesic, and used a higher concentration of lidocaine, leading to a shorter duration of injection. Cantiello et al. also found that pelvic plexus block under Doppler guidance provided better analgesia than periprostatic nerve block and the reduced pain was noticeable up to 30 min after the procedure. Although the results seem encouraging, more studies are needed to determine the long-term safety of pelvic plexus injections. Possible complications such as adhesion formation in the periplexus area could potentially interfere with erectile function, urinary continence, or even future pelvic surgeries [43].

Sedation

The use of sedatives has also been explored as a possible option for pain relief for prostate biopsy patients. The benefits of general anesthesia, although the best practice for pain control for procedures, are generally felt to be outweighed by the risks given the relatively short duration of the prostate biopsy technique.

Entonox, a 50 % oxygen and 50 % nitrous oxide mixture, is an appealing inhaled analgesic because it provides analgesia within 3 min of inhalation and the effects disappear less than 4 min after cessation [14]. Masood et al. performed a short-term, placebo-controlled, double-blind trial evaluating the effectiveness of Entonox during transrectal ultrasound-guided prostate biopsy. The group found a highly significant reduction in pain for patients who inhaled Entonox versus those that inhaled normal air. The chief complaint was that 7 of the 51 patients on Entonox became drowsy, but this resolved by the end of the procedure. The authors thus recommend it as a safe and effective method of pain control. In addition, it is so well tolerated that patients can even drive the same day, unlike with propofol [44]. Manikandan et al. compared Entonox versus periprostatic injection of lidocaine versus placebo and found both analgesic methods to be significantly better at controlling pain from prostate biopsy compared to placebo. When they compared Entonox to periprostatic injection, they did not find a statistical difference in pain control, though the trend was in favor of periprostatic injection over Entonox ($p = 0.08$) [45].

Turgut et al. compared periprostatic lidocaine injection versus intravenous midazolam versus no anesthetic and found that both anesthetics were significantly better at controlling pain compared to no intervention. They also found that patients who received midazolam intravenously were significantly less likely to complain about moderate to severe pain than those who had periprostatic lidocaine injection (3 % vs. 29 %, respectively, $p < 0.05$) [46]. Peters et al. examined the effects of propofol on pain due to prostate biopsy and found a significant decrease in pain with the drug as well as an increase in patient satisfaction. The mean score on the visual analogue scale for patient discomfort with sedation was 1.5 compared with 3.5 with no sedation. Although the use of propofol resulted in good control of pain, it has significant drawbacks in its convenience. While an anesthesiologist is not strictly required, it is recommended that one should be present at the time of administration, thus raising the cost of the procedure significantly. Patients are also not allowed to drive for 24 h after the procedure and are required to have someone accompany them [47].

Bleeding

Number of Cores

When Raaijmakers et al. looked at 5,802 biopsy procedures they found that in patients with sextant biopsies, the main complications were hematospermia, which occurred in 50.4 % of patients, and hematuria, which lasted longer than 3 days in 22.6 % [11]. Hematuria was significantly correlated with larger prostate volume. Hematospermia was seen less often in older patients possibly because of fewer sexual encounters, in those with a previous transurethral resection of prostate (TURP) possibly because of retrograde ejaculation resulting in bloody semen hiding in the bladder, and patients with larger transitional zone volume/total volume. Rodriguez et al. found that the rate of rectal bleeding during biopsy increased with the number of cores taken, but no difference was found hours or days after the procedure [3, 6]. When Naughton et al. directly compared 6 core versus 12 core biopsies, they found a statistically significant increase in the report hematochezia and hematospermia in the latter group compared to the former. However, patients did not differ in terms of how problematic they found the bleeding [20]. Berger et al. retrospectively looked at patients who underwent 6, 10, or 15 core biopsies and found that the only difference in bleeding complications was an increase in hematospermia following 10 and 15 cores compared to 6 cores [12].

No significant increase in bleeding complications has been found from the added number of injections that go along with injection of periprostatic analgesia [24, 26, 28, 30, 33, 35].

First Versus Repeat Biopsies

When Djavan et al. compared the rates of bleeding-related complications associated with first-time prostate biopsies to those for repeat prostate biopsies, they found no significant differences. Immediate morbidity was minor for both groups and included rectal bleeding (2.1 % vs. 2.4 %, respectively, $p=0.13$), mild hematuria (62 % vs. 57 %, $p=0.06$), and severe hematuria (0.7 % vs. 0.5 %, $p=0.09$). Delayed morbidity included hematospermia (9.8 % vs. 10.2 %, respectively, $p=0.1$) and recurrent mild hematuria (15.9 % vs. 16.6 %, $p=0.06$) [4].

Anticoagulants

When patients are scheduled for a prostate biopsy they are often told to hold aspirin and other anticoagulants, such as warfarin and Plavix, at least 7 days before the procedure in order to avoid possible bleeding-related complications. A prospective study of 128 patients found no bleeding complications that were related to previous aspirin or nonsteroidal anti-inflammatory drug use, whether ingested within 3 days, 1 week, 10 days, or 2 weeks prior to prostate biopsy [3]. Another study of 1,966 patients found no significant difference in the rates of bleeding-related complications between patients taking aspirin (2/54, 3.7 %) and those not taking aspirin (44/1,756, 2.5 %) [5]. Finally, Kariotis et al. also found no significant difference in the incidence of hematuria or rectal bleeding relating to the use of aspirin, but they did reveal that aspirin extended the mean duration of the bleeding. Compared to the control group, patients on aspirin had hematuria for 4.45 ± 2.7 days versus 2.4 ± 2.6 days ($p=0.001$) and rectal bleeding for 3.3 ± 1.3 days versus 1.9 ± 0.7 days ($p<0.001$). In addition, only younger patients (mean age 60.1 years ±5.8 years) with a lower body mass index (<25 kg/m^2) taking aspirin were at a higher risk for bleeding-related complications (odds ratio $=3.46$, $p=0.047$) [7].

Infection

Epidemiology

Since most prostate biopsies are performed via a transrectal approach, the potential introduction of rectal bacteria into prostate tissue, the bloodstream, or the urinary tract is an important source of severe infectious complications. The most common organism responsible for these infectious complications is *Escherichia coli* [48]. Patients can experience symptoms as mild as dysuria, frequency, or urgency and as serious as life-threatening hemodynamic instability due to septic shock. Between 0.6 and 4.1 % of patients who have been biopsied require immediate admission to the hospital for antibiotics and hemodynamic monitoring [49].

Interestingly, the use of prophylactic antibiotics has not always been standard. In a study from 1997, before the trend of increasing infectious complications from prostate biopsy, Enlund et al. evaluated the infectious complication rates of patients undergoing prostate biopsy without any antibiotic prophylaxis [13]. Of the 415 patients in this prospective study, 12 (2.9 %) patients out of 415 had a fever. Of these 12 patients, 11 sought medical attention and the 12th recovered without treatment. One patient had sinusitis, eight were treated as outpatients, three were admitted to the hospital, and all patients recovered completely. The authors of this study concluded that antibiotics were not necessary given the rarity of infectious complications.

However, over time the use of prophylactic antibiotics became adopted as the standard of care despite a lack of a clear consensus [13]. With the current widespread use of pre- and peri-procedure antibiotics, sepsis remains a rare but significant problem, which has actually worsened in recent years. This is likely due, at least in part, to bacterial resistance to fluoroquinolones, the antibiotic class that has been most heavily used for prostate biopsies [48]. In fact, in the United States, fluoroquinolone resistance in *E. coli* blood stream isolates increased from 0 to 12 % from 1998 to 2007 [50]. Resistance occurs when bacteria are exposed to antimicrobials below the minimum inhibitory concentration (MIC), which can occur when patients are underdosed or treated with the same antibiotic multiple times [49]. The most common risk factor appears to be exposure to these antimicrobials within 6 months prior to biopsy. A previous history of prostatitis has also been linked to increased likelihood of infectious complications post-biopsy, possibly due to an

infectious organism residing asymptomatically in the prostate until the trauma from a needle biopsy re-exposes it [10, 11].

Other factors that may contribute to sepsis following prostate biopsy include residual bacteria in lubricants or improperly cleaned non-disposable needle guards that are reused between patients [49]. Some studies have shown that up to 22 % of men who receive a prostate biopsy have positive cultures of fluoroquinolone resistant bacteria from their rectums, and that these same men were also likely to have taken a fluoroquinolone within the previous 6 months [51]. Kamdar et al. found that hospital employees may become asymptomatically colonized with high-risk multidrug resistant bacteria from their work environments and subsequently contribute to the colonization of their family members. These employees and their family members are then at high risk of developing multidrug resistant complications following a prostate biopsy [52].

Hospital Admissions

The hospital admission rate for complications following transrectal ultrasound-guided prostate biopsies has increased at an alarming rate over the past decade primarily due to the increasing rate of infectious complications [10]. When stratified by year, one study found that the incidence of infectious complications was three times higher in 2006 compared to that in 2004 and 2005 and that the incidence of fluoroquinolone-resistant urinary tract infection (UTI) was 4.3 and 3.3 times higher in 2006 compared to 2004 and 2005, respectively ($p < 0.05$) [48]. In their study, Nam et al. revealed that 1.9 % of patients (781/41,482) were readmitted to the hospital less than 30 days after a prostate biopsy and the admission rate increased from 1 to 4 % between 1996 and 2005. The vast majority of these patients were admitted due to infection (71.6 %) [10].

In an analysis that identified Medicare patients who underwent a prostate biopsy using data from SEER (Surveillance, Epidemiology, and End Results), they compared 17,472 biopsy patients to a random sample of 134,977 controls and found that older age, non-white race, and higher comorbidity scores were significantly associated with an increased risk of infectious but not noninfectious complications [53]. Further examination of hospitalizations between 1991 and 2007 revealed that the frequency of infectious complications increased with time in men who underwent biopsy ($p=0.001$), although the rate remained stable in the control group (Fig. 1). In this study, the overall rate of hospitalization for biopsy patients was twice that of the control population.

Finally, when preoperative prophylactic antibiotics (trimethoprim-sulfamethoxazole or ciprofloxacin) were administered for 5,802 biopsy procedures, 200 patients (3.5 %) developed fever after biopsy and 27 (0.5 %) were hospitalized. Twenty-five of the 27 patients admitted to the hospital had signs of prostatitis and/or urosepsis [11].

Number and Patterns of Biopsy Cores

No study to date has identified significant differences in infection rates based solely on the number of core biopsies taken. Naughton et al. found no difference between 6 and 12 core biopsies in terms of fever or hospitalizations [20]. Furthermore, Berger et al. did not find significant differences when comparing patients who underwent 6, 10, or 15 core biopsies [12].

Preoperative Antibiotics

In 1998 Kapoor et al. studied the effects of ciprofloxacin prophylaxis on patients undergoing prostate biopsy by running a prospective, randomized, double-blind, multi-center study with 537 patients. They gave a 500 mg dose of ciprofloxacin to the study group and found that 6 ciprofloxacin recipients (3 %) and 12 placebo recipients (5 %) had clinical signs and symptoms of UTI ($p=0.15$). Even more striking, none of the patients in the ciprofloxacin group were admitted to the hospital compared to four patients (2 %) in the placebo group who were

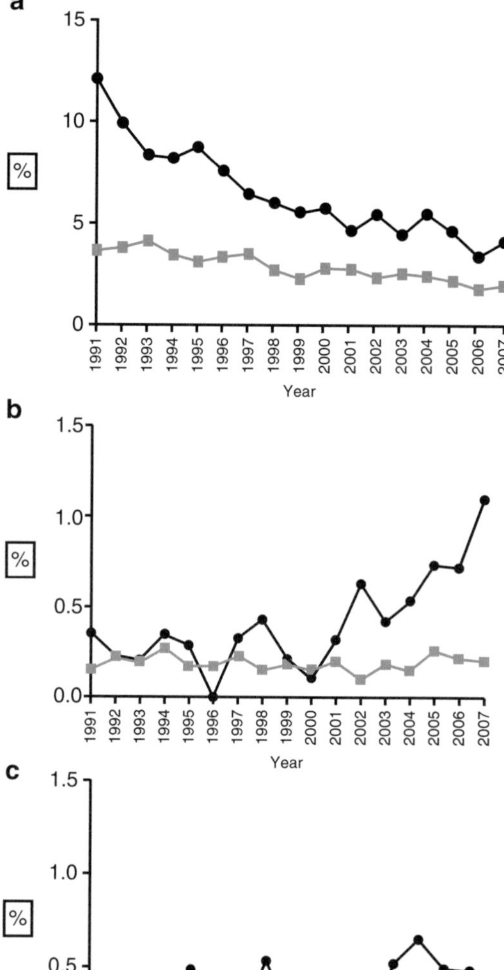

Fig. 1 Overall hospitalizations (**a**), hospitalizations with infection as primary diagnosis (**b**), and hospitalizations with noninfectious biopsy-related complications as primary diagnosis (**c**) within 30 days in biopsy (*circles*) and control (*squares*) groups. Reproduced with permission from [53]

admitted for febrile UTI after the biopsy [54]. Sabbagh et al. and Shigemura et al. both compared the use of fluoroquinolones as prophylaxis as a 1 day versus 3 day dose and found no significant differences in the rates of complications with duration of prophylaxis [55, 56].

Table 1 Adapted from AUA Best Practice Policy Statement on Urologic Surgery Antimicrobial Prophylaxis (2008) (reviewed and validity confirmed 2011, updated February 2012)

Procedure	Organisms	Prophylaxis	Antimicrobial of choice	Alternative antimicrobial	Duration of therapy
Transrectal prostate biopsy	Intestine	All	Fluoroquinolone 1st/2nd/3rd generation cephalosporin	Aminoglycoside (Aztreonam) + metronidazole or clindamycin	Less than or equal to 24 h

Furthermore, a Cochrane review from 2011 concluded that there was no definitive proof that 3-day courses or multiple-dose courses of antibiotics are superior to 1-day courses or single-dose courses. The review also concluded that antibiotic prophylaxis is indeed effective in preventing infectious complications following transrectal prostate biopsy and should be widely used [57].

The AUA Best Practice Policy Statement recommends the use of a fluoroquinolone or 1st/2nd/3rd generation cephalosporin for a duration of less than or equal to 24 h as antibiotic prophylaxis for prostate biopsy. For patients with allergies, the alternative recommended first-line antibiotic is an aminoglycoside (can be substituted with aztreonam if there is renal dysfunction) plus metronidazole or clindamycin (Table 1) [58].

Adibi et al. reported a rise in hospital admissions related to infection in their prostate biopsy patients who received ciprofloxacin or Bactrim DS prophylaxis. After the addition of a dose of gentamicin intramuscularly to their standard prophylaxis, the rates of hospitalization dropped from 3.8 % (11 patients among 290 biopsies) to 0.6 % (2 patients among 310 biopsies) [59]. Two different observational studies revealed that fluoroquinolones plus amikacin significantly decreased the rate of bloodstream infections compared to fluoroquinolone alone (0.3 % from 2.5 %, $p = 0.003$, and 1.7 % from 8.0 %, $p < 0.001$) [60, 61]. While utilization of various regimens of antibiotics may initially contribute to lower levels of infectious complications, caution must be taken in order to promote the development of antibiotic-resistant bacteria [62].

The AUA best practice statement also states that the risk of antimicrobial-associated adverse events related to prophylaxis for infectious endocarditis exceeds the benefit in genitourinary procedures. However, patients who have a history of prosthetic heart valves, previous infectious endocarditis, or certain forms of congenital heart disease may benefit from the addition of agents against enterococci such as amoxicillin or ampicillin [63].

Post-complication Antibiotics

Patients must be instructed that the development of fever, lethargy, difficulty voiding, testicular swelling, or symptoms suggestive of a urinary tract infection should be followed by an immediate call to their physician [49]. Signs or symptoms of sepsis should result in intravenous hydration as well as intravenous broad-spectrum antibiotics that cover *E. coli*, the most common cause of infectious complications following prostate biopsy. A urine culture should be obtained before the start of antibiotics, as well as blood cultures if the patient has a fever. When deciding on the broad-spectrum antibiotic to be employed, the physician must be aware that the bacteria responsible may be resistant to ampicillin and/or fluoroquinolones.

In a retrospective study of 1,273 patients who underwent prostate biopsy within the Veterans Affairs New York Harbor Healthcare System, 31 (2.4 %) patients presented with infectious symptoms within a month of the biopsy. Of these 31 patients, 23 had positive cultures, 18 of which were fluoroquinolone-resistant *E. coli*. The cultured *E. coli* also tended to have moderate to high resistance to ampicillin, trimethoprim/sulfamethoxazole, piperacillin, and gentamicin but were still susceptible to cephalosporins, ticarcil-

Table 2 Susceptibility of fluoroquinolone resistant *E. coli* to antibiotics in 18 samples (adapted from [48])

Antibiotic	% Susceptible
Trimethoprim/sulfamethoxazole	56
Ampicillin	6
Ampicillin/sulbactam	50
Peperacillin	28
Ticarcillin/clavulanate	94
Aztreonam	94
Imipenem	94
Cefazolin	100
Cefotaxime	100
Cefotetan	100
Cefuroxime	94
Ceftazidime	100
Ceftriaxone	100
Gentamicin	78
Amikacin	100
Tobramycin	94

lin/clavulanate, imipenem, aztreonam, tobramycin, and amikacin (see Table 2) [48]. Two additional studies, one from Israel and one from Egypt, found similar resistance and susceptibility patterns to these antibiotics, highlighting how widespread the antibiotic resistance problem has become [64, 65]. The authors of the Veteran Affairs study recommended empirical treatment with ceftriaxone, ceftazidime, or amikacin, antibiotics that they found to have 100 % susceptibility, until culture-specific therapy be implemented.

We have recently shown that immediate intervention by emergency department physicians can determine the eventual length of stay for a prostate biopsy patient with infectious complications. When we looked retrospectively at 17 patients who were admitted for infectious symptoms after having prostate biopsy with ciprofloxacin prophylaxis, we found that the patients who were given ceftriaxone by the emergency room personnel while in the emergency department were on average admitted for 2.8 days compared to 3.8 days for patients who were given an antibiotic other than ceftriaxone ($p = 0.029$) (unpublished results). A similar trend may occur in emergency departments that use other well-

established antibiotics that are effective against fluoroquinolone-resistant bacteria such as amikacin and carbapenems [1, 48].

Preparation of the Patient Prior to Biopsy

Rectal Swab

Taylor et al. tailored pre-biopsy antibiotics for 112 patients undergoing prostate biopsy based on rectal culture results [66]. They compared the targeted prophylaxis group to a group of 345 patients who were not swabbed and received standard empirical ciprofloxacin prophylaxis. Of the patients who received targeted prophylaxis, 22 (19.6 %) grew fluoroquinolone-resistant organisms and none experienced an infectious complication. In the control group there were nine cases of infectious complications, seven of which were due to fluoroquinolone-resistant organisms and one of which was sepsis. Although the targeted antimicrobial prophylaxis resulted in a notable decrease in the incidence of infectious complications caused by fluoroquinolone-resistant organisms compared to empiric therapy, the difference was not statistically significant ($p = 0.12$).

Iodine Suppositories, Laxatives, Enemas, and Bowel Prep

While intuitively it would seem that cleansing the rectum before a biopsy would reduce the rate of infectious episodes, results supporting this notion are mixed. For example, Carey et al. reported no difference in the rate of hospitalization due to infections in patients who had a pre-procedure enema versus those who did not and the authors did express concern about the possible added cost and discomfort from enemas [67]. Similarly, Ruddick et al. sought to determine the benefits of enemas. In addition to an established antibiotic regimen that both groups adhered to, the first group had nothing by mouth starting at midnight the night before the biopsy. Group two, on the other hand, received nothing by mouth for 24 h before biopsy and underwent an enema the night before biopsy and another the morning of the procedure. The study found that the rate of infection in the first group of 190 patients was approximately 2.11 % (confidence interval, ±2.04 %). Of the 217 patients who underwent the enemas and the 24-h diet of clear fluids, only one case of sepsis was reported, resulting in a 0.46 % infection rate (confidence interval, ±1.32 %). The difference in infection rates was suggestive but lacked statistical significance ($p=0.189$) [68].

Huang et al. performed a retrospective study in which all patients received the same antibiotics pre- and post-procedure. Patients in group 1 self-administered a phosphate enema the day before biopsy while patients in group 2 received a phosphate enema and rectal povidone-iodine on the day of the procedure performed by a doctor at the hospital. In group 1, 9.23 % were found to have a symptomatic infection with leukocytosis or chills while none were found in group 2 ($p=0.001$) [69]. This study attributed the difference to the povidone-iodine preparation, but the difference could also be attributed to the timing of the phosphate enema (day before versus day of biopsy). Park et al. also looked at povidone-iodine preparation, but as a suppository. The group took cultures from the rectum before and after the suppository and found that the mean number of colony-forming units decreased 99.9 % after the rectal povidone-iodine preparation. The researchers administered a suppository to 360 patients, while 121 patients received none, with a resulting infectious complication rate of 0.3 % and 6.6 %, respectively [70].

Association Between Infection and Periprostatic Analgesia

Despite the extra injection sites that result from local anesthetic injection, no study has found an association with increased risk of serious infection [24, 26, 28, 30, 33]. However, Öbek et al. did report that the incidence of bacteriuria was significantly higher in the anesthesia group. High fever and hospitalization due to infectious complications were also more common in the local anesthesia group, although this was not statistically significant [71].

Risk of Repeat Biopsies and Infection

When Nam et al. examined the hospital admission rates for patients who underwent repeat prostate biopsy, the admission rates were not higher than those with first-time biopsies. However both groups did show an increase in the rate of infectious complications in recent years [10]. Similarly, a study of SEER and Medicare databases from 1991 to 2007 in which 13,883 men were identified who had undergone a single prostate biopsy and 3,640 who had undergone multiple biopsies showed no significant difference between their rates of hospitalization, serious urological infections, or noninfectious urological complications [72].

Risk of Erectile Dysfunction After Prostate Biopsy

In a study 211 men who were to undergo prostate biopsy, 7 % reported erectile dysfunction attributed to anxiety in anticipation of the procedure. In addition, up to 15 % of men who were potent prior to prostate biopsy reported erectile dysfunction at days 7 and 30 after the procedure. Taken together, a total of 42 patients who were previously potent reported acute erectile dysfunction either before or after the prostate biopsy. Of the 42 episodes of erectile dysfunction, only 21 were resolved by post-op day 30 [2]. Klein et al. also found a change in erectile function. Their study consisted of three groups of patients. The first group included men who received a saturation biopsy, where 20 biopsy cores were obtained. The saturation biopsy was performed after a previous negative prostate biopsy. Groups two and three both consisted of men who underwent 10 core biopsies, one of which received a periprostatic lidocaine injection. All three groups reported a statistically significant decrease in their International Index of Erectile Function (IIEF) score at the end of the first week. The decrease in IIEF score persisted into week 4 in the two groups receiving the 10-core biopsies. Notably, by week 12, there were no longer any significant decreases in potency for any of the three groups [8].

Fujita et al. found that an increased number of core biopsies as well as an increased number of biopsy procedures were associated with a decrease in Sexual Health Inventory for Men (SHIM) score ($p=0.04$ and $p=0.02$, respectively). Fujita et al. also found that patients without preexisting erectile function (SHIM score 22–25) had a steeper decrease in SHIM score after three or more biopsies compared to men with mild to moderate erectile dysfunction (SHIM score 8–21) [73].

The potential reasons for transient erectile dysfunction are debatable and remain uncertain. From a physiological standpoint, erectile dysfunction may be secondary to anatomical disruption of the neurovascular bundle or nerve compression from a hematoma or edema [2]. Beyond the impact of the physical effects of the biopsy there are certainly possible psychological causes of erectile dysfunction in men concerned over the potential diagnosis of a prostatic malignancy.

Voiding Dysfunction

Zisman et al. performed a study looking at 204 patients who voided via urethra at biopsy. The average number of cores taken was 8.4 ± 1.7. The group noted that 52 (25 %) of patients reported subjective voiding impairment on post-op day number 7, including 12 % who rated the difficulty as mild (1–2 points on a 0–5 scale), 8 % as moderate (3/5), and 5 % as severe (4–5/5). Five patients (2.5 %) went into acute urinary retention that required a urethral catheter for relief. Patients with a transitional zone volume greater than 42 ml were at a significantly higher risk of acute urinary retention ($p=0.03$). Finally, patients with a baseline International Prostate Symptom Score (IPSS) greater than 20 points reported an increase in their IPSS on post-op day 7 [9].

A study by Raaijmakers et al. of 5,802 biopsy procedures found that 0.4 % of patients who underwent sextant biopsies developed urinary retention [11]. They found that characteristics of prostate hyperplasia, such as prostate volume and higher IPSS, were predictors of urinary retention. Berger et al. performed a retrospective study on 5,957 biopsy procedures on 4,303 men in Austria, where the number of biopsies per patient increased from 6 to 10 to 15 over the span of almost 10 years and found that the rate of urinary retention remained steady at 0.2 % [12]. Fujita et al. also found no correlation between biopsy number and IPSS [73].

Klein et al. were interested in the effect on voiding of 10-core prostate biopsy alone, 10-core biopsy with periprostatic nerve blockade, and 20-core saturation biopsy with periprostatic nerve block. This study found that in every group the IPSS was significantly higher at week 1, and for the saturation biopsy group the increased IPSS lasted into weeks 2 and 12. Furthermore, the impact on quality of life (QOL) due to urinary symptoms (measured on a scale of 0-delighted to 6-terrible) demonstrated that the 20 biopsy core saturation biopsies caused an impairment to QOL for up to 12 weeks post-biopsy [8].

Conclusions

Transurethral prostate biopsies are generally well tolerated and only rarely result in complications requiring hospitalization. However, it is clear that many patients suffer increased anxiety around the time of the biopsy. Furthermore, there is significant risk of both transient urinary and sexual function decline surrounding the biopsy procedure. Clinicians need to be aware of these complications and advise their patients accordingly. Additional precautions should be considered for patients who are at risk for serious infectious complications, including those with diabetes, depressed immune function, or a history of resistant organisms [35].

References

1. Loeb S. Antimicrobial prophylaxis for transrectal ultrasound biopsy. AUA update series. 2013 Volume 32, Lesson 1.
2. Zisman A, Leibovici D, Kleinmann J, Siegel YI, Lindner A. The impact of prostate biopsy on patient well-being: a prospective study of pain, anxiety and erectile dysfunction. J Urol. 2001;165(2):445–54.
3. Rodriguez LV, Terris MK. Risks and complications of transrectal ultrasound guided prostate needle biopsy:

a prospective study and review of the literature. J Urol. 1998;160(6):2115–20.

4. Djavan B, Waldert M, Zlotta A, Dobronski P, Seitz C, Remzi M, Borkowski A, Schulman C, Marberger M. Prospective European prostate cancer detection study. J Urol. 2001;166(3):856–60.

5. Herget EJ, Saliken JC, Donnelly BJ, Gray RR, Wiseman D, Brunet G. Transrectal ultrasound-guided biopsy of the prostate: relation between ASA use and bleeding complications. Can Assoc Radiol J. 1999; 50(3):173–6.

6. Ghandi KR, Dundas D, Patel U. Bleeding after transrectal ultrasonography-guided prostate biopsy: a study of 7-day morbidity after six-, eight- and 12-core biopsy protocol. BJU Int. 2004;94(7):1014–20.

7. Kariotis I, Philippou P, Volanis D, Serafetinides E, Delakas D. Safety of ultrasound-guided transrectal extended prostate biopsy in patients receiving low-dose aspirin. Int Braz J Urol. 2010;36(3):308–16.

8. Zisman A, Leibovici D, Kleinmann J, Cooper A, Siegel Y, Lindner A. The impact of prostate biopsy on patient well-being: a prospective study of voiding impairment. J Urol. 2001;166(6):2242–6.

9. Klein T, Palisaar RJ, Holz A, Brock M, Noldus J, Hinkel A. The impact of prostate biopsy and periprostatic nerve block on erectile and voiding function: a prospective study. J Urol. 2010;184(4):1447–52.

10. Nam RK, Saskin R, Lee Y, Liu Y, Law C, Klotz LH, Loblaw DA, Trachtenberg J, Stanimirovic A, Simon AE, Seth A, Urbach D, Narod SA. Increasing hospital admission rates for urological complications after transrectal ultrasound guided prostate biopsy. J Urol. 2010;183(3):963–9.

11. Raaijmakers R, Kirkels WJ, Roobol MJ, Wildhagen MF, Schrder FH. Complication rates and risk factors of 5802 transrectal ultrasound-guided sextant biopsies of the prostate within a population-based screening program. Urology. 2002;60(5):826–30.

12. Berger AP, Gozzi C, Steiner H, Frauscher F, Varkarakis J, Rogatsch H, Bartsch G, Horninger W. Complication rate of transrectal ultrasound guided prostate biopsy: a comparison among 3 protocols with 6, 10, and 15 cores. J Urol. 2004;171(4):1478–81.

13. Enlund AL, Varenhorst E. Morbidity of ultrasound-guided transrectal core biopsy of the prostate without prophylactic antibiotic therapy. A prospective study in 415 cases. Br J Urol. 1997;79(5):777–80.

14. Autorino R, De Sio M, Di Lorenzo G, Damiano R, Perdona S, Cindolo L, D'Armiento M. How to decrease pain during transrectal ultrasound guided prostate biopsy: a look at the literature. J Urol. 2005;174(6):2091–7.

15. Mehta KM, Simonsick EM, Penninx BWJH, Schulz R, Rubin SM, Satterfield S, Yaffe K. Prevalence and correlates of anxiety symptoms in well-functioning older adults: findings from the health aging and body composition study. J Am Geriatr Soc. 2003;51(4):499–504.

16. Dale W, Bilir P, Han M, Meltzer D. The role of anxiety in prostate carcinoma. Cancer. 2005;104(3): 467–78.

17. Peyromaure M, Ravery V, Messas A, Toublanc M, Boccon-Gibod L, Boccon-Gibod L. Pain and morbidity of an extensive prostate 10-biopsy protocol: a prospective study in 289 patients. J Urol. 2002; 167(1):218–21.

18. Gustafsson O, Theorell T, Norming U, Perski A, Öhström M, Nyman CR. Psychological reactions in men screened for prostate cancer. Br J Urol. 1995; 75(5):631–6.

19. Prostate biopsy and specimen handling workgroup. AUA/Optimal Technique of Prostate Biopsy and Specimen Handling. AUA. 2013.

20. Naughton CK, Ornstein DK, Smith DS, Catalona WJ. Pain and morbidity of transrectal ultrasound guided prostate biopsy: a prospective randomized trial of 6 versus 12 cores. J Urol. 2000;163(1):168–71.

21. Vaidya A, Soloway MS. Periprostatic local anesthesia before ultrasound-guided prostate biopsy: an update of the Miami experience. Eur Urol. 2001;40(2): 135–8.

22. Hollabaugh RS, Dmochowski RR, Steiner MS. Neuroanatomy of the male rhabdosphincter. Urology. 1997;49(3):426–34.

23. Nash PA, Bruce JE, Indudhara R, Shinohara K. Transrectal ultrasound guided prostatic nerve blockade eases systematic needle biopsy of the prostate. J Urol. 1996;155(2):607–9.

24. Berger AP, Frauscher F, Halpern EJ, Spranger R, Steiner H, Bartsch G, Horninger W. Periprostatic administration of local anesthesia during transrectal ultrasound-guided biopsy of the prostate: a randomized, double-blind, placebo-controlled study. Urology. 2003;61(3):585–8.

25. Davis M, Sofer M, Kim SS, Soloway MS. The procedure of transrectal ultrasound guided biopsy of the prostate: a survey of patient preparation and biopsy technique. J Urol. 2002;167(2 Pt 1):566–70.

26. Seymour H, Perry MJ, Lee-Elliot C, Dundas D, Patel U. Pain after transrectal ultrasonography-guided prostate biopsy: the advantages of periprostatic local anesthesia. BJU Int. 2001;88(6):540–4.

27. Rodriguez A, Kyriakou G, Leray E, Lobel B, Guillé F. Prospective study comparing two methods of anaesthesia for prostate biopsies: apex periprostatic nerve block versus intrarectal lidocaine gel: review of the literature. Eur Urol. 2003;44(2):195–200.

28. Taverna G, Maffezzini M, Benetti A, Seveso M, Giusti G, Graziotti P. A single injection of lidocaine as local anesthesia for ultrasound guided needle biopsy of the prostate. J Urol. 2002;167(1):222–3.

29. Özden E, Yaman Ö, Göğüs C, Özgencil E, Soygür T. The optimum doses of and injection locations for periprostatic nerve blockade for transrectal ultrasound guided biopsy of the prostate: a prospective, randomized, placebo controlled study. J Urol. 2003; 170(6 Pt 1):2319–22.

30. Lee-Elliott CE, Dundas D, Patel U. Randomized trial of lidocaine vs lidocaine/bupivacaine periprostatic injection on longitudinal pain scores after prostate biopsy. J Urol. 2004;171(1):247–50.

31. Mutaguchi K, Shinohara K, Matsubara A, Yasumoto H, Mita K, Usui T. Local anesthesia during 10 core biopsy of the prostate: comparison of 2 methods. J Urol. 2005;173(3):742–5.

32. Benoit G, Merlaud L, Meduri G, Moukarzel M, Quillard J, Ledroux M, Giuliano F, Jardin A. Anatomy of the prostatic nerves. Surg Radiol Anat. 1994; 16(1):23–9.

33. Lee HY, Lee HJ, Byun SS, Lee SE, Hong SK, Kim SH. Effect of intraprostatic local anesthesia during transrectal ultrasound guided prostate biopsy: comparison of 3 methods in a randomized, double-blind, placebo controlled trial. J Urol. 2007;178(2):469–72.

34. Cam K, Sener M, Kayikci A, Akman Y, Erol A. Combined periprostatic and intraprostatic local anesthesia for prostate biopsy: a double-blind, placebo controlled. Randomized trial. J Urol. 2008; 180(1):141–4.

35. Issa MM, Bux S, Chun T, Petros JA, Labadia AJ, Anastasia K, Miller LE, Marshall FF. A randomized prospective trial of intrarectal lidocaine for pain control during transrectal prostate biopsy: the Emory University experience. J Urol. 2000;164(2):397–9.

36. Desgrandchamps F, Meria P, Irani J, Desgrippes A, Teillac P, Le Duc A. The rectal administration of lidocaine gel and tolerance of transrectal ultrasonography-guided biopsy of the prostate: a prospective randomized placebo-controlled study. BJU Int. 1999;83(9):1007–9.

37. Chang SS, Alberts G, Wells N, Smith Jr JA, Cookson MS. Intrarectal lidocaine during transrectal prostate biopsy: results of a prospective double-blind randomized trial. J Urol. 2001;166(6):2178–80.

38. Cevik I, Ozveri H, Dillioglugil O, Akdaş A. Lack of effect of intrarectal lidocaine for pain control during transrectal prostate biopsy: a randomized prospective study. Eur Urol. 2002;42(3):217–20.

39. Obek C, Ozkan B, Tunc B, Can G, Yalcin V, Solok V. Comparison of local anesthesia techniques during transrectal ultrasound-guided biopsies. J Urol. 2004; 172(2):502–5.

40. Ragavan N, Philip J, Balasubramanian SP, Desouza J, Marr C, Javle P. A randomized, controlled trial comparing lidocaine periprostatic nerve block, diclofenac suppository and both for transrectal ultrasound guided biopsy of prostate. J Urol. 2005;174(2):510–3.

41. Wu CL, Carter HB, Naqibuddin M, Fleisher LA. Effect of local anesthetics on patient recovery after transrectal biopsy. Urology. 2001;57(5):925–9.

42. Akpinar H, Tüfek I, Atuğ F, Esen EH, Kural AR. Doppler ultrasonography-guided pelvic plexus block before systematic needle biopsy of the prostate: a prospective randomized study. Urology. 2009;74(2): 267–71.

43. Cantiello F, Cicione A, Autorino R, Cosentino C, Amato F, Damiano R. Pelvic plexus block is more effective than periprostatic nerve block for pain control during office transrectal ultrasound guided prostate biopsy: a single center, prospective, randomized double arm study. J Urol. 2012;188(2):417–22.

44. Masood J, Shah N, Lane T, Andrews H, Simpson P, Barua JM. Nitrous oxide (Entonox) inhalation and tolerance of transrectal ultrasound guided prostate biopsy: a double-blind randomized controlled study. J Urol. 2002;168(1):116–20.

45. Manikandan R, Srirangam SJ, Brown SC, O'Reilly PH, Collins GN. Nitrous oxide vs periprostatic nerve block with 1 % lidocaine during transrectal ultrasound guided biopsy of the prostate: a prospective, randomized, controlled trial. J Urol. 2003;170(5):1881–3.

46. Turgut AT, Ergun E, Koşar U, Koşar P, Ozcan A. Sedation as an alternative method to lessen patient discomfort due to transrectal ultrasonography-guided prostate biopsy. Eur J Radiol. 2006;57(1):148–53.

47. Peters JL, Thompson AC, McNicholas TA, Hines JE, Hanbury DC, Boustead GB. Increased patient satisfaction from transrectal ultrasonography and biopsy under sedation. BJU Int. 2001;87(9):827–30.

48. Feliciano J, Teper E, Ferrandino M, Macchia RJ, Blank W, Grunberger I, Colon I. The incidence of fluoroquinolone resistant infections after prostate biopsy—are fluoroquinolones still effective prophylaxis? J Urol. 2008;179(3):952–5.

49. AUA/SUNA white paper on the incidence, prevention and treatment of complications related to prostate needle biopsy. 2012 American Urological Association Education and Research, Inc.

50. Al-Hasan MN, Lahr BD, Eckel-Passow JE, Baddour LM. Antimicrobial resistance trends of Escherichia coli bloodstream isolates: a population-based study, 1998–2007. J Antimicrob Chemother. 2009;64(1): 169–74.

51. Liss MA, Peeples AN, Peterson EM. Detection of fluoroquinolone-resistant organisms from rectal swabs by use of selective media prior to a transrectal prostate biopsy. J Clin Microbiol. 2011;49(3): 1116–8.

52. Kamdar C, Mooppan UM, Gulmi FA, Kim H. Multi-drug-resistant bacteremia after transrectal ultrasound guided prostate biopsies in hospital employees and their relatives. Urology. 2008;72(1):34–6.

53. Loeb S, Carter HB, Berndt SI, Ricker W, Schaeffer EM. Complications after prostate biopsy: data from SEER-Medicare. J Urol. 2011;186(5):1830–4.

54. Kapoor DA, Klimberg IW, Malek GH, Wegenke JD, Cox CE, Patterson AL, Graham E, Echols RM, Whalen E, Kowalsky SF. Single-dose oral ciprofloxacin versus placebo for prophylaxis during transrectal prostate biopsy. Urology. 1998;52(4):552–8.

55. Sabbagh R, McCormack M, Péloquin F, Faucher R, Perreault JP, Perrotte P, Karakiewicz PI, Saad F. A prospective randomized trial of 1-day versus 3-day antibiotic prophylaxis for transrectal ultrasound guided prostate biopsy. Can J Urol. 2004;11(2): 2216–9.

56. Shigemura K, Tanaka K, Yasuda M, Ishihara S, Muratani T, Deguchi T, Matsumoto T, Kamidono S, Nakano Y, Arakawa S, Fujisawa M. Efficacy of 1-day prophylaxis medication with fluoroquinolone for prostate biopsy. World J Urol. 2005;23(5):356–60.

57. Zani EL, Clark OA, Rodrigues Netto N Jr. Antibiotic prophylaxis for transrectal prostate biopsy. Cochrane Database Syst Rev. 2011;(5).
58. Wolf Jr JS, Bennett CJ, Dmochowski RR, Hollenbeck BK, Pearle MS, Schaeffer AJ. Best practice policy statement on urologic surgery antimicrobial prophylaxis. J Urol. 2008;179(4):1379–90.
59. Adibi M, Hornberger B, Bhat D, Raj G, Roehrborn CG, Lotan Y. Reduction in hospital admission rates due to post-prostate biopsy infections after augmenting standard antibiotic prophylaxis. J Urol. 2013; 189(2):535–40.
60. Batura D, Rao GG, Bo Nielsen P, Charlett A. Adding amikacin to fluoroquinolone-based antimicrobial prophylaxis reduces prostate biopsy infection rates. BJU Int. 2011;107(5):760–4.
61. Kehinde EO, Al-Maghrebi M, Sheikh M, Anim JT. Combined ciprofloxacin and amikacin prophylaxis in the prevention of septicemia after transrectal ultrasound-guided biopsy of the prostate. J Urol. 2013;189(3):911–5.
62. Kibel AS. To biopsy or not to biopsy: minimizing the risk of prostate needle biopsy. J Urol. 2013;189(3): 796–7.
63. Dajani AS, Bisno AL, Chung KJ, Durack DT, Freed M, Gerber MA, Karchmer AW, Millard HD, Rahimtoola S, Shulman ST, et al. Prevention of bacterial endocarditis. JAMA. 1990;264(22):2919–22.
64. Tal R, Livne PM, Lask DM, Baniel J. Empirical management of urinary tract infections complicating transrectal ultrasound guided prostate biopsy. J Urol. 2003;169(5):1762–5.
65. Mosharafa AA, Torky MH, El Said WM, Meshref A. Rising incidence of acute prostatitis following prostate biopsy: fluoroquinolone resistance and exposure is a significant risk factor. Urology. 2011;78(3): 511–4.
66. Taylor AK, Zembower TR, Nadler RB, Scheetz MH, Cashy JP, Bowen D, et al. Targeted antimicrobial prophylaxis using rectal swab cultures in men undergoing transrectal ultrasound guided prostate biopsy is associated with reduced incidence of postoperative infectious complications and cost of care. J Urol. 2012;187(4):1275–9.
67. Carey JM, Korman HJ. Transrectal ultrasound guided biopsy of the prostate. Do enemas decrease clinically significant complications? J Urol. 2001;166(1):82–5.
68. Ruddick F, Sanders P, Bicknell SG, Crofts P. Sepsis rates after ultrasound-guided prostate biopsy using a bowel preparation protocol in a community hospital. J Ultrasound Med. 2011;30(2):213–6.
69. Huang YC, Ho DR, Wu CF, Shee JJ, Lin WY, Chen CS. Modified bowel preparation to reduce infection after prostate biopsy. Chang Gung Med J. 2006;29(4):395–400.
70. Park DS, Oh JJ, Lee JH, Jang WK, Hong YK, Hong SK. Simple use of the suppository type povidone-iodine can prevent infectious complications in transrectal ultrasound-guided prostate biopsy. Adv Urol. 2009;2009:750598.
71. Obek C, Onal B, Ozkan B, Onder AU, Yalçin V, Solok V. Is periprostatic local anesthesia for transrectal ultrasound guided prostate biopsy associated with increased infectious or hemorrhagic complications? A prospective randomized trial. J Urol. 2002; 168(2):558–61.
72. Loeb S, Carter HB, Berndt SI, Ricker W, Schaeffer EM. Is repeat prostate biopsy associated with a greater risk of hospitalization? Data from SEER-Medicare. J Urol. 2013;189(3):867–70.
73. Fujita K, Landis P, McNeil BK, Pavlovich CP. Serial prostate biopsies are associated with an increased risk of erectile dysfunction in men with prostate cancer on active surveillance. J Urol. 2009;182(6):2664–9.

The Future of Prostate Ultrasound

Imaging the Prostate with Quantitative Ultrasound: Implications for Guiding Biopsies, Targeting Focal Treatment, and Monitoring Therapy

Ernest J. Feleppa

E.J. Feleppa, Ph.D., F.A.I.U.M., F.A.I.M.B.E. (✉)
Biomedical Engineering Laboratory, Lizzi Center for
Biomedical Engineering, Riverside Research
Institute, 156 William Street, 9th Floor, New York,
NY 10038, USA
e-mail: efeleppa@riversideresearch.org

Introduction

The American Cancer Society estimates that 233,000 new cases of prostate cancer will be detected in men in the United States during 2014, which continues to make prostate cancer the most commonly detected male cancer in the United States, excluding skin cancers [1]. The Society also estimates that more than 29,480 men in the United States will die of prostate cancer during 2014, which continues to make prostate cancer the second-leading cause of death by cancer in the United States. Accordingly, prostate cancer will account for 27 % of the newly detected cancers and 10 % of the cancer deaths for men in the United States during 2013.

Current Needs

Definitive diagnosis of prostate cancer is performed using core-needle biopsies obtained transrectally or transperineally, and the most-common means of guiding prostate biopsies is conventional transrectal "B-mode" ultrasound (TRUS) imaging. However, TRUS does not reliably distinguish between cancerous and noncancerous tissue in the prostate. Therefore, TRUS-guided biopsies rely upon relatively well-imaged anatomical structures, such as the interface between the gland and periprostatic fibroadipose tissues, as spatial references for placing core needles in the gland—primarily in lateral and medial portions of the peripheral zone. Because cancerous lesions are not reliably depicted on conventional images, biopsy sampling is done essentially blindly with respect to actual cancer foci, and a positive biopsy cannot be assured even if prostate cancer foci actually are present.

The probability of a positive core in a gland having small scattered cancer foci is unacceptably small. In fact, our analysis of published repeat-biopsy data for traditional sextant biopsies suggests that the actual sensitivity of the TRUS-guided biopsy procedure may be as low as 50 %; other studies draw similar conclusions [2–4]. In other words, a significant fraction of the population of patients who actually have prostate cancer have a false-negative biopsy result because of an inability to image suspicious regions reliably, and therefore to target biopsy needles to cancerous tissue. Furthermore, all negative procedures, whether they are true or false, impose an unwarranted health risk as well as cost to the patient. This risk is associated with various side effects of the biopsy, including hemorrhage and infection [5, 6]. In addition, recent reports express concern that drug resistance is developing among the common pathogens associated with biopsy-related infections [7].

C.R. Porter and E.M. Wolff (eds.), *Prostate Ultrasound: Current Practice and Future Directions,*
DOI 10.1007/978-1-4939-1948-2_11, © Springer Science+Business Media New York 2015

Therefore, reducing the number of true-negative biopsies would be beneficial to patients from the standpoint of reducing risk and cost.

A second concern regarding current ultrasonic imaging methods is the difficulty encountered in justifying focal therapy and planning therapy with confidence that no clinically significant cancer foci are missed. Many current forms of ablative therapy are amenable to a focal approach, e.g., external-beam radiation therapy, brachytherapy, cryo-ablation, and high-intensity focused ultrasound (commonly termed HIFU). Approaches to focal surgery emphasize hemi-therapy, which excludes either the left or right side of the gland and attempts to spare the ure-thra, bladder, rectum, and the contralateral neuro-vascular bundle. If no significant cancer foci are present in the untreated portion of the gland, then obvious benefits of focal therapy are reduction of side effects and maintenance of gland function (e.g., retention of reproductive capability). Justification and planning of focal therapy now rely heavily on saturation transperineal biopsies that utilize 24–80 needle cores to provide a reasonably good sense of the regions, if any, that can be spared from treatment. The availability of a reliable means of imaging cancer in the prostate would reduce or even eliminate the need for saturation biopsies and would markedly improve means of patient selection for focal therapy and planning the therapy itself.

An additional concern regarding ultrasonic imaging of prostate cancer is the inability of TRUS to provide a reliable means of staging or estimating the aggressiveness of detected prostate cancer. Because conventional ultrasound (US) does not reliably distinguish cancerous from non-cancerous prostate tissue, TRUS images based upon conventional, B-mode US cannot depict the degree of tumor aggressiveness, tumor proximity to the capsule, extracapsular extensions, or seminal-vesicle invasion with certainty. Therefore, TRUS imaging does not contribute useful information for estimating disease grade or stage. Improved clinical staging is desirable in surgical planning because 20–30 % of radical prostatectomies show evidence of disease that is not gland confined. If surgeons were aware of the specific areas of the gland harboring more dangerous extracapsular disease, then appropriate intraoperative measures could be applied, resulting in improved patient outcomes [8, 9].

Indolent forms of prostate cancer are becoming more common and a consensus is developing that many men with low-risk prostate cancer could avoid definitive therapy and benefit from an active surveillance approach [10–12]. If a noninvasive method were available to monitor untreated prostate cancer with confidence, then changes indicating disease progression, such as tumor growth or micro-architectural tissue changes, would provide a basis for initiating treatment; a static cancer could continue to be monitored with confidence.

Although some advanced methods mentioned in this chapter show promise for overcoming existing limitations, all currently used conventional imaging modalities are deficient in their ability to identify cancerous regions of the gland with sufficient certainty.

Quantitative Ultrasound

Ultrasonic spectrum analysis is an advanced method of exploiting the information that is present in the raw "radio-frequency" (RF) echo signals derived from tissue during an US scan. The "video" signals that comprise the gray-scale B-mode images routinely viewed on an US scanner discard or distort much of the information present in the original RF signals. In other words, a large amount of potentially useful information is not utilized for patient assessment when reliance is placed on conventional, B-mode US imaging.

Our group has investigated effective, quantitative methods of utilizing all the information available in the RF signal. Our focus for the past four decades has been on spectrum analysis of linearly processed RF signals as a way of extracting and presenting much of the information that is ordinarily discarded in producing B-mode images. Although knowing in advance whether the captured information can be of use for tissue typing and imaging is not possible, our research has shown that spectrum analysis of RF signals can be useful in distinguishing among tissue types of interest in the eye, liver, blood vessels, lymph nodes, and prostate gland [13–30]. Because the methods used to compute spectra retain and exploit quantitative information present in the original RF signals, the methods have been termed quantitative ultrasound or "QUS."

Although the term QUS was originally applied to spectrum analysis and estimates of parameter values associated with spectra, the term QUS is becoming more generalized to include any signal processing approach that quantitatively exploits the information contained in the original, RF echo signals, such as methods that derive estimates from the statistics of envelope signals computed from linearly processed RF data. Examples of the use of envelope statistics to characterize tissue are studies to detect metastatic foci in lymph nodes as described by Mamou et al. [31].

Background

Spectrum Analysis

When used to characterize or type tissue, QUS based on spectrum analysis seeks to exploit the fact that different types of tissues may have different US-scattering properties. If those differences exist in tissues that need to be distinguished from each other or in tissues that change over time, such as during the course of surveillance or in response to treatment, then sensing those differences and expressing them quantitatively may have great medical value. Spectrum analysis provides a convenient, easy-to-implement method for representing the properties of tissues of interest as they are expressed in backscattered ultrasonic echo signals.

Spectrum analysis as the basis for the prostate QUS methods of tissue-type imaging described here can trace its origins to the work of investigators in the 1960s and 1970s, including, perhaps most notably, the research of Purnell and Sokulu [32]. Purnell and Sokulu coined the term "spectracolor" for an ultrasonic imaging technique that used color to depict the frequency content of echo signals compared to those in the incident US pulse.

However, spectrum analysis subsequently matured as a method of tissue typing largely through the work of Lizzi and other pioneering investigators such as Nicholas, Zagzebski, Insana, Hall, and Wagner [33–41]. Hosokowa et al. attempted to validate the theory underlying spectrum analysis using widely spaced, spherical cell clusters cultured in a collagen-based medium to represent ideal scatterers and obtained results that matched theoretical predictions over a limited range of scatterer (i.e., cell cluster) sizes [42]. More recently, investigators, such as Kolios, Czarnota, Oelze, Mamou, and Bigelow, have made valuable contributions to spectral methods by advancing insights into underlying mechanisms and by extending and refining the scattering theory associated with spectral behaviors [43–52].

Spectrum analysis takes advantage of the fact that a pulse of US that is sufficiently brief to provide acceptable axial spatial resolution contains a range of frequencies. A 10-MHz US probe does not transmit pulses that contain only 10-MHz signals. A "good" 10-MHz probe would contain useful signal content over a band of frequencies extending from approximately 5 to 15 MHz. The band of usable frequencies, i.e., the frequencies that provide ample signal compared to noise, is termed the effective bandwidth of the system. A figure of merit for a transducer is its fractional bandwidth, which is defined as the usable bandwidth divided by the center frequency and expressed as a percent; in this example, the fractional bandwidth is 10/10, which results in an excellent 100 % figure of merit.

When an US pulse enters tissue, it is scattered by heterogeneity in the tissue, e.g., collagen strands, capillaries, vacuoles, melanin deposits, and cell nuclei. A fraction of the scattered energy returns and is converted to a small voltage by the transducer of the US scanner. These received signals are termed "backscatter" signals. (For further information see the section on scattering in the chapter on the physics of US in this book.) The basic theories of scattering in tissue assume that scattering is weak; i.e., that the total field does not include any contribution from the scattered US. The theoretical framework first published by Lizzi in 1983 states that the spectrum of the backscattered US echo signals received at the transducer is dependent upon the acoustic properties of the scatterers themselves, the properties of the incident-beam profile, and the properties of the window used to select backscattered signals for spectral processing [34–37]. The fundamental equation derived by Lizzi et al. for a normalized (system-corrected) spectrum is described and discussed in additional detail in the Appendix at the end of this chapter.

"Normalization" or "calibration" of the spectrum is traditionally performed by computing the spectrum of a "perfectly" reflecting surface (such as an optically flat glass plate) placed parallel to the planar wave front of the US pulse at the transducer focal point. However, our group has recently been using a weakly reflecting water-oil interface to reduce reflected-signal amplitude and allow the use of identical instrument power and gain settings for acquiring calibration and actual tissue echo-signal data. (The oil has a density greater than that of water, so an US beam can be directed downward toward the planar water-oil interface through weakly attenuating water.) The reflectivity of the oil-water interface is well known so that calibration data acquired from it can be referenced to a perfect reflector.

In practice, the Lizzi theory is applied using assumed mathematical functions to describe the acoustic properties of the effective scatterers. For most reasonable functions, the theory predicts a gently curving power spectrum when the spectrum is expressed in logarithmic form with respect to a perfectly reflecting calibration target. When approximated by a straight line over the effective system bandwidth, the linear fit to a calibrated spectrum has two basic, independent defining parameters: (1) a slope value that theoretically depends only on scatter size and on attenuation in the intervening medium and (2) an intercept value that theoretically depends on scatterer size, concentration, and acoustic impedance relative to the environment of the scatterers but is independent of intervening-tissue attenuation. An additional spectral parameter is the midband (or midband fit), which is the value of the straight-line approximation at the center of the effective noise-limited bandwidth, i.e., the average value of the amplitude of the straight-line approximation over the usable frequency band. The midband parameter is equivalent to the integrated-backscatter parameter developed by Miller and his coworkers [54–57].

If attenuation is negligible or can be estimated, then an attenuation-corrected slope value can be computed easily, and from it, the effective size, d, of scatterers can be estimated. Once d is estimated using the attenuation-corrected slope value, then the combination of concentration, C, and relative acoustic impedance, Q, can be derived from the intercept value. Q is defined as $(z_2-z_1)/(z_2+z_1)$ where z_2 and z_1 are the acoustic impedances of the scatterers and the surrounding medium respectively. (See the chapter on US physics in this book and note the similarity of the expression for Q to the expression for the reflection coefficient.) The combination CQ^2 often is simply termed "acoustic concentration." Only two of the three spectral parameters—slope, intercept, and midband— are independent of each other. Their relationship is expressed by $y=af+y_0$ where y is the amplitude of a straight line, a is the slope of the line, f is frequency, and y_0 is its intercept value (i.e., the value of the line at zero frequency).

The central premise underlying application of QUS to tissue evaluation is that different tissues scatter US differently; in doing so, each tissue may have a distinct spectral signature. This signature depends on the micro-architectural properties of the scattering components of the tissue, which are conveyed in the RF echo signal that returns to the probe. Based on differences in their spectral parameters, different tissue types can be classified, e.g., to distinguish cancerous from noncancerous tissue in the prostate.

Tissue-type Classification

Once spectral parameter values are computed for known tissue types, e.g., cancerous and noncancerous tissues in biopsied regions of the prostate, a classifier can be trained to assign a score for the likelihood of an unknown tissue being in one or the other tissue-type category. If the "truth" is known, e.g., if biopsy histology is available to serve as the gold standard, then the scores generated by the classifier can be compared to the true tissue type to determine the performance of the classifier. The most-accepted method of expressing classifier performance is the ROC curve, where ROC originally stood for "receiver-operator characteristics" when the method was first developed for technical purposes, e.g., to assess the ability to extract usable signals from noise. The ROC curve shows how effective a system is in classifying an unknown correctly into either of two possible groups, e.g., cancerous or noncancerous tissue in the prostate [58]. The ROC curve expresses system performance as the trade-off between the true-positive fraction (sensitivity) as a function of the false-positive fraction (1 minus specificity). By reversing the abscissa, the curve directly expresses sensitivity as a function of specificity. This rarely used "reversed ROC curve" is perhaps a more appropriate representation for clinical evaluations.

A perfect classifier is one that has a sensitivity of 1.0 with a specificity of 1.0, i.e., a value of 1.0 for sensitivity at a value of 0.0 for 1 minus specificity. The sensitivity value of the ROC curve for such a classifier would be 1.0 for all values of 1 minus specificity, and the area under that curve (AUC) would be 1.0. A classifier that is purely random in its determinations would have an ROC curve that begins at the origin and linearly goes to a value of 1.0 for sensitivity at a value of 1.0 for 1 minus specificity, and the AUC value for that classifier would be 0.5. *In other words, an AUC value of 1 indicates a perfect classifier and an AUC value of 0.5 indicates an entirely random classifier.* Real classifier systems, including humans reading images such as X-ray, US, or magnetic-resonance images, typically produce AUCs in the range of 0.6–0.9.

To utilize determinations made by classifiers such as linear discriminant analysis methods, nearest-neighbor methods, artificial neural networks, or support-vector machines as inputs for ROC curve calculations, the computations by the classifier produce a score for the likelihood of a positive finding. This score is compared to a gold standard, such as the biopsy histology results in our prostate studies. Such scores can

be "continuous" over a range determined by the classification software, but typically scores are normalized to a range extending from 0 to +1 or −1 to +1. To utilize reader interpretations as inputs for ROC curve calculations, reader determinations often are expressed as a "discrete" level of suspicion (LOS) for positives using 5 or more integer values. As an example, on a scale of 1–5, 1 would indicate the reader's virtual certainty of a negative finding, 5 would indicate virtual certainty of a positive finding, and 3 would indicate an indeterminate case with an equal likelihood of a positive or a negative finding. These LOS scores for cancer are compared to a gold standard to compute the ROC curve.

In our studies, we use the LOS values assigned by the urologist performing a TRUS-guided prostate biopsy to establish a baseline ROC curve for comparing the classifier being developed to the available conventional image-based classification method. Most available ROC-computing software accommodates discrete and continuous types of likelihood assignment. Such software also typically provides considerable information in addition to the AUC values, such as the standard error in the AUC estimate and the 95 % confidence interval AUC values.

When only a single parameter is needed for classification of two tissue types, then a simple histogram can be used to display the distributions of parameter values for the two types of interest. A decision threshold value can be selected for assigning tissue type based on the values of that parameter, and a sensitivity and specificity can be computed for the distributions and the threshold point. Alternatively, an ROC curve can be generated from the parameter-value distributions; the overall classification performance of the single parameter can be determined from the AUC value and the trade-off between sensitivity and specificity can be determined from the curve shape [58]. In our experience, a single parameter is rarely sufficient for reliable differentiation of tissue types, and this is emphatically the case in identifying prostate cancer.

Typically, two or more parameters are required to differentiate between two tissue types. Because only two independent parameters are associated with the linear-regression approximation, the best two parameters are usually all that is needed for classification. For example, if effective scatterer size is an important tissue property, i.e., if scatterer size is significantly different in the two tissue types, then slope and intercept or slope and midband would be useful parameter combinations.

For clinical decision making, a single number is desirable for a decision threshold, and in the case of two or more relevant parameters, linear discriminant analysis provides a single discriminant-function value for the threshold [59]. Linear-discriminant methods work well when the categories of interest occupy different but linearly separable regions in the distributions of parameter values. However, when the two categories of interest, e.g., cancerous and noncancerous prostate tissue, include many subcategories (e.g., mixed Gleason grades of prostate cancer and various types of benign tissues such as atrophic, hyperplastic, calcified, acutely inflamed, chronically inflamed), then the distributions of parameter values of different tissue types can overlap to the extent that *linear methods have little hope of performing effective classification.*

When linear methods are not adequate, nonlinear methods of classification may be better for distinguishing different tissue types. Examples of such nonlinear methods are nearest-neighbor analyses (NNAs), artificial neural networks (ANNs), and support-vector machines (SVMs) [60–64]. Our prostate classification and imaging studies to date have investigated the use of all three classification methods and we have had the most success using SVMs, as discussed below. *These nonlinear methods produce scores that express the relative likelihood of an unknown tissue being cancerous or noncancerous*; the scores have a distribution for each tissue type, and classification performance can be expressed as the area under an ROC curve.

As shown by the results summarized below in this chapter, nonlinear classifiers applied to QUS parameter estimates show great promise for reliably distinguishing cancerous from noncancerous tissue in the prostate. Such differentiation is possible only because the micro-architectural properties of cancerous prostate tissue differ sufficiently from those of noncancerous tissue, allowing backscattered US signals to be distinguished by these advanced QUS-based tissue classification methods. Once a classification method is available to distinguish effectively between cancerous and noncancerous prostate tissue, it can be used to generate clinically essential, two-dimensional (2D) or three-dimensional (3D) images depicting regions of high versus low suspicion of being cancerous.

Tissue-type Imaging

A classifier that is trained to distinguish between cancerous and noncancerous tissue based on QUS estimates can be used to generate an image that depicts tissue properties or type in a 2D or 3D tissue-type image (TTI). The classifier can be applied to an entire image volume or image plane or to a subset of voxels or pixels in a user-defined region of interest (ROI) within the volume or plane. In the case of TRUS examinations of the prostate, data tend to be acquired in sets of planes rather than in 3D over a volume; however, a 3D depiction can be generated from signals acquired, analyzed in individual planes, and then rendered into a 3D volume.

To generate a TRUS-derived image that depicts tissue type or relative likelihood of prostate cancer, spectrum analysis is performed over an ROI in each scan plane; the ROI can be limited to a portion of the scan plane (e.g., the region the biopsy needle will sample) or can encompass the entire scanned area. Spectral-parameter values computed at each pixel location in the ROI are translated by the classifier to a cancer-likelihood score, and the score is expressed in the image as a gray-scale or color-encoded pixel to generate a two-dimensional (2D) TTI. Then 3D TTI renderings can be generated from sets of properly registered, component 2D TTIs.

A lookup table (LUT) can be used to expedite translation of parameter values to cancer-likelihood values. A table of "artificial" parameter values is generated to span the range of values found in the data, e.g., the spectral-parameter values for cancerous and noncancerous prostate tissue. These artificial parameter values then serve as test values and are assigned cancer-likelihood scores by the trained classifier. The output is an LUT that contains a likelihood score for each of the combinations of parameter values likely to be encountered in actual tissue. To generate a TTI during a TRUS examination, spectral parameters can be computed at a pixel location within the specified ROI, and parameter values can be referred to the matching parameter-value-combination location in the LUT to obtain the corresponding likelihood score at each pixel location. Each pixel then can be grayscale or color encoded to indicate relative cancer likelihood within the ROI.

As discussed below, we have found that locally computed intercept and midband spectral-parameter values combined with the value of the patient's serum prostate-specific antigen (PSA) level provide good classification using either an ANN or an SVM. The combination of local parameter values is translated into TTI pixel values using a multidimensional LUT. For the practicing urologist, the result is an image that shows the relative likelihood of prostate cancer throughout the specified ROI, possibly the entire gland, in 2D or 3D.

Prostate Tissue-type Images

Database Development

Our first step toward generating TTIs of the prostate was to build a database of spectral-parameter values for digitized RF echo signals acquired from tissue that was sampled by TRUS-guided core-needle biopsies. The RF signals were digitized immediately prior to firing the spring-loaded biopsy-needle gun and removing tissue. This method prevented corruption of the RF signals either by the needle itself or by the subsequent tissue trauma and hemorrhage along the needle track.

A key feature of our studies was that the acquired RF data were spatially related to the actual site of the tissue sample with high accuracy.

Acquired RF data and subsequently computed spectral-parameter values were directly correlated with the histologically determined tissue type in each biopsy tissue sample.

To provide a baseline for comparing the performance of the computer machine-learning classifiers to conventional methods for determining the presence of cancer, the urologist performing the biopsy assigned a LOS for the tissue being biopsied. The urologist based the LOS primarily on its appearance in the conventional B-mode, US image used to direct the needle. The examining urologist also consciously combined the B-mode impression with all other available information regarding the patient, e.g., the results of the palpation performed during the digital rectal examination (DRE), PSA level, gland size estimated from the B-mode image, and family history. The LOS values ranged from 1 for virtual certainty of noncancerous tissue to 5 for virtual certainty of cancerous tissue, with 3 indicating an entirely indeterminate tissue.

Subsequently, the actual tissue type of each biopsy core was provided by the pathologist. Pathology reports specified the biopsy-core location as described above, which enabled matching the results of RF spectrum analysis to the tissue type determined by the pathologist. We used the pathologists' determinations as our gold standard.

Classifier Development

The complex and interwoven expressions of healthy and unhealthy prostate tissue make linear methods of classification unable to distinguish cancerous from noncancerous prostate tissues with adequate reliability. For example, a range of grades exist for prostate cancer, with higher grades associated with a greater loss of differentiation and normal tissue architecture. Therefore, as expected, our attempts to use linear methods to distinguish cancerous from noncancerous prostate tissue based on the values of spectral parameters and clinical variables such as PSA level failed to produce acceptable results. However, our early investigations of nonlinear methods, such as NNAs, showed promise and encouraged us to apply more powerful ANN methods that included a multilayer perceptron (MLP).

The MLP was developed using PSA along with intercept and midband parameter values computed within a 15.0 mm×1.5 mm ROI that matched the biopsied region. Classifier training was performed by using a leave-one-patient-out approach as well as a leave-one-biopsy-out approach. In the leave-one-biopsy-out approach, the MLP was trained using 90 % of the data and validated using 10 % of the data while a single biopsy was tested (i.e., assigned a score for the likelihood of cancer) by the trained MLP. This was repeated for every biopsy in the data set, and the scores for all the biopsies, along with their true tissue types, were input to the ROC software. As a specific example, our data set from the Washington DC Veterans Affairs Medical Center included 64 patients and 617 TRUS-guided biopsies. We ran our MLP using a leave-one-patient-out approach 64 times using the set of data for a different single patient each time and we randomly divided the remaining data into a training set (90 %) and a validation set (10 %). The scores and true tissue types were input to any one of a variety of ROC software packages, including ROCkit by Charles Metz (http://xray.bsd.uchicago.edu/krl/KRL_ROC/software_index6.htm), MedCalc by Frank Schoonjans (http://www.medcalc.be/), or our own custom MATLAB-based ROC software.

For all methods, computed ROC AUC values essentially were identical, and our best-performing MATLAB MLP classifier gave AUCs of 0.844±0.018 (95 % confidence interval: 0.806, 0.877) for the classifier and 0.638±0.031 (95 % confidence interval: 0.576, 0.697) for the corresponding B-mode-based classification using LOS assignments, as shown in Fig. 1. The standard errors (0.018 and 0.031) in the AUC estimates are very small compared to the AUC difference (0.206) between these ROC curves, and the lower 95 % confidence interval value (0.806) of the MLP ROC is significantly greater than the upper value (0.697) of the LOS ROC. For the likely values of sensitivity for B-mode-guided biopsies of approximately 0.50, the corresponding sensitivity of the

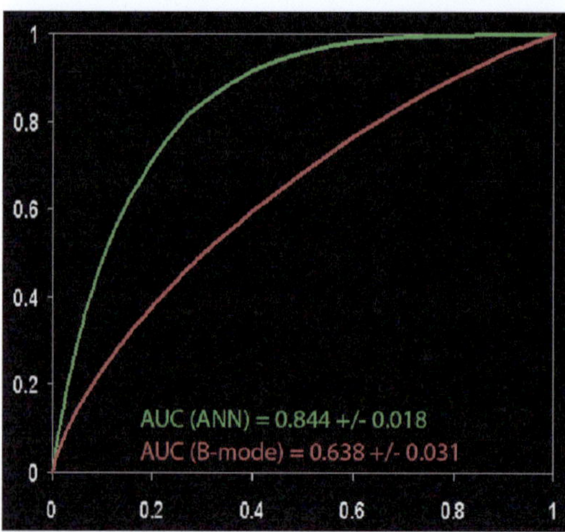

Fig. 1 ROC curves produced (1) by an MLP ANN using a leave-one-patient-out approach (*upper curve*) and (2) by LOS assignments primarily based on B-mode appearance (*lower curve*). The vertical axis is True-positive Fraction (TPF), which is equivalent to sensitivity; the horizontal axis is False-positive Fraction (FPF), which is equivalent to 1 minus specificity

MLP ROC curve is approximately 0.80, i.e., the MLP sensitivity is superior to the B-mode-based sensitivity by approximately 60 %.

This means that if this classification improvement could be translated into real-time images used for biopsy guidance by the urologist during a biopsy procedure, then a marked improvement in biopsy yield would be possible. Similarly, such images, whether generated in real time or offline, could make targeted or focal treatments a clinical reality.

A similar approach was used for developing and assessing the SVM classifier, which has the advantage of being less vulnerable with respect to false minima, overtraining, and excessive dimensionality. As was the case with ANN development, the data, consisting of intercept, midband, and PSA values plus the actual, histologically determined tissue type (cancerous vs. noncancerous), were analyzed using SVM methods. An ROC analysis showed the SVM-based classification performance to be equivalent to the performance of the MLP ANN. However, the advantages of SVMs in terms of robustness to false minima, etc., mitigate in favor of using SVMs for prostate-tissue classification.

Tissue-type Image Development

TTIs represent the likelihood of cancer at each pixel or voxel within an ROI. To provide the most-rapid processing, we chose to use a LUT to assign values to pixels within the ROI.

Figure 2 shows an SVM-based LUT surface plot for a PSA level of 7.5. The surface plot depicts the relative likelihood of cancer on the vertical axis for the given PSA value. As PSA value increases, all likelihood values increase, but with less emphasis in any particular region of the midband-intercept space, i.e., the LUT surface plot tends to flatten as it rises with increasing PSA values.

The computed spectral parameter values of midband and intercept are entered into the TTI software for each pixel location along with the patient's PSA level. The combination of midband, intercept, and PSA-level values for each pixel falls on a specific step in the LUT. The value for the relative cancer likelihood at that step in the

LUT is returned, and the likelihood value is translated into a color-encoded or gray-scale value for the corresponding pixel in the TTI image. Figure 3 shows an example of a TTI for a prostate that was scanned in situ immediately prior to prostatectomy while the patient was in the operating room. Subsequent prostatectomy histology showed a 12-mm, previously unrecognized, anterior tumor as well as smaller cancer foci and some PIN tissue. The left image in Fig. 3 is the gray-scale TTI; the center image is a midband-parameter image of the same scan plane with superimposed TTI color encoding to display the regions of highest relative likelihoods for cancer; the right image is the approximately corresponding whole-mount histology section, which clearly shows the demarcated anterior tumor and some smaller foci of cancerous and PIN tissue. The planes of the US scans and whole-mount histology are not necessarily identical, but are at the widest gland cross section and clearly overlap in the region of the anterior tumor.

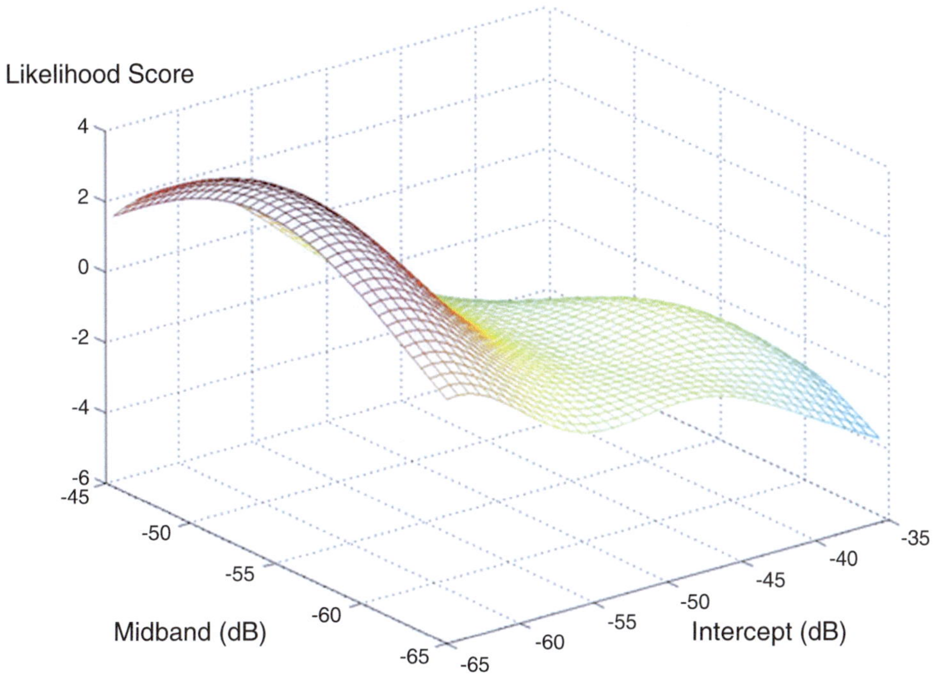

Fig. 2 An SVM-based LUT for a PSA value of 7.5 showing a broad peak in the score value for relative cancer likelihood at low (negative) intercept and intermediate midband parameter values. The vertical axis is the cancer-likelihood score; the horizontal axis on the *left* is the midband axis, with decreasing values toward the viewer; the horizontal axis on the *right* is the intercept axis with decreasing values toward the viewer

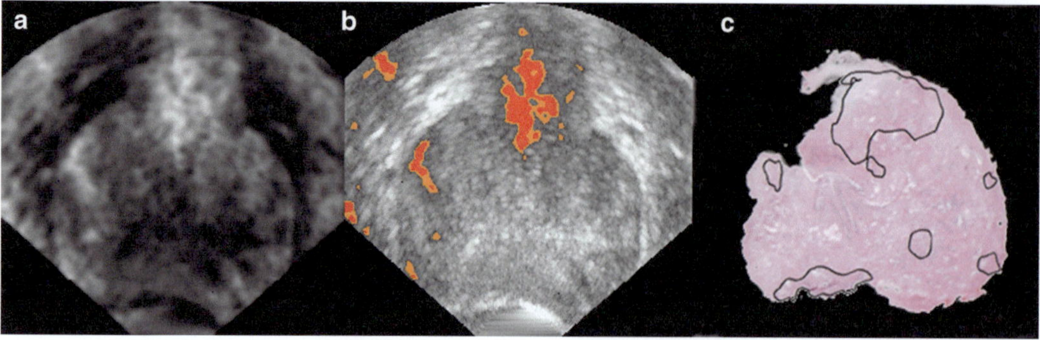

Fig. 3 TTI images compared to postsurgical histology. Gray-scale TTI image (*left image*) and a color-overlay TTI on a midband image (*center image*) show a high suspicion of cancer in a large anterior tumor and smaller nearby foci. (In the color image, *red* depicts the highest cancer likelihood and *orange* the second-highest likelihood.) Whole-mount prostatectomy histology (*right image*) shows demarcations made by the pathologist to indicate cancerous and precancerous neoplastic tissue, particularly a large (12-mm) anterior tumor that was not detected previously by conventional imaging or palpation. All views are from the apex: the patient's right is the viewer's left; his anterior is up (reprinted with permission from *Ultrasonic Imaging* [28])

Fig. 4 3D TTI of the gland shown in Fig. 3. Cancerous regions warranting dose escalation in ablative treatments or a conservative (wide) surgical margin are clearly indicated; regions that could be spared in ablative treatments or safely could undergo nerve-sparing surgery also are apparent. All views are from the base; i.e., the gland is rotated around its vertical axis compared to Fig. 3 (reprinted with permission from *Ultrasonic Imaging* [28])

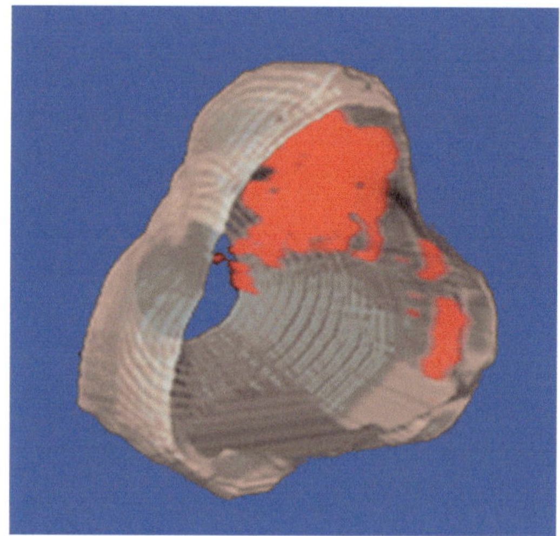

Additional examples of TTIs are the 3D versions of this same prostate, as shown in Fig. 4, and the biopsy-search-window ROI in the TTIs of Fig. 5. In Fig. 4, the most highly suspicious volumes are depicted in red. The representation of the gland in Fig. 4 was generated from a set of parallel scan planes acquired at 5-mm plane separations; 2D TTIs were generated for each plane. The set of 2D TTIs was assembled into a 3D rendering using manual demarcation of the gland surface and TTI color-encoding to demarcate the tumor surfaces automatically. In Fig. 4, the gland is rotated so that it is viewed through the base rather than viewing it more conventionally from the apex as shown in Fig. 3. This 3D rendering could be extremely useful in planning therapy. For example, the rendering clearly shows that a nerve-sparing approach could be applied with a tight margin on the right portion of the gland, but a more generous and cautious one on the left side. The 3D TTI could also provide input for planning focal or differential radiation, cryo-ablation, or HIFU treatments. The illustrative biopsy-guidance TTI windows of Fig. 5 were generated from two separate scans of the same biopsy patient. In this figure five levels of relative

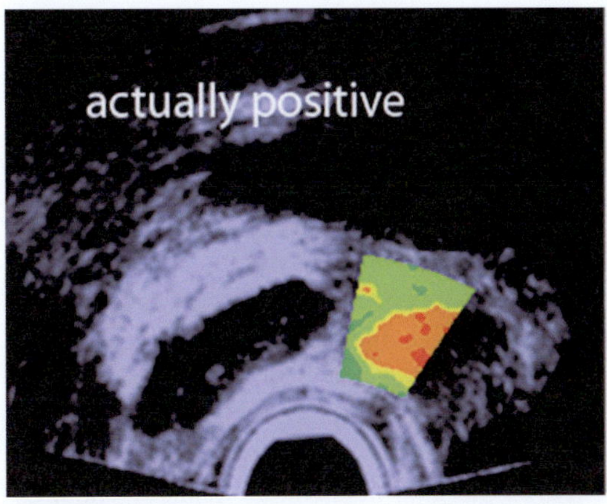

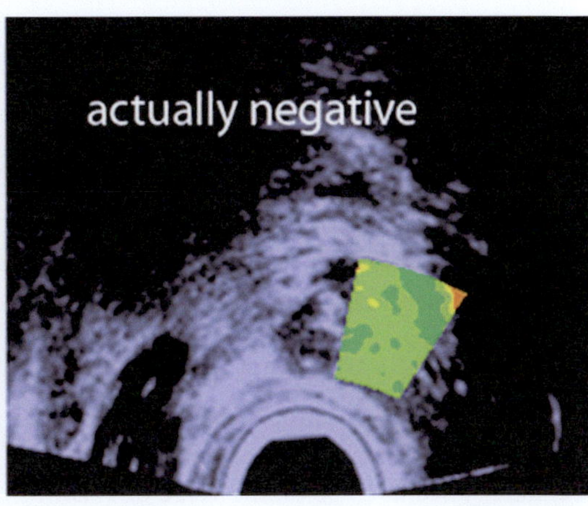

Fig. 5 Illustrative biopsy-guidance images with a small TTI ROI window. Two planes from the same patient are shown. Color encoding is used to depict cancer likelihood; the highest likelihood is depicted in *red* and the lowest in *green*; the background gray-scale image is a midband image. The actual biopsy histology was positive in the *left* image and negative in the *right* one. This type of search-window TTI could be used to guide biopsies more effectively (reprinted with permission from *Ultrasonic Imaging* [26])

cancer likelihood are shown, with green indicating the lowest likelihood, yellow-green a slightly higher likelihood, yellow an intermediate likelihood, orange a moderately high likelihood, and red the highest likelihood. The left image in Fig. 5 was generated from a plane in which the biopsy subsequently proved to be positive; the right image was from a plane that had a negative biopsy. If such images had been available to guide the biopsies in real time, the biopsy needle certainly could have been targeted into the red and orange regions shown in the left image, but the green and yellow-green regions in the right image might have been spared.

Summary

Focal treatments for prostate cancer may reduce treatment toxicity without degrading treatment efficacy as long as regions of the gland that harbor cancer are effectively treated. Therefore, a key requirement for focal treatment is reliable imaging of the cancer within the gland. Similarly, biopsies that are guided by images that present the likelihood of cancer can improve the positive yields of core-needle biopsies while simultaneously reducing or eliminating the current need to insert the needle blindly into the gland.

The studies described here use sophisticated, nonlinear methods of classification to distinguish cancerous from noncancerous tissues based on spectrum analysis RF echo signals. At present, these methods rely on ANNs and SVMs, and although more than 600 samples are available from more than 60 patients in the data set cited above, only 17 % of the samples in our most-recent data set are cancerous. Considering the range of possible expressions of cancerous and noncancerous prostatic tissues, further study certainly is required to increase the number of independent samples and to assure that the classifier has sufficient generality. Furthermore, a conservative perspective would consider the patients, and not the biopsy cores, to be the independent samples; to take that perspective into account, a much larger data set is required to fully validate the method and allay concerns regarding the generality of the classifier.

Confidence in reliable ultrasonic TTIs, such as the ones under development and described here, can enable detection and treatment of prostate cancer to advance dramatically. The ultrasonic TTIs illustrated in this chapter can be applied clinically either as pure US techniques using existing digital technology to generate TTIs in real time or they can be used alone or in combination with other modalities (e.g., magnetic resonance imaging) to produce even more powerful methods of imaging prostate cancer. As an example, the mechanical properties sensed by US and exploited in US-based TTIs also can be applied in conjunction with spatially matching chemical properties sensed by magnetic resonance spectroscopy methods, with perfusion and diffusion properties sensed by contrast-enhanced magnetic resonance, or with metabolic properties sensed by positron emission methods. Admittedly, such hybrid methods require reliable means of spatial co-registration, but modern image-processing technology seems to be on the verge of enabling such co-registration to be performed quickly and accurately. The practicing urologist would then have a hybrid TTI based upon real-time US with co-registration of the MRI to produce a fused image that indicates regions of the gland likely to be harboring disease.

The inability of current imaging methods to depict suspicious regions reliably is well recognized and it prevents many patients from choosing the option of active surveillance. A reliable means of imaging cancerous foci would give patients confidence that their diseases can be monitored safely and non-invasively, and consequently, unnecessary treatment of indolent disease could be avoided. Once these QUS-based TTI methods are more fully validated by the ongoing studies cited in the acknowledgments below, clinical implementation should be straightforward.

Acknowledgements The studies described in this chapter were inspired, guided, and encouraged by the late Edgar A. Parmer, William R. Fair, and Frederic L. Lizzi. Roslyn Raskin provided invaluable assistance in preparing the manuscript, particularly her meticulous proofreading. Paul Lee, Stella Urban, and Ronald Silverman made vital contributions to the classification aspects of the studies. The original prostate TTI research was supported in part by NIH/NCI grant CA053561 and the Riverside Research Fund for Biomedical Engineering. Current studies to integrate TTIs with prostate-HIFU instruments and to integrate US TTIs with MR methods are supported by NIH/NCI grants CA135089 and CA140772, respectively. Current studies applying envelope statistics in combination with spectrum-analysis methods to distinguish cancerous from noncancerous tissue in lymph nodes are supported by NIH/NCI grant CA100183. Some images are shown with permission from *Ultrasonic Imaging*, as indicated in their figure legends.

Appendix

The basic theories of scattering in tissue assume that scattering is weak and the Born approximation applies [53]. In essence, this approximation considers scattering behavior to depend solely on the interaction between scatterers and the incident field; i.e., it assumes that the total field, which includes contributions that result from scattering, can be replaced by the incident field alone because the contribution of the scattered field to the total field can be ignored. The theoretical framework first published by Lizzi in 1983 expresses the spectrum of the backscattered echo signals received at the transducer as an integral over three spatial autocorrelation functions: the three-dimensional autocorrelation function of spatial variations in relative acoustic impedance, which defines the acoustic properties of the scatterers themselves; the two-way beam-directivity autocorrelation function, which specifies the behavior of the incident-beam profile in two dimensions transverse to the beam-propagation direction; and the one-dimensional autocorrelation function of the time-domain window used to select backscattered signals for spectral processing [34–37]. The fundamental equation derived by Lizzi et al. for a normalized (system-corrected) spectrum is

$$S = 4k^2 \iiint R_\zeta \left(\Delta \mathbf{x} \right) R_\mathrm{D} \left(\Delta y, \Delta z \right) R_\mathrm{G} \left(\Delta x \right) \mathrm{e}^{j2k\Delta x} \mathrm{d}\Delta x \, \mathrm{d}\Delta y \, \mathrm{d}\Delta z$$

where S is the normalized power spectrum (i.e., the spectrum that is corrected for the acoustical and electronic properties of the system), k is the wave number ($2\pi/\lambda$ where λ is the wavelength of the US), $R_\zeta(\Delta \mathbf{x})$ is the spatial autocorrelation function of the distribution of the relative acoustic impedance of the scatterers, $R_\mathrm{D}(\Delta y, \Delta z)$ is the autocorrelation function of the two-way US beam-directivity function, and $R_\mathrm{G}(\Delta x)$ is the autocorrelation function of the gating function (typically a Hamming or Hanning window, which resembles a squared cosine function) [34].

The power spectrum is computed by digitizing RF echo signals over some or all of a scanned plane or volume; defining an ROI for analysis within that plane or volume; gating a portion the RF signals within the ROI by multiplying a gating function times the selected RF data; computing the squared magnitude of the Fourier transform of the gated RF signals; and converting the result to decibels (dB) (i.e., ten times the log of the squared magnitude of the Fourier transform). Because of the randomness of a typical spectrum derived from tissue echo signals, ample averaging is required and is performed by shifting the gating window, repeating the spectral computation, and averaging the results computed over the entire ROI. Once the average power spectrum is computed, normalization is performed to correct for system properties, and parameters representing the spectrum are calculated and related by theory to tissue properties.

In practice, the Lizzi equation is applied using assumed autocorrelation functions for the scatterer acoustic impedance. For most reasonable functions, such as the autocorrelation function for a sphere or a Gaussian autocorrelation function, the equation predicts a gently curving spectrum when the power spectrum is expressed in dB with respect to a perfectly reflecting calibration target. When approximated by a straight line over the available, effective, noise-limited bandwidth, the linear fit to a calibrated spectrum has two basic, independent defining parameters: (1) a slope value that theoretically depends only on scatter size and on attenuation in the intervening medium, and (2) an intercept value that theoretically depends on scatterer size, concentration, and acoustic impedance relative to the environment of the scatterers. An additional spectral parameter is the midband (or midband fit), which is the value of the straight-line approximation at the center of the effective noise-limited bandwidth, i.e., the average value of the amplitude of the straight-line approximation over the usable frequency band. The midband parameter is equivalent to the integrated-backscatter parameter developed by Miller and his coworkers [54–57].

The theory relating spectral parameters to tissue properties was further developed and published in the 1990s by Insana and Hall who applied the concept of form factors to tissue-property assessment [40, 41]. Form factors, which pertain to the "shape" of the relative acoustic impedance of the scatterer, are the Fourier transform of the autocorrelation functions described by Lizzi. The most commonly used form factor is the Gaussian, and it provides a better approximation to the empirical spectrum and, presumably, more accurately estimates effective scatterer properties than the simpler linear approximation.

References

1. Cancer facts & figures 2014. Atlanta, GA: American Cancer Society; 2012. p. 12.
2. Haas GP, Delongchamps NB, Jones RF, Chandan V, Serio AM, Vickers AJ, Jumbelic M, Threatte G, Korets R, Lilja H, de la Roza G. Needle biopsies on autopsy prostates: sensitivity of cancer detection based on true prevalence. J Natl Cancer Inst. 2007; 99(19):1484–9.
3. Applewhite J, Matlaga B, McCullough D. Results of the 6-region prostate biopsy method: the repeat biopsy population. J Urol. 2002;168(2):500–3.
4. Feleppa EJ, Ketterling JA, Kalisz A, Urban S, Schiff PB, Ennis RD, Wuu CS, Porter CR, Fair WR, Gillespie JW. Application of spectrum analysis and neural-network classification to imaging for targeting and monitoring treatment of prostate cancer. In: Schneider S, Levy M, McAvoy B, editors. Proceedings of the 2001 ultrasonics symposium. Piscataway: IEEE; 2002. p. 1269–72.
5. Feliciano J, Teper E, Ferrandino M, Macchia RJ, Blank W, Grunberger I, Colon I. The incidence of fluoroquinoline-resistant infections after prostate biopsy—are fluoroquinolines still effective prophylaxis? J Urol. 2008;179:952–5.
6. Loeb S, van den Heuvel S, Zhu X, Bangma CH, Schröder FH, Roobol MJ. Infectious complications and hospital admissions after prostate biopsy in a European randomized trial. Eur Urol. 2012;61(6): 1110–4.
7. Macchia R. Resistant infections after prostate biopsy: are fluoroquinolones still effective prophylaxis. Presented on November 11, 2007 at the 2007 annual meeting of the New York section of the AUA in Buenos Aires, Argentina.
8. Epstein JI, Walsh PC, Carmichael M, Brendler CB. Pathologic and clinical findings to predict tumor extent of nonpalpable (stage T1c) prostate cancer. JAMA. 1994;271(5):368–74.
9. Partin AW, Kattan MW, Subong EN, Walsh PC, Wojno KJ, Oesterling JE, Scardino PT, Pearson JD. Combination of prostate-specific antigen, clinical stage, and Gleason score to predict pathological stage

of localized prostate cancer. A multi-institutional update. JAMA. 1997;277:1445–51.

10. Ahmed HU, Emberton M, Kepner G, Kepner J. A biomedical engineering approach to mitigate the errors of prostate biopsy. Nat Rev Urol. 2012;9(4):227–31.

11. Ahmed HU, Kirkham A, Arya M, Illing R, Freeman A, Allen C, Emberton M. Is it time to consider a role for MRI before prostate biopsy? Nat Rev Clin Oncol. 2009;6(4):197–206.

12. Wei JT. Limitations of a contemporary prostate biopsy: the blind march forward. Urol Oncol. 2010; 28(5):546–9.

13. Coleman DJ, Silverman RH, Rondeau MJ, Boldt HC, Lloyd HO, Lizzi FL, Weingeist TA, Chen X, Vangveeravong S, Folberg R. Noninvasive in-vivo detection of prognostic indicators for high risk uveal melanoma: ultrasound parameter imaging. Ophthalmology. 2004;111(3):558–64.

14. Silverman RH, Folberg R, Rondeau MJ, Boldt HC, Lloyd HO, Chen X, Lizzi FL, Weingeist TA, Coleman DJ. Spectral parameter imaging for detection of prognostically significant histologic features in uveal melanoma. Ultrasound Med Biol. 2003;29(7):951–9.

15. Lizzi FL, Feleppa EJ, Astor M, Kalisz A. Statistics of ultrasonic spectral parameters for prostate and liver examinations. IEEE Trans Ultrason Ferroelect Freq Contr. 1997;44:935–42.

16. Lizzi FL, King DL, Rorke MC, Hui J, Ostromogilsky M, Yaremko MM, Feleppa EJ, Wai P. Comparison of theoretical scattering results and ultrasonic data from clinical liver examinations. Ultrasound Med Biol. 1988;14(5):377–85.

17. Lee DJ, Sigel B, Swami VK, Justin JR, Gahtan V, O'Brien SP, Dwyer-Joyce L, Feleppa EJ, Roberts AB, Berkowitz HD. Determination of carotid-plaque risk by ultrasonic tissue characterization. Ultrasound Med Biol. 1998;24(9):1291–9.

18. Noritomi T, Sigel B, Gahtan V, Swami V, Justin J, Feleppa EJ, Shirouzu K. In vivo detection of carotid plaque thrombus by ultrasonic tissue characterization. J Ultrasound Med. 1997;16(2):107–11.

19. Noritomi T, Sigel B, Swami V, Justin J, Gahtan V, Chen X, Feleppa EJ, Roberts AB, Shirouzu K. Carotid plaque typing by multiple-parameter ultrasonic tissue characterization. Ultrasound Med Biol. 1997;23(5): 643–50.

20. Kolecki RV, Sigel B, Justin J, Feleppa EJ, Parsons RE, Kitamura H, Machi J, Hayashi J, Taylor P, McGann L, Roberts AB. Determining the acuteness and stability of deep venous thrombosis by ultrasonic tissue characterization. J Vasc Surg. 1995;21(6):976–84.

21. Feleppa EJ, Machi J, Noritomi T, Tateishi T, Oishi R, Yanagihara E, Jucha J. "Differentiation of metastatic from benign lymph nodes by spectrum analysis *in vitro*. In: Schneider S, Levy M, McAvoy B, editors. Proceedings of the 1997 ultrasonics symposium. Piscataway: Institute of Electrical and Electronics Engineers; 1998. p. 1137–42.

22. Tateishi T, Machi J, Feleppa EJ, Oishi RH, Jucha J, Yanagihara E, McCarthy LJ, Noritomi T, Shirouzu K. In vitro diagnosis of axillary lymph node metastases in breast cancer by spectrum analysis of radio frequency echo signals. Ultrasound Med Biol. 1998; 24(8):1151–9.

23. Noritomi T, Machi J, Feleppa EJ, Yanagihara E, Shirouzu K. In vitro investigation of lymph node metastasis of colorectal cancer using ultrasonic spectral parameters. Ultrasound Med Biol. 1998;24: 235–43.

24. Dasgupta S, Feleppa EJ, Ramachandran S, Ketterling JA, Kalisz A, Haker S, Tempany C, Porter C, Lacrampe M, Isacson C, Sparks D. Spatial co-registration of magnetic resonance and ultrasound images of the prostate as a basis for multi-modality tissue-type imaging. In: Yuhas MP, editor. Proc. 2007 IEEE-Int. ultrasonics symp. Piscataway: Institute of Electrical and Electronics Engineers; 2007. p. 641–3.

25. Feleppa EF, Porter CR, Ketterling J, Dasgupta S, Ramachandran S, Sparks D. "Recent advances in ultrasonic tissue-type imaging of the prostate: improving detection and evaluation". In: Andre MP, editor. Acoustical imaging, vol. 28. Dordrecht: Springer; 2007. p. 331–9.

26. Feleppa EJ, Porter CR, Ketterling JA, Lee P, Dasgupta S, Urban S, Kalisz A. Recent developments in tissue-type imaging (TTI) for planning and monitoring treatment of prostate cancer. Ultrason Imaging. 2004; 26:71–84.

27. Feleppa EJ, Ennis RD, Schiff PB, Wuu CS, Kalisz A, Ketterling JA, Urban S, Liu T, Fair WR, Porter CR, Gillespie JR. Ultrasonic spectrum-analysis and neural-network classification as a basis for ultrasonic imaging to target brachytherapy of prostate cancer. J Brachytherapy Int. 2002;1(1):1–6.

28. Feleppa EJ, Ennis RD, Schiff PB, Wuu CS, Kalisz A, Ketterling J, Urban S, Liu T, Fair WR, Porter CR, Gillespie JW. Spectrum-analysis and neural networks for imaging to detect and treat prostate cancer. Ultrason Imaging. 2001;23:135–46.

29. Feleppa EJ, Fair WR, Liu T, Kalisz A, Balaji KC, Porter CR, Tsai H, Reuter V, Gnadt W, Miltner MJ. Three-dimensional ultrasound analyses of the prostate. Mol Urol. 2000;4(3):133–41.

30. Feleppa EJ, Liu T, Kalisz A, Shao MC, Fleshner N, Reuter V. Ultrasonic spectral-parameter imaging of the prostate. Int J Imaging Syst Technol. 1997;8:11–25.

31. Mamou J, Coron A, Oelze ML, Saegusa-Beecroft E, Hata M, Lee P, Machi J, Yanagihara E, Laugier P, Feleppa EJ. Three-dimensional high-frequency backscatter and envelope quantification of cancerous human lymph nodes. Ultrasound Med Biol. 2011; 37(3):345–57.

32. Jones JP, Holasek E, Jennings WD, Purnell EW. Two dimensional display of spectral information and its application to diagnostic medicine. Proc 1976 Ultrasonics Symposium, IEEE, vol. 1; 1976. p. 58–9.

33. Nicholas D. Evaluation of backscattering coefficients for excised human tissues: results, interpretation and associated measurements. Ultrasound Med Biol. 1982;8:17–28.

34. Lizzi FL, Greenebaum M, Feleppa EJ, Elbaum M, Coleman DJ. Theoretical framework for spectrum

analysis in ultrasonic tissue characterization. J Acoust Soc Am. 1983;73(4):1366–73.

35. Zagzebski JA, Lu ZF, Yao LX. Quantitative ultrasound imaging: *in vitro* results in normal liver. Ultrason Imaging. 1983;15:335–51.

36. Feleppa EJ, Lizzi FL, Coleman DJ, Yaremko MM. Diagnostic spectrum analysis in ophthalmology: a physical perspective. Ultrasound Med Biol. 1986;12(8):623–31.

37. Lizzi FL, Ostromogilsky M, Feleppa E, Rorke MC, Yaremko MM. Relationship of ultrasonic spectral parameters to features of tissue microstructure. IEEE Trans Ultrason Ferroelect Freq Contr. 1987; UFFC-34:319–29.

38. Nassiri DK, Hill CR. The use of angular scattering measurements to estimate structural parameters of human and animal tissues. J Acoust Soc Am. 1990; 87:179–92.

39. Lizzi FL, Astor M, Liu T, Deng C, Coleman DJ, Silverman RH. Ultrasonic spectrum analysis for tissue assays and therapy evaluations. Int J Imaging Syst Technol. 1997;8:3–10.

40. Insana MF, Wagner RF, Brown DG, Hall TJ. Describing small-scale structure in random media using pulse-echo ultrasound. J Acoust Soc Am. 1990; 87:179–92.

41. Insana MF, Hall TJ. Parametric ultrasound imaging from backscatter coefficient measurements: image formation and interpretation. Ultrason Imaging. 1990;12:245–67.

42. Hosokowa T, Sigel B, Machi J, Kitamura H, Kolecki RV, Justin JR, Feleppa EJ, Tuszynski G, Kakegawa T. Experimental assessment of spectrum analysis of ultrasonic echoes as a method for estimating scatterer properties. Ultrasound Med Biol. 1994;20(5): 4763–470.

43. Bigelow TA, O'Brien WD. Scatterer size estimation in pulse-echo ultrasound using focused sources: theoretical approximations and simulation analysis. J Acoust Soc Am. 2004;116(1):578–93.

44. Bigelow TA, O'Brien WD. Scatterer size estimation in pulse-echo ultrasound using focused sources: calibration measurements and phantom experiments. J Acoust Soc Am. 2004;116(1):594–602.

45. Bigelow TA, O'Brien WD. Evaluation of the spectral fit algorithm as functions of frequency range and Δka_{eff}. IEEE Trans Ultrason Ferroelect Freq Contr. 2005;52(11):2003–10.

46. Bigelow TA, O'Brien WD. Impact of local attenuation approximations when estimating correlation length from backscattered ultrasound echoes. J Acoust Soc Am. 2006;120(1):546–53.

47. Mamou J, Oelze ML, O'Brien WD, Zachary JF. Ultrasound characterization of three animal mammary tumors from three-dimensional acoustic tissue models. Proc 2005 ultrasonics symposium, IEEE, vol. 2; 2005. p 866–9.

48. Oelze ML, Zachary JF, O'Brien WD. "Ultrasonic quantification of the tissue microstructure of spontaneous mammary tumors in rats.Proc 2002 ultrasonics symposium, IEEE, vol. 4; 2002. p. 1369–72.

49. Oelze M, Zachary J. Examination of cancer in mouse models using high-frequency quantitative ultrasound. Ultrasound Med Biol. 2006;32(11):1639–48.

50. Oelze ML, Zachary JF, O'Brien WD. Characterization of tissue microstructure using ultrasonic backscatter: theory and technique for optimization using a Gaussian form factor. J Acoust Soc Am. 2002; 112:1202–11.

51. Kolios MC, Czarnota GJ, Hussain M, Foster FS, Hunt JW, Sherar MD. Analysis of ultrasound backscatter from ensembles of cells and isolated nuclei. Proc 2001 ultrasonics symposium, IEEE, vol. 2; 2001. p. 1257–60.

52. Kolios MC, Czarnota GJ, Lee M, Hunt JW, Sherar MD. Ultrasonic spectral parameter characterization of apoptosis. Ultrasound Med Biol. 2002;28(5):589–97.

53. Wu T, Ohmura T. Quantum theory of scattering. Upper Saddle River, NJ: Prentice Hall; 1962.

54. O'Donnell M, Bauwens D, Mimbs JW, Miller JG. Broadband integrated backscatter: an approach to spatially localized tissue characterization *in vivo*. Proceedings of the IEEE ultrasonics symposium; 1979. p. 1482–9, 175–8.

55. Lanza GM, Trousil RL, Wallace KD, Rose JH, Hall CS, Scott MJ, Miller JG, Eisenberg PR, Gaffney PJ, Wickline SA. In vitro characterization of a novel, tissue-targeted ultrasonic contrast system with acoustic microscopy. J Acoust Soc Am. 1998;104:3665–72.

56. Lanza GM, Wallace K, Scott MJ, Cachetis C, Abendschein D, Christy D, Sharkey A, Miller J, Gaffney P, Wickline S. A novel site-targeted ultrasonic contrast agent with broad biomedical applications. Circulation. 1996;94:3334–40.

57. Miller JG, Perez JE, Wickline SA, Baldwin SL, Barzilai B, Davila-Roman V, Fedewa RJ, Finch-Johnston AE, Hall CS, Handley SM, Huckett FD, Holland MR, Kovacs A, Lanza GM, Lewis SS, Marsh JN, Mobley J, Sosnovik DE, Trousil RL, Wallace KD, Waters KR. Backscatter imaging and myocardial tissue characterization. Proceedings of the IEEE ultrasonics symposium. Sendai Japan, 1998. p. 1373–83.

58. Metz CE, Herman BA, Shen J-H. Maximum likelihood estimation of receiver operating characteristic (ROC) curves from continuously-distributed data. Stat Med. 1998;17(9):1033–53.

59. McLachlan GJ. Discriminant analysis and statistical pattern recognition. New York: John Wiley & Sons, Inc.; 1992.

60. Shawe-Taylor J, Cristianini N. Support vector machines and other kernel-based learning methods. New York: Cambridge University Press; 2000.

61. Shakhnarovish D, Indyk E, editors. Nearest-neighbor methods in learning and vision. Cambridge, MA: MIT Press; 2005.

62. Keller JM, Gray MR, Givens JA. A k-nearest neighbor algorithm. IEEE Trans Syst Man Cybern. 1985; SMC-15:580–5.

63. Cortes C, Vapnik V. Support-vector networks. Mach Learn. 1995;20:273–97.

64. Theodoridis S, Koutroumbas K. Pattern Recognition. 4th ed. New York: Academic Press; 2009.

Prostate Elastography

Stephen Rosenzweig, Zachary Miller,
Thomas Polascik, and Kathryn Nightingale

Introduction

Conventional B-mode transrectal ultrasound (TRUS) generates images of the acoustic properties of tissues (density and sound speed). TRUS is used extensively to aid in visualizing the prostate gland and needle during biopsy. However, TRUS has limited sensitivity and specificity for prostate cancer (PCa) detection/visualization [1, 2], and therefore advanced ultrasonic methods are currently being investigated to improve PCa detection. One promising approach, called elastography, generates images of the elastic properties of tissues (i.e., tissue stiffness), providing complementary information to B-mode images. This approach has promise for PCa imaging due to the inherent differences in stiffness between normal and pathologic tissues in the prostate.

The digital rectal exam (DRE) is used extensively to diagnose PCa; however, this technique is limited to palpation of the posterior region of the prostate. In essence, elastography is an extension of the digital rectal exam, portraying variations in stiffness throughout the gland. Elastographic imaging techniques introduce a mechanical excitation and use either MRI or ultrasound to monitor the tissue response, thereby creating an image of the tissue stiffness.

There are many elastographic methods that have been used to visualize structures in the prostate:

1. Strain imaging [3–6].
2. Acoustic radiation force impulse (ARFI) imaging [7–10].
3. Shear wave imaging [2, 11, 12].
4. Vibration elastography imaging [13, 14].
5. Vibration amplitude sonoelastography [15–17].

Although there are a multitude of elastographic techniques, they are all based on the same concept of applying a force and imaging the resulting tissue response. Common forces employed in prostate elastography include compressing the tissue, using a vibrating piston or other mechanical actuator, or using acoustic radiation force. The induced tissue deformation, or displacement, is related to the mechanical properties of the tissue through the principles of elasticity.

There are two general types of elastographic images, qualitative and quantitative. Qualitative images are generated by compressive strain imaging and ARFI imaging, and they portray the relative stiffness, strain, or displacement response of the tissue. Quantitative images are generated

S. Rosenzweig, Ph.D. (✉) • Z. Miller, B.S.E.
K. Nightingale, Ph.D.
Department of Biomedical Engineering, Duke University, Room 136, Hudson Hall, Box 90281, Durham, NC 27708, USA
e-mail: Stephen.rosenzweig@duke.edu; kathy.nightingale@duke.edu

T. Polascik, M.D.
Department of Urology, Duke Cancer Institute, Duke University Medical Center, Yellow Zone, Erwin Road, Durham, NC 27710, USA
e-mail: Polas001@mc.duke.edu

C.R. Porter and E.M. Wolff (eds.), *Prostate Ultrasound: Current Practice and Future Directions,*
DOI 10.1007/978-1-4939-1948-2_12, © Springer Science+Business Media New York 2015

by shear wave-based methods, which utilize the principles of elasticity to derive the underlying elastic material properties of the tissue. The quality of the images depends on the imaging modality being used, the magnitude and type of force being applied, the signal processing of the data, and the validity of the assumptions used to reconstruct the images.

Governing Principles of Elasticity

In order to appreciate elastography images and the data that they contain, a brief overview of the governing principles of elasticity is necessary. Elastographic imaging methods measure the displacement (u), or strain (ε), of the tissue in response to an applied force (or stress, σ). The strain is the spatial gradient of the displacement $\left(\varepsilon = \dfrac{du}{dx} \right)$ and represents the change in displacement with depth (i.e., how tissue compresses). Strain is related both to the applied stress (σ, i.e., force per unit area) and the inherent tissue mechanical properties (E, the elastic, or Young's modulus), and under simplifying assumptions is described by the equation:

$$\varepsilon = \frac{\sigma}{E}. \tag{1}$$

The elastic modulus describes the stiffness of tissue; stiffer tissues have a higher elastic modulus than softer tissues. Since strain is inversely proportional to the elastic modulus, for a given stress, stiffer structures exhibit smaller strain, or displacement, and softer tissues exhibit larger strains (Fig. 1). Both MRI and ultrasound can be used to measure tissue motion; thus, in compressive strain imaging methods, tissue displacement in response to an applied stress is measured, and images of tissue displacement or strain are generated that reflect relative differences in tissue stiffness.

In addition to compressing the tissue, it is possible to generate shear waves in the tissue. These shear waves propagate in a direction orthogonal to the applied stress and are similar in concept to the ripples that propagate away from a pebble dropped in water. The spatial and temporal behavior of a shear wave in tissue is governed by the wave equation:

$$\nabla^2 \boldsymbol{u} = \frac{1}{c_s^2} \frac{\delta^2 \boldsymbol{u}}{\delta t^2}, \tag{2}$$

where $\boldsymbol{u}$ is the displacement of the tissue, c_s is the wave speed, and ∇^2 is the Laplacian operator.

Equation (2) relates the spatial behavior of the wave (left side of the equation) to the temporal behavior of the wave (right side of the equation). Additionally, there is a constant of proportionality, c_s, which is known as the shear wave speed. The shear wave speed can be related to the shear modulus through assumptions of linear elasticity and homogeneity, such that $\mu = \rho c_s^2$ where μ is the shear modulus and ρ is the density. Furthermore, under the assumption of incompressibility, which is considered reasonable in soft tissues such as the prostate, the shear modulus is directly proportional to the Young's modulus, such that $E = 3\mu = 3\rho c_s^2$. Therefore, if the shear wave speed is measured using elastographic techniques, it is common to directly estimate the corresponding shear and Young's moduli, which represent the inherent material elastic properties of the tissue. It is important to be aware of the specific stiffness parameter that is presented in quantitative elastographic images (i.e., c_s, E, or μ).

Elastic Properties of the Prostate

In order for elastography to successfully differentiate PCa from surrounding tissue, prostate lesions must have material properties distinct from healthy tissue. A number of studies have shown that PCa has substantially different biomechanical properties compared to healthy prostate tissue [18]. This seems reasonable because tumor formation involves a complex series of events including uncontrolled cell growth, angiogenesis/vascularization, and substantial changes in the underlying tissue microenvironment that set it apart from healthy tissue [19, 20]. In addition, PCa has been shown to have

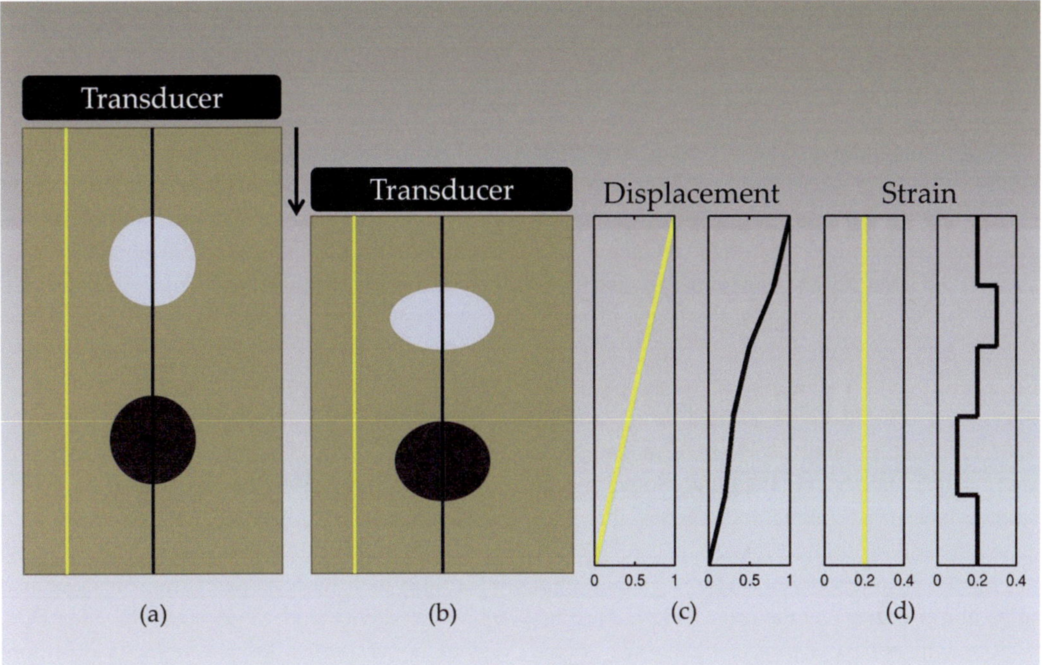

Fig. 1 Schematic representation of tissue with a soft circular inclusion (*top, light gray*) and stiff circular inclusion (*bottom, dark gray*) prior to compression (**a**), post-compression (**b**), the induced displacements (**c**), and the computed strain (**d**). The background has linearly varying displacement throughout depth due to the applied force at the top of the tissue and fixed bottom boundary; thus, the background has constant strain, as represented by the *yellow line*. The displacement in the region with the two inclusions is piecewise linear, with different slopes in the lesions and the background. The soft lesion displaces more than the background and the stiff inclusion displaces less than the background; thus, the strain provides information about the relative stiffnesses of the lesions compared to the background

increased cell density and collagen deposition (implying an immune response), increased microvessel density, and changes in stromal to glandular ratios relative to healthy peripheral zone tissues [16, 21].

Taken together, these biomechanical changes result in tumor tissues that tend to be stiffer than surrounding tissue, which has been demonstrated in a number of studies. Zhang et al. performed a study on ex vivo prostates and found that the Young's moduli of normal posterior and cancerous prostatic tissue were 15.9 ± 5.9 and 40.4 ± 15.7 kPa, respectively [22]. Zhai et al. utilized quantitative shear wave-based elastography methods in ex vivo samples and reported that the Young's moduli of normal peripheral zone and cancerous prostatic tissues were 12.3 ± 2.4 and 30 ± 3.0 kPa, respectively [11]. Although the stiffness differed between the studies, both found that there is approximately a 2.5× increase in the stiffness of the cancerous regions as compared to the prostatic peripheral zone tissue.

Elastographic Imaging Methods in Prostate

Strain Imaging

The vast majority of prostate elastography clinical studies have employed strain imaging (i.e., compression elastography) because this method has been commercially available for the past decade [1, 3, 5, 23–29]. Strain imaging requires the user to obtain a B-mode image of the prostate, then compress the organ and obtain a second

B-mode image. The tissue displacement is estimated using correlation-based techniques and the strain between the two states is then computed [27, 30].

Strain imaging assumes that the operator applies a uniform stress across the prostate and out-of-plane motion is negligible. Stiffer regions can then be identified by their relatively low strain compared to the surrounding tissue as shown in Fig. 1. Elastography is typically performed as a free-hand technique with the operator gently compressing the prostate with the ultrasound transducer. A skilled technician is needed to obtain adequately uniform compression, which can be challenging. Some recent studies have used inflatable balloons that surround the endorectal transducer and can be filled or emptied by the operator, thereby generating a more uniform stress on the prostate [27, 31, 32].

Researchers have also investigated the potential use of strain imaging to obtain quantitative information about the tissue. To accomplish this, the inverse problem is solved using models of the tissue structure and displacement data. While this method holds promise, it has not been used clinically to date due to challenges with implementation [33, 34].

Transrectal ultrasound (TRUS) is widely used for prostate visualization during systematic prostate biopsies, but it is not typically used for targeting regions of suspicion since tumors are often not visualized by TRUS [1, 2, 25]. The primary use of strain imaging investigated in the clinical literature is for biopsy guidance. As will be reviewed below, many studies have employed conventional biopsy techniques, and then used strain imaging to identify and target additional regions [1, 3, 23, 24, 29, 31]. Some studies have acquired elastographic strain imaging data and retrospectively compared suspicious regions with those that were biopsied [5] or with whole-mount histology after the prostate was excised [28].

Cochlin et al. demonstrated a significant improvement using strain imaging as compared to TRUS for PCa biopsy guidance. The authors studied 100 patients and using elastography identified five cancers that would not have otherwise been biopsied. Additionally, of these five cancerous regions, three were in patients whose other biopsies showed no cancer; thus, cancer detection was only achieved through the use of elastography. For elastography, the reported sensitivity and specificity for PCa were 51 and 83 %, respectively [23].

In 2007 Nelson et al. studied targeting biopsies using TRUS, color Doppler, and elastography in addition to the traditional sextant biopsy. The authors concluded that color Doppler and elastography both improve cancer detection, but that the detection is not sufficient to replace the standard sextant biopsy. Additionally, the authors demonstrated that cancer detection in gray-scale ultrasound, color Doppler, and elastography images are all correlated with Gleason score [1].

Kamoi et al. studied 107 patients using both power Doppler ultrasound and elastography, indicating that elastographic strain imaging had 68 % sensitivity and 81 % specificity for PCa. The authors reported that elastography was more successful at detection of high Gleason score tumors, with 100 % of the tumors with a Gleason score 8 being detected. The authors indicated that their primary difficulty with elastography was the image quality variability between users due to the user-dependent nature of compression [3].

Although the previous studies used both Doppler ultrasound and strain imaging, other groups have evaluated strain imaging exclusively. A 311 patient study by Miyagawa et al. reported a 90 % diagnostic sensitivity for PCa using the combination of TRUS and elastography. The authors reported that elastography was most successful in detecting cancer in the anterior prostate. They also noted that the sensitivity of elastography decreased as prostate volume increased, which they attributed to the confounding effects of BPH [24].

The observation that the diagnostic utility of elastography differs in various regions of the prostate was expanded upon by Tsutsumi et al. The authors divided the prostate into three regions, anterior, middle, and posterior and analyzed the utility of elastography for PCa detection. While elastography improved cancer detection in all regions of the prostate, the largest benefit was seen with anterior tumors, with decreasing improvement for middle and posterior tumors [29].

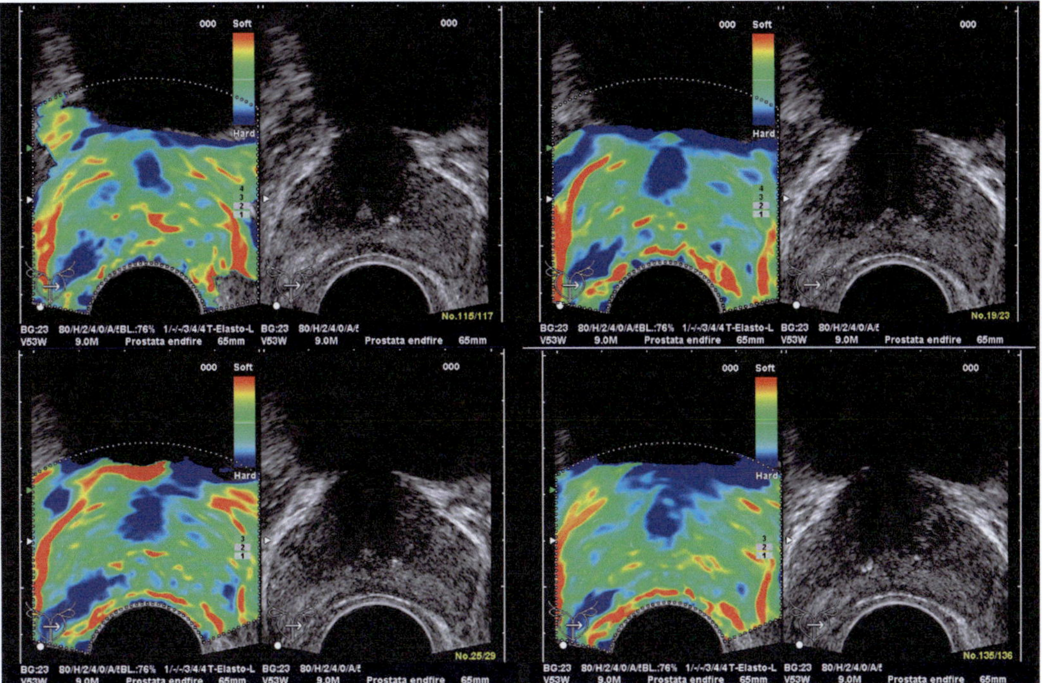

Fig. 2 Patient (picture series) with histologically confirmed prostate cancer in the right mid-gland of prostate. The elastographic examination showed a well-defined lesion with low strain (*dark blue*, patient *right*, peripheral zone near *bottom* of images). The peripheral zone on the patient *left side* showed normal stiffness. Figure reproduced with permission [5]

Pallwein et al. studied 492 patients, who had elastograms of the prostate recorded prior to receiving a systematic 10 core biopsy. The urologist performing the biopsy was blinded to the results of the elastography study. The authors found a whole organ sensitivity of 86 % and specificity of 72 % in the retrospective analysis of suspicious regions in the elastograms. Cancer detection in the basal region was compromised due to a high false positive rate associated with chronic inflammation and atrophy. A representative series of elastograms is reproduced from their work in Fig. 2 [5].

Kapoor et al. performed a 50 patient study specifically focused on determining the utility of elastography in targeting biopsies. The authors reported the sensitivity and specificity of 91.7 and 86.8 %, respectively, as compared to their reported sensitivity and specificity of TRUS at 16.7 and 89 %, respectively. They noted that the primary challenges in using elastography are the inability to differentiate between cancer and prostatitis, very large prostates, and lack of operator experience [31].

Salomon et al. studied prostate elastography in 109 patients undergoing radical prostatectomy, in which the preoperative elastography data was correlated with whole-mount histology data. The authors reported 75 % sensitivity and 77 % specificity for elastography. The authors found that elastography detection of PCa was positively correlated with Gleason score [28].

One of the common challenges reported for strain imaging of the prostate is achieving uniform compression of the organ. To address this challenge, Tsutsumi et al. inflated a water balloon surrounding the transducer to compress the tissue, which reduced the operator dependence of the image quality. Using this method, the authors detected 71 % of histology confirmed PCa lesions [32].

Overall, the multitude of studies performed using strain imaging has demonstrated great promise for guidance of targeted biopsies. The primary benefits have been reported for detecting PCa in the peripheral zone, where approximately 80 % of cancers are located [25]. Although the studies have demonstrated higher sensitivity than with TRUS alone, challenges have also been identified. The studies using free hand compression noted that an experienced operator was needed to obtain high-quality images. Additionally, many studies demonstrated a high false positive rate due to the confounding effects of BPH, which looks similar to cancer in strain images. Finally, the studies determined that targeted biopsies are not sufficient and that standard sextant or 10-core biopsies are necessary in addition to elastography targeted biopsies.

Acoustic Radiation Force Impulse (ARFI)-Based Techniques

Unlike compressive strain imaging methods, ARFI-based imaging methods do not rely on external compression from an outside source. Instead, ARFI methods remotely palpate tissue through ultrasonic energy absorption. Tissues act as low-pass filters, trapping high-frequency wave energy as heat and momentum. The momentum transfer from the wave results in a force on the tissue, which then displaces the tissue on the order of 10 µm and induces shear waves that radiate out from the force focus. Both tissue displacement (qualitative ARFI imaging) and shear wave propagation (quantitative shear wave elastography, vibroacoustography, etc.) can be monitored using traditional B-mode imaging as described below.

Shear Wave Imaging

Shear wave elastography (SWE™) is an elastography technique in which the tissue stiffness is interrogated by exciting a shear wave and monitoring the speed of propagation away from the excitation, thus measuring c_s, as given in Eq. (2). To generate shear waves in vivo, ARFI excitations are used, either with a single focus or in a multifocal "supersonic" configuration [35]. An image of the tissue is then generated by estimating the shear wave speed in small regions that are assumed to be uniform [27]. SWE™ methods have recently been introduced commercially for prostate imaging (Fig. 3).

Barr et al. evaluated SWE™ imaging alone compared to TRUS biopsy in 53 patients. They reported a sensitivity of 96.2 % (25/26), a specificity of 96.2 % (281/292), a positive predictive value of 69.4 %, and a negative predictive value of 99.6 % [36]. The negative predictive value suggests that SWE™ could find application as an initial screening tool. In another study, Ahmad et al. imaged and biopsied 50 patients, 33 of which had at least one positive biopsy [12]. He found similarly high sensitivity and specificity values (0.90 and 0.88, respectively). Correas replicated Barr's and Ahmad's results in two feasibility studies with 21 and 31 patients, respectively [2]. Although the above results are exciting, further studies in larger patient populations are necessary.

Acoustic Radiation Force Impulse (ARFI) Imaging

ARFI imaging applies short duration (<1 ms) focused ultrasound pushing pulses that displace the tissue on the order of 10 µm; the displacement response is then measured where the force is applied (in the focal region) with the same ultrasonic transducer. Images reflect relative differences in displacement response, and, as such, the images are qualitative (similar to compressive strain images). Regions of decreased displacement are assumed to represent stiffer tissues in the same way that regions of decreased strain represent stiffer tissues in strain imaging [37].

ARFI imaging has been used in preliminary feasibility studies to detect PCa. Zhai et al. acquired three-dimensional volumes of ARFI data and correlated their results to whole-mount histology in both ex vivo and in vivo studies. The initial ex vivo studies demonstrated that ARFI images portrayed zonal anatomy, BPH, and PCa with considerably higher contrast than matched B-mode images [8]. In a follow-up study of 19 patients, the same group acquired

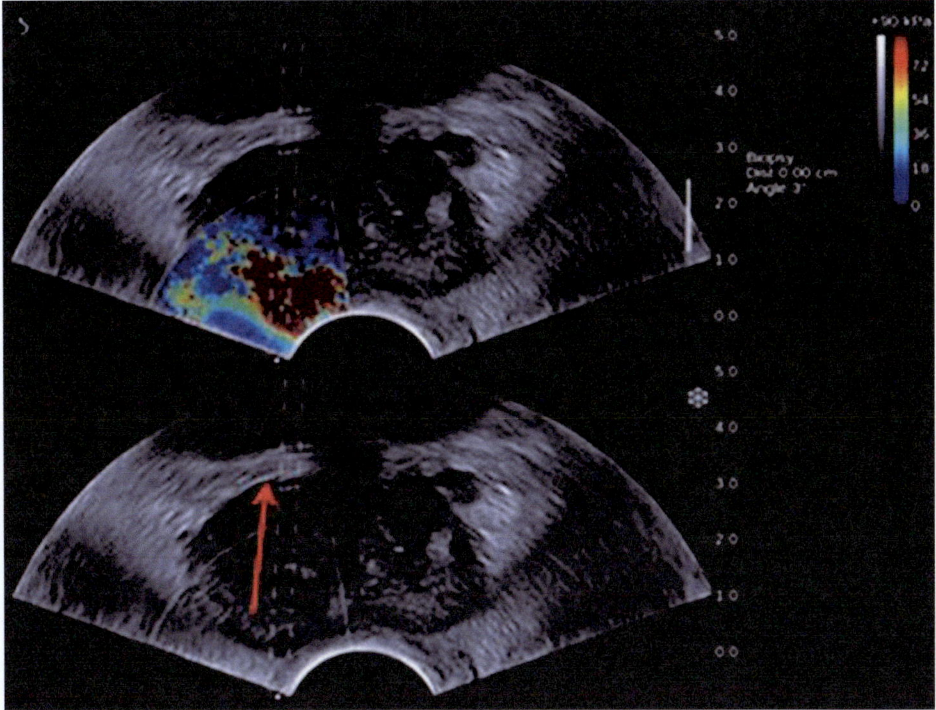

Fig. 3 Comparison of gray-scale TRUS (B-mode; *bottom row*) and overlaid SWE images (*top row*). Representative images showing abnormal area (*red* indicates high stiffness) detected only by SWE. Note the *red arrow* showing needle guide for the real-time biopsy of an abnormal area seen only on SWE images. The abnormal area was Gleason 3+4 adenocarcinoma on histopathology. Figure reproduced with permission [12]

three-dimensional volumes in vivo using an end-fire endocavity transducer prior to radical prostatectomy. The images were then correlated with histologic results. As with strain imaging, when visible, cancers appeared as stiffer regions, corresponding to decreased displacement in the ARFI images. In addition, regions of BPH within the central gland were well visualized with a nodular appearance. Representative ARFI images and corresponding histology slide are shown in Fig. 4 [7, 10]. This technology is not yet commercially available for prostate imaging.

Vibro-elastography

Vibro-elastography is an elastography technique that uses external vibratory actuators to excite the tissue at many frequencies simultaneously. The displacement of the tissue is then monitored using ultrasound and the biomechanical properties of the tissue are calculated from the induced displacement. This method is equivalent to a strain image, but is calibrated to the frequency and amplitude of motion, and therefore it can be used to obtain quantitative values for stiffness, density, and viscosity [38].

Vibro-elastography has been used in a pilot study by Salcudean et al. to demonstrate the potential utility in detecting PCa and brachytherapy seed placement. The tissue is excited using a mechanical actuator coupled to a transrectal ultrasound transducer to generate displacements within the tissue, which are subsequently observed using correlation-based techniques. The authors showed the ability to generate repeatable, operator independent images that revealed stiff regions in the prostates they studied [13, 14].

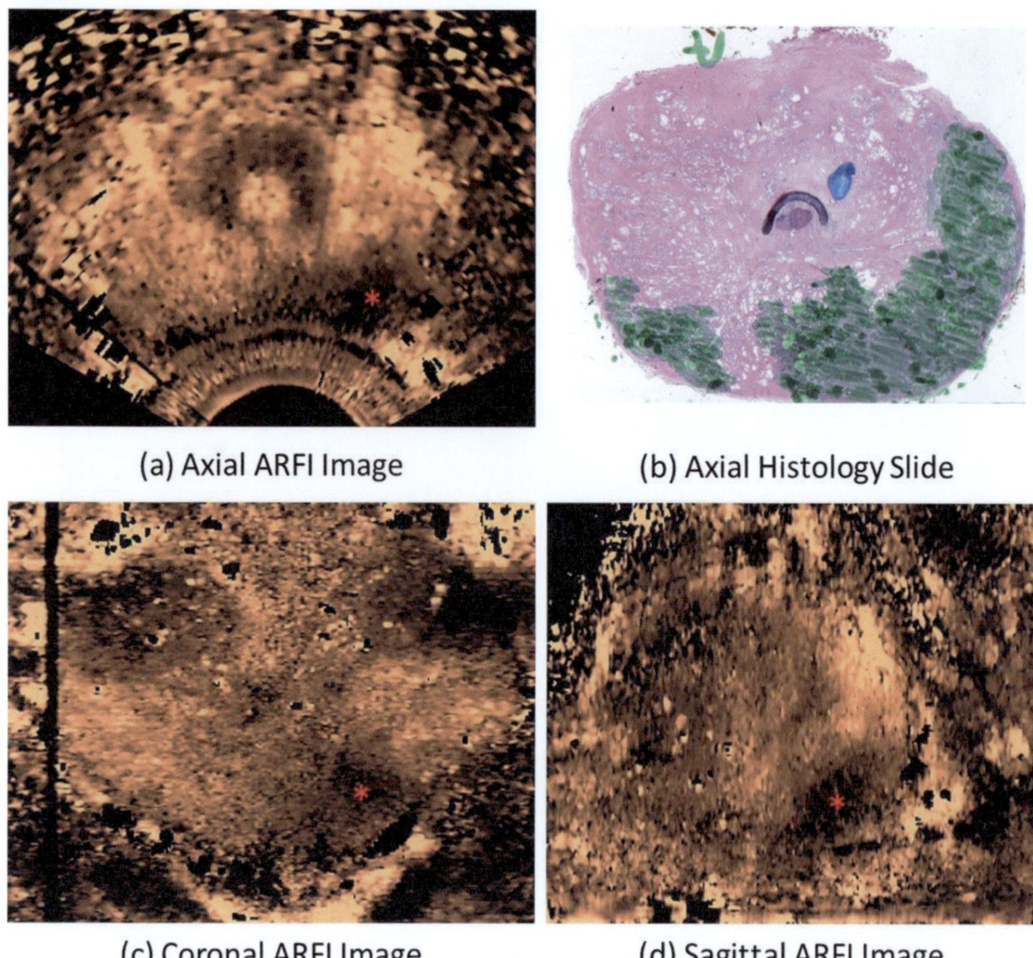

(a) Axial ARFI Image   (b) Axial Histology Slide

(c) Coronal ARFI Image   (d) Sagittal ARFI Image

Fig. 4 Axial, coronal, and sagittal sections of ARFI images in vivo and the corresponding histological slide. The base of the prostate is at the *top* of the coronal image, and the apex is at the *bottom*; the *red asterisk* indicates where the orthogonal views intersect. Images were obtained in vivo immediately prior to radical prostatec-tomy surgery. In the histological slide, cancerous regions were masked in *green* by a pathologist. The stiff structure (*dark*) in the apical region on patient *left* shown in the ARFI images at the *red asterisk* corresponds to the large cancerous region

Vibration Amplitude Sonoelastography

Another ultrasound-based elastographic method that has been used to evaluate PCa in vivo is vibration amplitude sonoelastography. Two external mechanical actuators positioned beneath the patient's pelvis vibrate at a low frequency (70–200 Hz), generating vibrations within the prostate. These vibrations are monitored using a specially designed ultrasound Doppler processing mode. Regions of decreased amplitude are associated with stiffer structures in the tissue [15–17, 27].

Castaneda et al. imaged ten patients prior to radical prostatectomy and correlated the results with whole-mount histology. Twelve of 19 cancerous lesions were identified (average diameters: 7.4 mm visualized, 3.8 mm missed), and 12 false positive regions were identified, 6 of which corresponded to BPH. The primary challenges associated with this method are the inability to detect small tumors and difficulty in coupling enough vibration energy into the tissue [15, 16].

Conclusions

Empirical evidence and quantitative experiments have demonstrated that cancerous regions in the prostate can be stiffer than healthy tissue. Strain imaging, which is available on multiple commercial ultrasound scanners, has been investigated for targeted biopsy guidance. Reports generally indicate improved sensitivity (70–90 %) and specificity (72–87 %) for PCa as compared to TRUS alone using compression elastography. However, several challenges have been identified for this method of elastography, including operator-dependent image quality; difficulty in differentiating between BPH, prostatitis, atrophy, and PCa; reduced image quality in larger prostates; and limitations of cancer sensitivity in the basal region of the prostate.

Compared to compressive strain imaging, SWE™ and ARFI have reduced user dependence. When limited to evaluation of the peripheral zone, SWE™ has shown high sensitivity, specificity, PPV, and NPV values in initial feasibility studies. While these results are promising, larger studies are needed to confirm these results. ARFI imaging is a novel technology that has only recently been investigated in the prostate in vivo, and the visibility of structures, zonal anatomy, and regions of pathology such as PCa and BPH appear promising for procedural guidance and image fusion.

Given these promising initial findings, elasticity imaging could find application for guidance of targeted biopsy procedures, guidance of prostatic focal therapies, and for facilitating watchful waiting and monitoring therapeutic treatment response.

References

1. Nelson ED, Slotoroff CB, Gomella LG, Halpern EJ. Targeted biopsy of the prostate: the impact of color Doppler imaging and elastography on prostate cancer detection and Gleason score. Urology. 2007;70(6):1136–40.
2. Correas J-M, Tissier AM, Khairoune A, Khoury G, Eiss D, Hélénon O. Ultrasound elastography of the prostate: State of the art. Diagn Interv Imaging. 2013;94(5):551–60.
3. Kamoi K, Okihara K, Ochiai A, Ukimura O, Mizutani Y, Kawauchi A, Miki T. The utility of transrectal real-time elastography in the diagnosis of prostate cancer. Ultrasound Med Biol. 2008;34(7):1025–32.
4. Miyanaga N, Akaza H, Yamakawa M, Oikawa T, Sekido N, Hinotsu S, Kawai K, Shimazui S, Shiina T. Tissue elasticity imaging for diagnosis of prostate cancer: a preliminary report. Int J Urol. 2006;13(12): 1514–8.
5. Pallwein L, Aigner F, Faschingbauer R, Pallwein Pinggera G, Bartsch G, Schaefer G, Struve P, Frauscher F. Prostate cancer diagnosis: value of real-time elastography. Abdom Imag. 2008;33(6):729–35.
6. Eggener S, Salomon G, Scardino PT, De la Rosette J, Polascik TJ, Brewster S. Focal therapy for prostate cancer: possibilities and limitations. Eur Urol. 2010;58(1):57–64.
7. Zhai L, Dahl J, Madden J, Mouraviev V, Polascik T, Palmeri M, Nightingale K. Three-dimensional acoustic radiation force impulse (ARFI) imaging of human prostates in vivo. IEEE ultrasonics symposium. 2008. pp 540–3.
8. Zhai L, Madden J, Foo WC, Mouraviev V, Polascik TJ, Palmeri ML, Nightingale KR. Characterizing stiffness of human prostates using acoustic radiation force. Ultrason Imag. 2010;32(4):201–13.
9. Zhai L, Madden J, Foo WC, Palmeri ML, Mouraviev V, Polascik TJ, Nightingale KR. Acoustic radiation force impulse imaging of human prostates ex vivo. Ultrasound Med Biol. 2010;36(4):576–88.
10. Zhai L, Polascik TJ, Foo WC, Rosenzweig S, Palmeri ML, Madden M, Nightingale KR. Acoustic radiation force impulse imaging of human prostates: initial in vivo demonstration. Ultrasound Med Biol. 2012; 38(1):50–61.
11. Zhai L, Madden J, Mouraviev V, Polascik T, Nightingale K. Correlation between SWEI and ARFI image findings in ex vivo human prostates. Ultrasonics symposium (IUS) IEEE international. 2009. pp 523–6.
12. Ahmad S, Cao R, Varghese T, Bidaut L, Nabi G. Transrectal quantitative shear wave elastography in the detection and characterisation of prostate cancer. Surg Endosc. 2013;20:3280.
13. Salcudean SE, French D, Bachmann S, Zahiri-Azar R, Wen X, Morris WJ. Viscoelasticity modeling of

the prostate region using vibro-elastography. Med Image Comput Comput Assist Interv. 2006;9(Pt 1):389–96.

14. Mahdavi S, Moradi M, Wen X, Morris WJ, Salcudean SE. Evaluation of visualization of the prostate gland in vibro-elastography images. Med Image Anal. 2011;15(4):589–600.

15. Castaneda, B, Hoyt K, Westesson K, An L, Yao J, Baxter L, Joseph J, Strang J, Rubens D, Parker K. Performance of three-dimensional sonoelastography in prostate cancer detection: a comparison between ex vivo and in vivo experiments. In Ultrasonics Symposium (IUS), 2009 IEEE International. 2009:519–22.

16. Hoyt K, Castaneda B, Zhang M, Nigwekar P, di Sant'agnese PA, Joseph JV, Strang J, Rubens DJ, Parker KJ. Tissue elasticity properties as biomarkers for prostate cancer. Cancer Biomark. 2008;4(4–5): 213–25.

17. Taylor LS, Rubens DJ, Porter BC, Wu Z, Baggs RB, di Sant'Agnese PA, Nadasdy G, Pasternack D, Messing EM, Nigwekar P, Parker KJ. Prostate cancer: Three-dimensional sonoelastography for in Vitro Detection 1. Radiology 2005;237(3):981–985.

18. Chung LW, et al. Molecular insights into prostate cancer progression: the missing link of tumor microenvironment. J Urol. 2005;173(1):10–20.

19. Gout S, Huot J. Role of cancer microenvironment in metastasis: focus on colon cancer. Cancer Microenviron. 2008;1(1):69–83.

20. Marx J. How cells cycle toward cancer. Science. 1994;263(5145):319–21.

21. Tuxhorn JA, et al. Reactive stroma in human prostate cancer induction of myofibroblast phenotype and extracellular matrix remodeling. Clin Cancer Res. 2002;8(9):2912–23.

22. Zhang M, Nigwekar P, Castaneda B. Quantitative characterization of viscoelastic properties of human prostate correlated with histology. Ultrasound Med Biol. 2008;34(7):1033–42.

23. Cochlin D, Ganatra R, Griffiths D. Elastography in the detection of prostatic cancer. Clin Radiol. 2002; 57(11):1014–20.

24. Miyagawa T, Tsutsumi M, Matsumura T, Kawazoe N, Ishikawa S, Shimokama T, Miyanaga N, Akaza H. Real-time elastography for the diagnosis of prostate cancer: evaluation of elastographic moving images. Jpn J Clin Oncol. 2009;39(6):394–8.

25. Pallwein L, Mitterberger M, Pelzer A, Bartsch G, Strasser H, Pinggera GM, Aigner F, Gradl J, Zur Nedden D, Frauscher F. Ultrasound of prostate cancer: recent advances. Eur Radiol. 2008;18(4): 707–15.

26. Pallwein L, Mitterberger M, Pinggera G, Aigner F, Pedross F, Gradl J, Pelzer A, Bartsch G, Frauscher F. Sonoelastography of the prostate: comparison with systematic biopsy findings in 492 patients. Eur J Radiol. 2008;65(2):304–10.

27. Parker KJ, Doyley MM, Rubens DJ. Imaging the elastic properties of tissue: the 20 year perspective. Phys Med Biol. 2011;56(2):513.

28. Salomon G, Kollerman J, Thederan I, Chun F, Budaus L, Schlomm T, Isbarn H, Heinzer H, Huland H, Graefen M. Evaluation of prostate cancer detection with ultrasound real-time elastography: a comparison with step section pathological analysis after radical prostatectomy. Euro Urol. 2008;54:1354.

29. Tsutsumi M, Miyagawa T, Matsumura T, Kawazoe N, Ishikawa S, Shimokama T, Shiina T, Miyanaga N, Akaza H. The impact of real-time tissue elasticity imaging (elastography) on the detection of prostate cancer: clinicopathological analysis. Int J Clin Oncol. 2007;12(4):250–5.

30. Ophir O. Elastography: a quantitative method for imaging the elasticity of biological tissues. Ultrasonic Imag. 1991;13(2):111–34.

31. Kapoor A, Mahajan G, Sidhu BS. Real-time elastography in the detection of prostate cancer in patients with raised PSA level. Ultrasound Med Biol. 2011; 37(9):1374–81.

32. Tsutsumi M, Miyagawa T. Real-time balloon inflation elastography for prostate cancer detection and initial evaluation of clinicopathologic analysis. Am J Roentgenol. 2010;194:471–6.

33. Barbone PE, Gokhale NH. Elastic modulus imaging: on the uniqueness and nonuniqueness of the elastography inverse problem in two dimensions. Inverse Probl. 2004;20(1):283–96.

34. Fehrenbach J. Influence of Poisson's ratio on elastographic direct and inverse problems. Phys Med Biol. 2007;52(3):707–16.

35. Bercoff J, Tanter JM, Fink M. Supersonic shear imaging: a new technique for soft tissue elasticity mapping. IEEE Trans Ultrason Ferroelectr Freq Control. 2004;51(4):396–409.

36. Richard G Barr, Richard Memo, and Carl R Schaub. Shear wave ultrasound elastography of the prostate: Initial results. Ultrasound Quarterly. 2012;28(1): 13–20.

37. Nightingale KR, Soo M, Nightingale R, Trahey GE. Acoustic radiation force impulse imaging: in vivo demonstration of clinical feasibility. Ultrasound Med Biol. 2002;28:227–35.

38. Turgay E, Salcudean S, Rohling R. Identifying the mechanical properties of tissue by ultrasound strain imaging. Ultrasound Med Biol. 2006;32(2):221–35.

Application of Prostate US for Advanced Techniques in Prostate Biopsy and Prostate Cancer Staging

Katsuto Shinohara

Abbreviations

ECE   Extracapsular extension
NPV   Negative predictive value
PPV   Positive predictive value
ROC   Receiver-operating characteristic
SVI   Seminal vesicle invasion
TRUS   Transrectal ultrasound

Introduction

Prostate cancer continues to be the most commonly diagnosed cancer in men. In 2014, the American Cancer Society estimates there will be 233,000 newly diagnosed cases and 29,480 deaths from prostate cancer [1]. Significant declines in prostate cancer mortality have been achieved in recent years, likely with screening efforts involving blood testing and with detection efforts in the form of ultrasound-guided biopsy of the prostate [2]. Transrectal ultrasound (TRUS) guided needle biopsy of the prostate is the current gold standard for the detection of prostate cancer and is the most commonly performed urological office procedure in the United States. The technique is well established and training programs have been incorporated during residency. However, occasionally unusual situations can be encountered during TRUS procedures. In the first part of this chapter, such unusual situations associated with TRUS-guided needle biopsy and solutions with advanced techniques will be discussed. The second part describes staging of prostate cancer using TRUS. TRUS staging has been underutilized due to previously published data suggesting it is of little value. However, the outcome of staging is highly dependent upon the operator. If TRUS imaging is carefully done, it will provide reliable information regarding staging of prostate cancer to help manage treatment in cost-effective ways.

Advanced Techniques in Prostate Biopsy

Anterior Tissue Biopsy

In 1989, Hodge et al. proposed the modern model of performing biopsy of defined areas of the prostate, namely the "sextant" method of prostate biopsy [3]. After the initial introduction of the sextant systematic prostate biopsy, little refinement of the technique was made until Stamey suggested moving the biopsies more laterally to better sample the anterior horns of the peripheral zone and avoid sampling error [4–6].

K. Shinohara, M.D. (✉)
Department of Urology and Helen Diller Family Comprehensive Cancer Center, University of California San Francisco, 1600 Divisadero St A634, San Francisco, CA 94143-1695, USA
e-mail: kshinohara@urol.ucsf.edu

C.R. Porter and E.M. Wolff (eds.), *Prostate Ultrasound: Current Practice and Future Directions*,
DOI 10.1007/978-1-4939-1948-2_13, © Springer Science+Business Media New York 2015

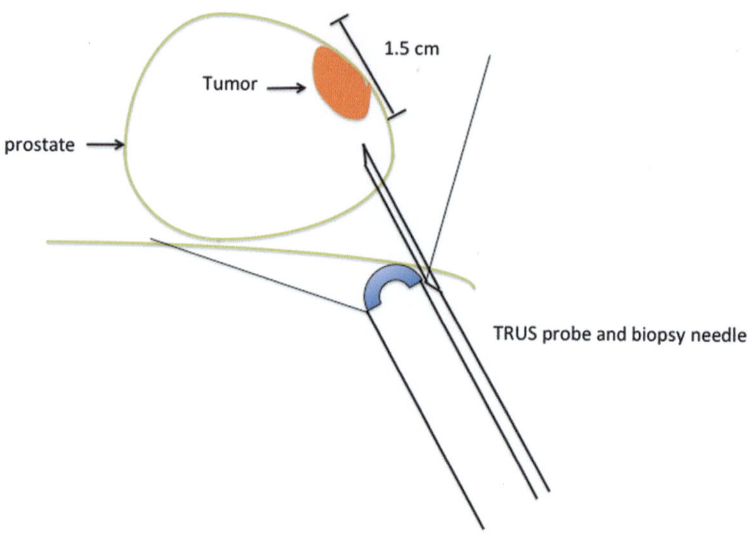

Fig. 1 Anterior tissue biopsy should be performed to obtain tissue along the anterior capsule. For random biopsy, a needle should be advanced about 1.5 cm from the anterior capsule

Such recommendations were supported by meticulous whole-mount analyses of radical prostatectomy specimens, which helped to further delineate the zonal anatomy of the prostate as well as the spatial origin of prostate cancers [7]. Extended sextant biopsy obtaining two specimens from each sextant totaling 12 samplings is common practice. Within each sextant, one biopsy is obtained from the medial part close to the median furrow of the gland and the other from the lateral part close to the lateral edge of the gland.

Anterior Apex Biopsy

Takashima et al. carefully examined radical prostatectomy specimens in 62 T1c cancer patients and reported that T1c cancer is densely located at the apex to midportion in the anterior half of the gland [8]. At UCSF, in addition to extended sextant biopsy, a pair of samples along the anterior capsule of the apex/midgland is routinely collected. With this biopsy scheme, two anterior biopsies are obtained not from the transition zone but from the peripheral zone located anterior to the urethra at the apex and extending anteriorly along the lateral edge of the midgland. Meng et al. reported that adding anterior apical biopsy to the extended sextant biopsy scheme increased cancer detection especially in patients with

normal digital rectal examination [9]. Biopsy in the middle of the transition zone is less likely to yield positive biopsy. Biopsy must be taken from the tissue along the anterior capsule. When the anterior part of the gland is biopsied, the needle tip must be located 1.5 cm from the anterior capsule in order to sample the tissue along the anterior capsule, where cancer is frequently located (Fig. 1).

In recent years, multiparametric MRI has been shown to detect prostate cancer previously not found by random needle biopsy. Those lesions are commonly located at the anterior part of the gland [10–12]. Urologists are asked to biopsy the anterior lesion more and more based on MRI findings (Figs. 2 and 3). Anterior cancer is commonly located along the capsule of the prostate. In order to obtain a useful sample of the anterior lesion, the biopsy needle must be advanced up to the edge of the lesion prior to triggering the automated biopsy device button. The biopsy needle is designed to take 15 mm tissue from the tip of the needle. However, it advances 23 mm from the needle tip. Biopsy of the anterior lesion, especially when located at the base of the gland, frequently results in the needle penetrating through the bladder wall due to the extra needle advancement (Fig. 4). This may result in significant hematuria. Careful observation of the biopsy site

Fig. 2 A 57-year-old man with PSA of 17. Two previous biopsies showed no evidence of cancer. T2 weighted MR image showed a low signal intensity area suspicious for cancer at *left* anterior base of the prostate (*arrows*)

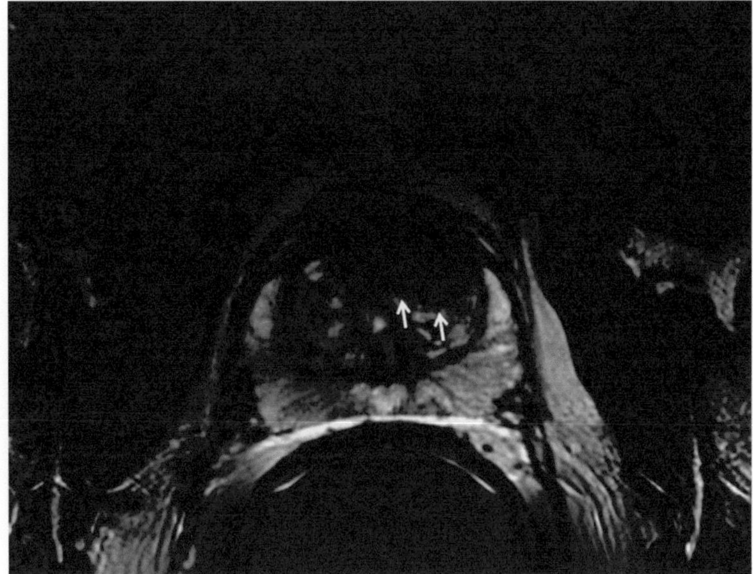

Fig. 3 Same patient on TRUS, a hypoechoic area was seen at *left* anterior base (*arrows*)

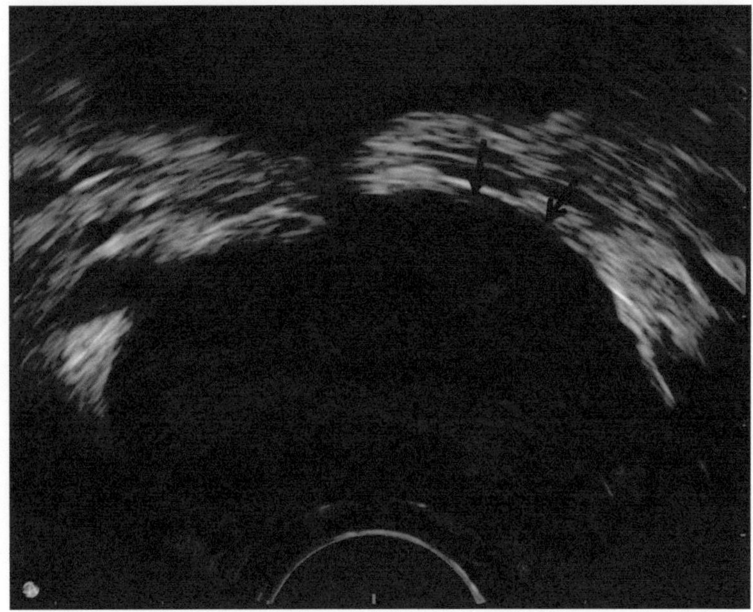

often shows the extent of the bladder wall bleeding. Mild oozing without pulsating bleeding seen by ultrasound generally stops by itself. However, persistent pulsating and pumping bleeding seen on ultrasound may need attention (Fig. 5). If bleeding persists after a few minutes of observation, a Foley catheterization with mild traction may be necessary to monitor and control the bleeding.

Midline Lesion Biopsy

A midline lesion may be missed by random biopsy, since a biopsy is commonly not taken from midline tissue. However, cancer can be found over the midline (Fig. 6). Biopsy of the midline, especially at the apex, is delicate because the biopsy needle may penetrate the urethra in a sagittal plane biopsy. In this setting, biopsy can

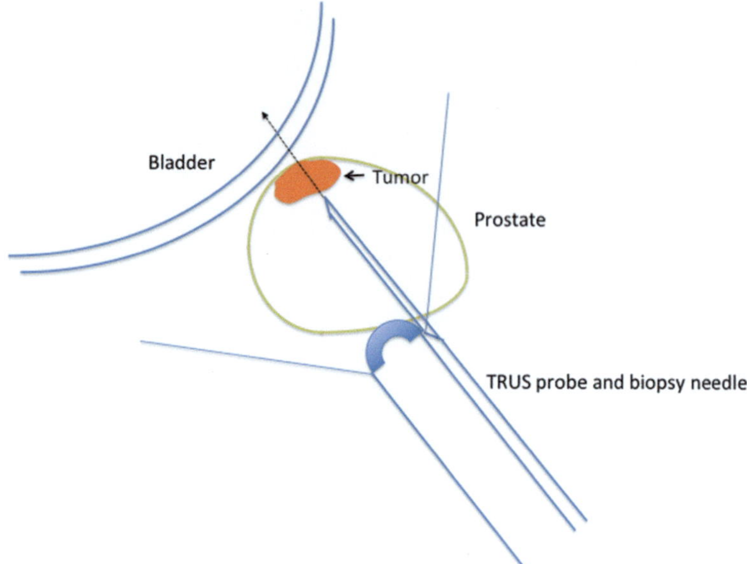

Fig. 4 In order to take an anterior base lesion, a biopsy needle has to be advanced just before the target area. Generally, the biopsy needle advances beyond the capsule and often results in penetration of the bladder wall

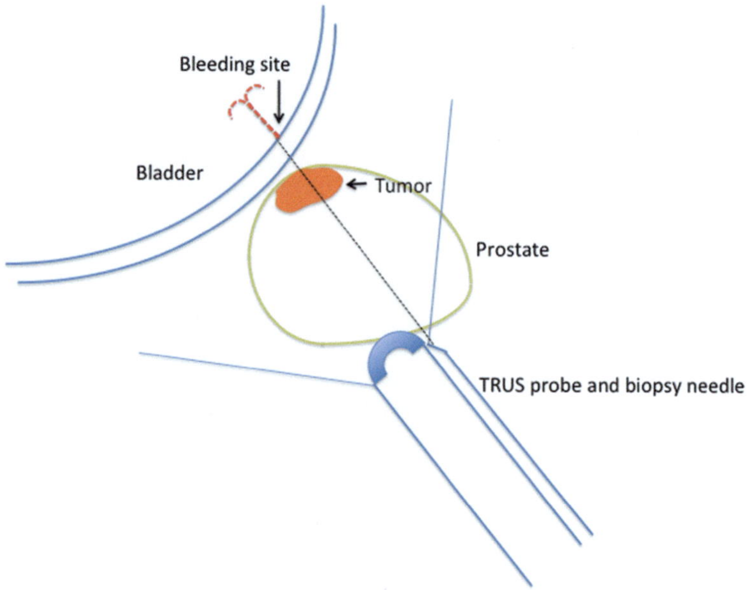

Fig. 5 Observation of the puncture site of the bladder wall by TRUS after biopsy is important. Pulsating bleeding can be seen if a small artery is injured

be performed in transverse view and the biopsy needle can be obliquely inserted in the midline apical nodule in order to prevent urethral injury (Fig. 7). The same strategy can be used for anterior midline lesion found on TRUS or MRI. Again, biopsy of the anterior midline lesion in sagittal view requires the needle to penetrate the urethral lumen. In order to avoid urethral injury, biopsy should be done in transverse view to avoid the needle entering into the urethral lumen (Fig. 8).

Extraprostatic Tissue Biopsy

Seminal Vesicle Biopsy

Routine seminal vesicle biopsy is usually not necessary. However, patients with significant disease found at the base of the prostate or abnormal seminal vesicle appearance should undergo seminal vesicle biopsy. Seminal vesicle abnormality is not apparent in patients previously treated with radiation therapy, but risk of seminal vesicle

Fig. 6 A 55-year-old man with previous biopsy by referring urologist showing 1 mm focus of Gleason grade 3 + 4 cancer. TRUS revealed a hypoechoic area over the midline at apex (*arrow*)

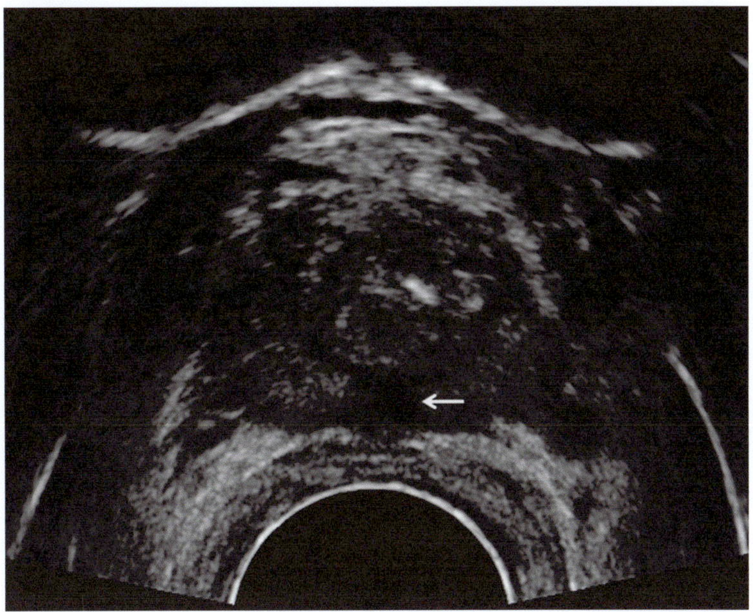

Fig. 7 A hypoechoic area over the midline at apex can be biopsied in transverse view in order to avoid urethral puncture

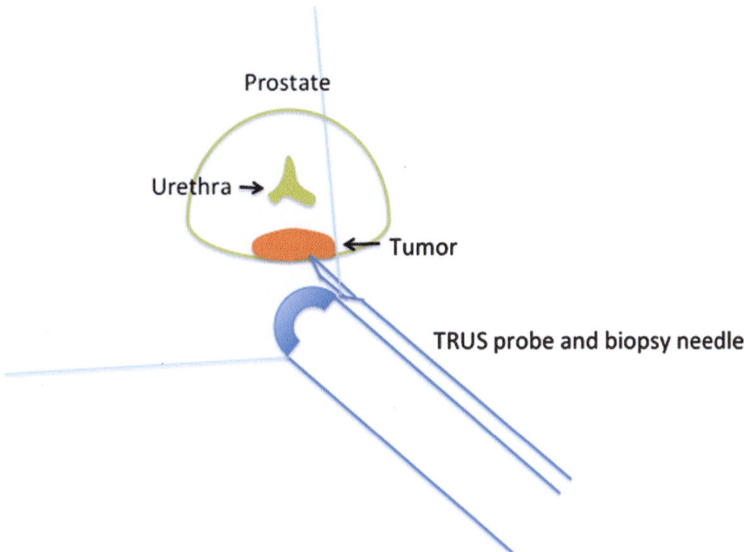

invasion is high for patients with local failure after radiation therapy [13]. In this population, seminal vesicle biopsy should be performed regardless of findings. In order to obtain a meaningful pathology specimen, the base of the seminal vesicle near the junction of the prostate should be biopsied, since tumor invasion always occurs from the base. In order to avoid confusion between cancer in the prostate next to seminal vesicle and seminal vesicle invasion, the needle tip must be advanced against the seminal vesicle base before taking the biopsy (Fig. 9).

Fig. 8 A lesion anterior to the urethra can also be biopsied in transverse view in order to avoid urethral penetration

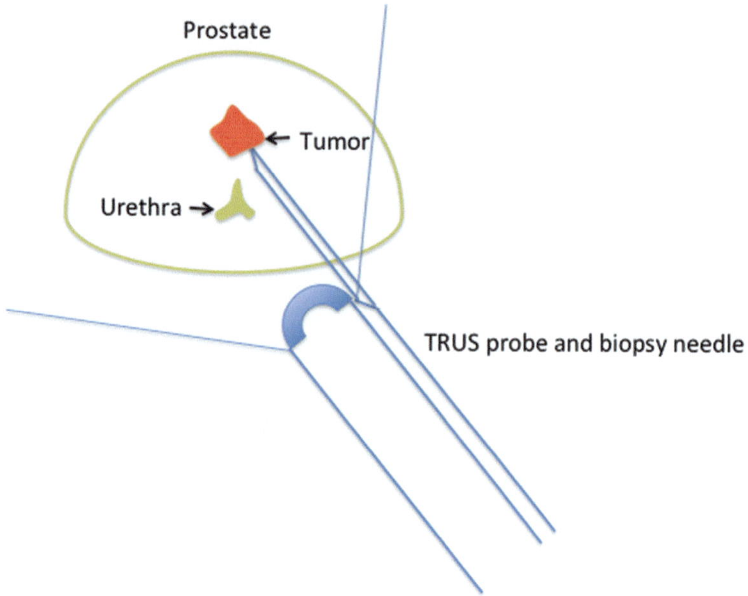

Fig. 9 Biopsy of the seminal vesicle should be aimed at the base of the seminal vesicle. Biopsy of the base of the prostate should be avoided

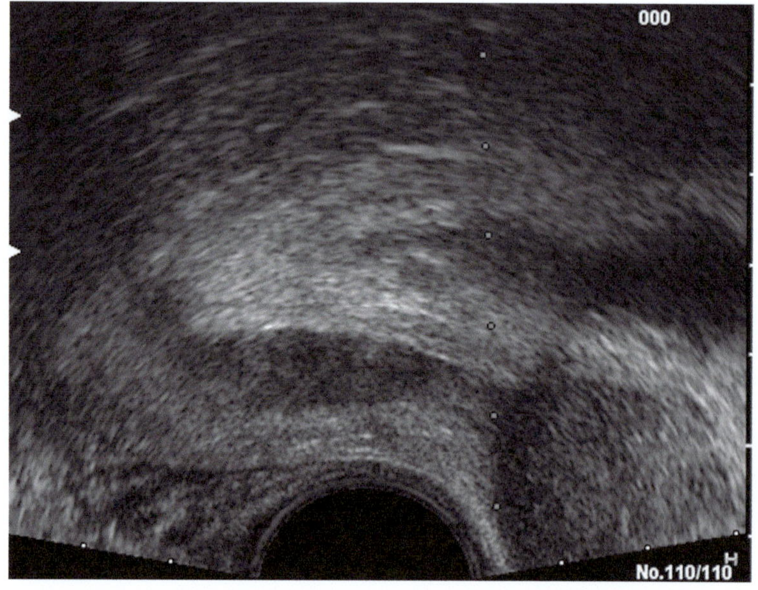

Bladder Neck Biopsy

In patients with locally extensive disease or patients with local recurrence after radiation therapy, bladder neck invasion can be observed on TRUS. If histological confirmation is necessary, the tissue diagnosis can be made by TRUS-guided biopsy of the bladder neck rather than cystoscopic biopsy (Fig. 10). A needle must be advanced right up to the suspicious tissue at the bladder neck; then the biopsy gun should be triggered. As with a base anterior lesion biopsy, the needle always penetrates the bladder mucosa. Careful observation of bladder wall bleeding from the biopsy site by TRUS is necessary.

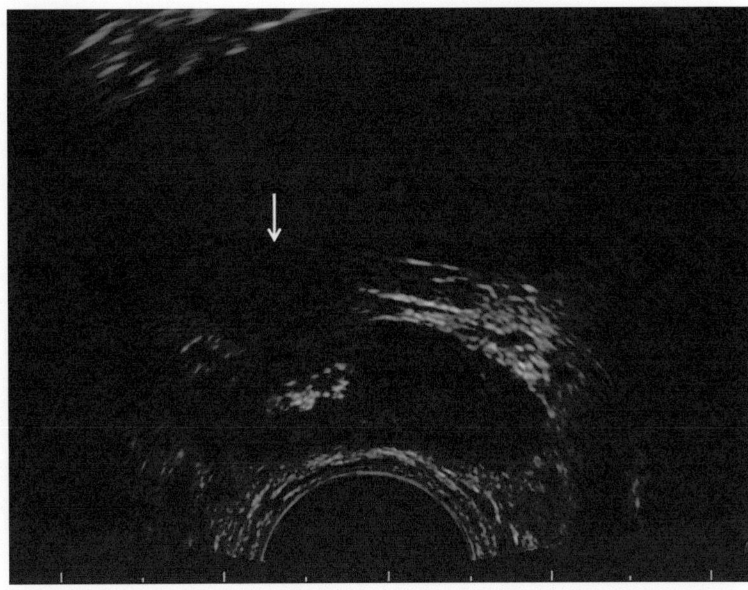

Fig. 10 A 49-year-old man status post radiation therapy for Gleason grade 4 + 5 cancer 3 years ago presented with rising PSA. TRUS revealed a mass extending from the right lobe of the prostate to the bladder neck (*arrow*). In order to biopsy this tissue, a needle has to be advanced beyond the prostate gland

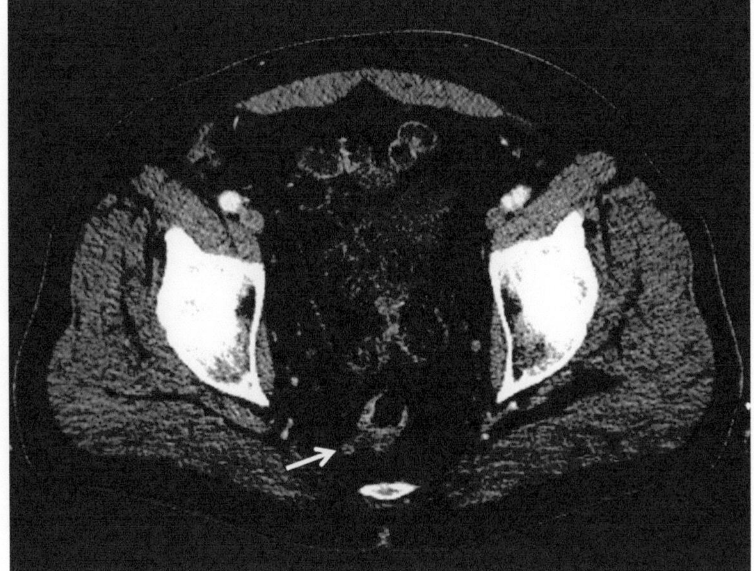

Fig. 11 A 78-year-old man status post high-dose rate radiation therapy for Gleason grade 4 + 4, PSA 22.3 ng/ml cancer 11 years ago presented with rising PSA to 1.398 ng/ml. CT scan revealed a 9 mm perirectal lymph node (*arrow*)

Periprostatic or Rectal Lymph Node

For advanced disease or post radiation patients with biochemical failure, sometimes enlarged lymph nodes can be seen in the perirectal space or periprostatic tissue. If it is noted, biopsy of the lymph node can be performed (Figs. 11 and 12). However since large pelvic vessels may be nearby laterally, only lymph nodes in a safe area, such as anterior to the prostate or posterior to the rectum, should be biopsied transrectally.

Mass Anterior to the Prostate

During TRUS, abnormal tissue anterior to the prostate may be encountered. Biopsy of those

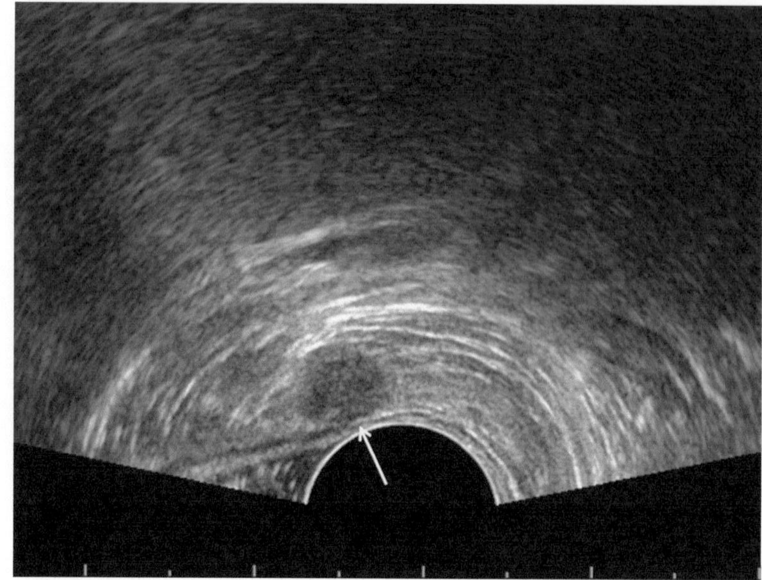

Fig. 12 Same patient. The perirectal lymph node was visualized by TRUS (*arrow*). Biopsy of the prostate and seminal vesicles did not show any evidence of local recurrence. However, biopsy of the lymph node revealed metastatic adenocarcinoma Gleason grade 4 + 4

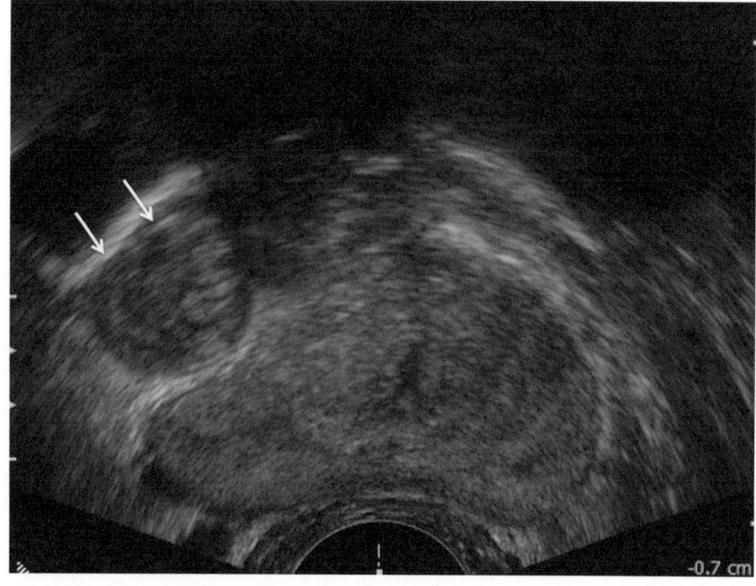

Fig. 13 A 62-year-old man with elevated PSA of 8.7 was found to have a round mass anterior to the right lobe of the prostate (*arrows*). Biopsy of the mass showed degenerated prostatic stroma only

lesions frequently requires a needle completely traversing through the prostate tissue to get to the anterior aspect of the prostate gland (Fig. 13).

Prostate cancer may recur in the rectal wall due to cancer cell seeding by previous biopsy (Fig. 14). Malignancy unrelated to the prostate gland can be also encountered in the rectal wall (Fig. 15). Needle biopsy of such lesions may be necessary. Of course, biopsy of the rectal wall requires the needle tip to be advanced shallowly just before the lesion prior to triggering the biopsy gun.

Biopsy of Local Recurrence After Radical Prostatectomy

Biochemical failure with detectable PSA after radical prostatectomy can be seen in 30–40 % of cases in follow-up. Patients with a slow PSA rise

Fig. 14 A 65-year-old man status post radical prostatectomy was found to have a palpable nodule in the prostatic fossa with elevating PSA. TRUS showed a mass in the rectal wall (*black arrows*). Biopsy of the mass revealed Gleason grade 4+4 adenocarcinoma of the prostate

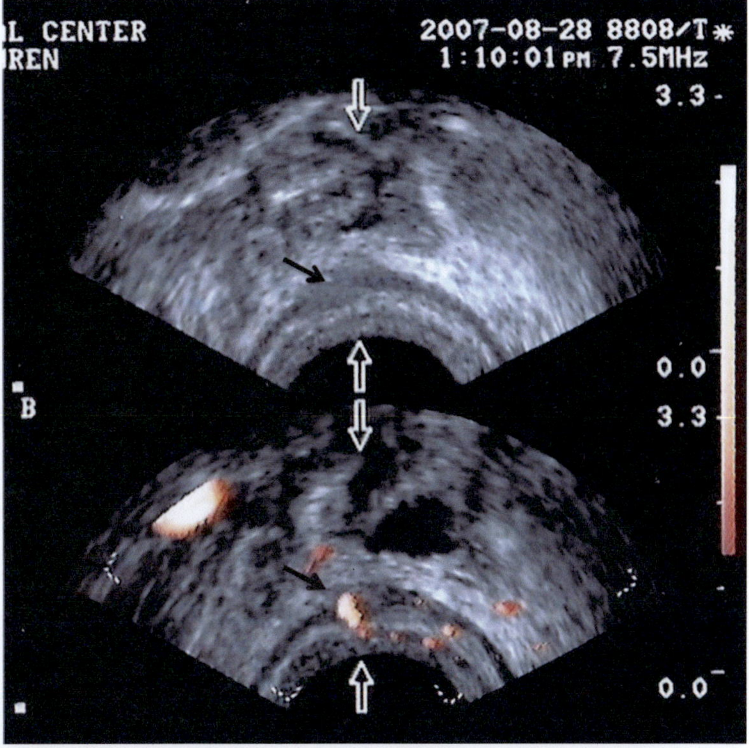

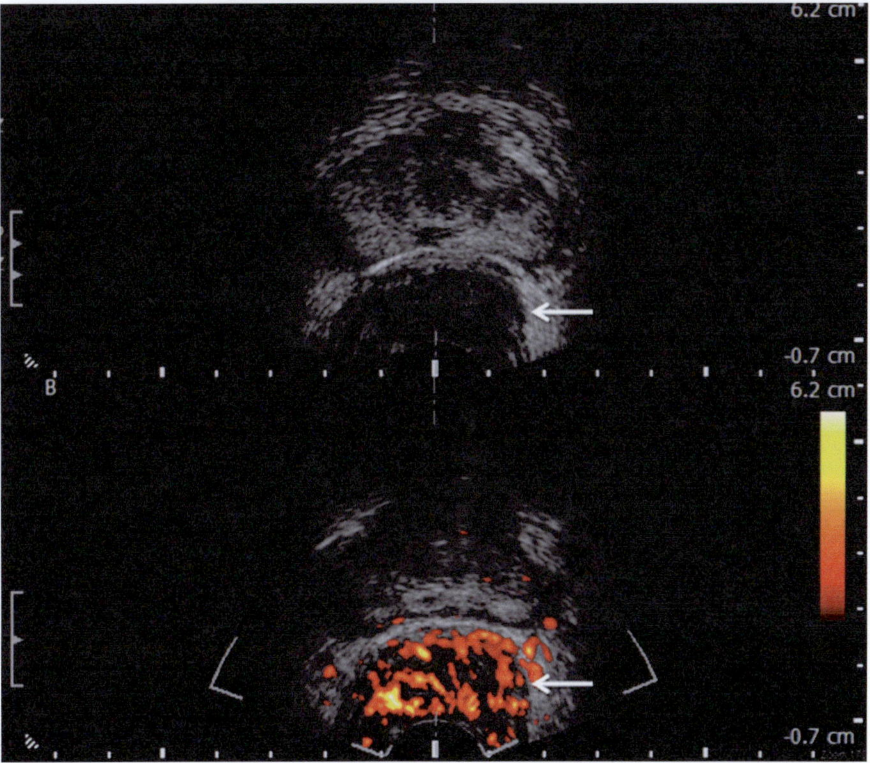

Fig. 15 A 45-year-old HIV positive man was found to have a rectal mass. Biopsy of the mass under proctoscope revealed only normal rectal mucosa. TRUS showed a hypervascular submucosal mass in the rectal wall. Biopsy revealed low-grade squamous cell carcinoma

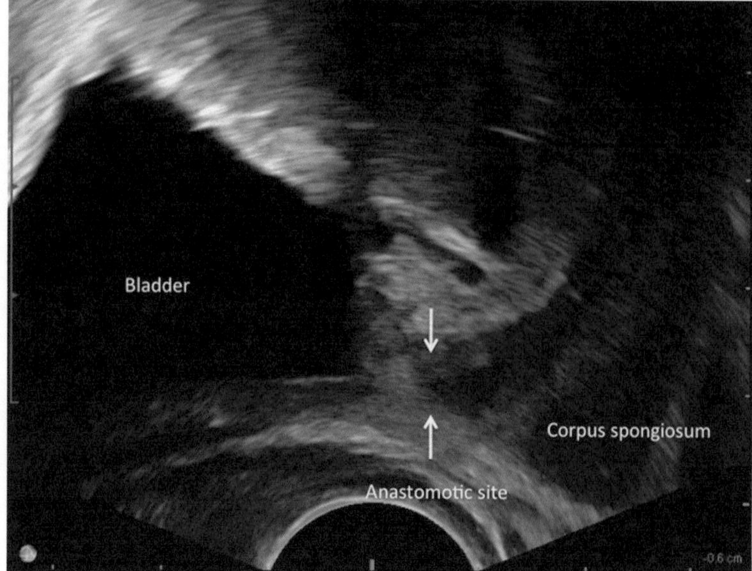

Fig. 16 Typical sagittal TRUS image of post radical prostatectomy patient. Anastomotic site is identifiable by the area where echogenicity changes from echogenic bladder neck to hypoechoic membranous urethra (*arrows*)

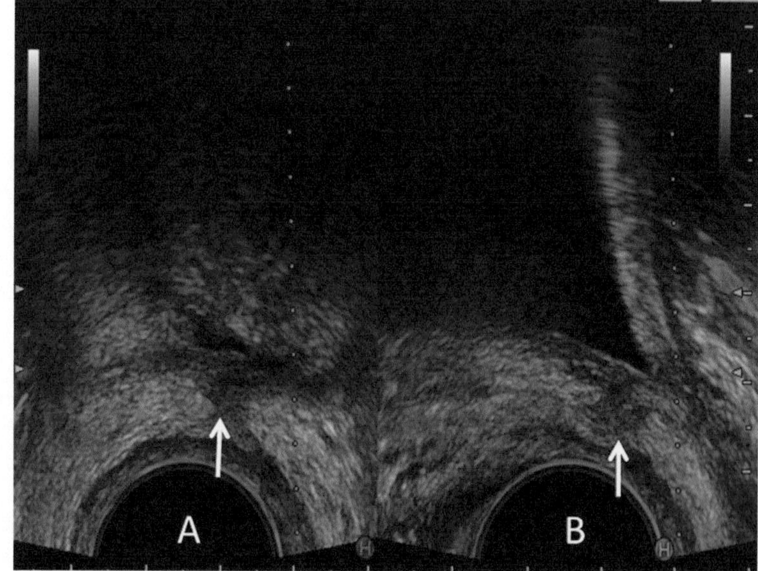

Fig. 17 A 61-year-old man status post radical prostatectomy with gradual rise of PSA to 0.52 ng/ml. TRUS showed a hypoechoic tissue suspicious for local recurrence at the posterior aspect of the bladder neck over midline (*arrows*). (**a**) Transverse view, (**b**) sagittal view

and evidence of a positive surgical margin at the time of radical prostatectomy are more likely to have local recurrence. Biopsy in this setting is not generally considered mandatory prior to radiation therapy. However, confirmation of pathology and fiduciary marker placement may help to improve outcome.

Anatomy of Anastomotic Site After Radical Prostatectomy

Recognition of TRUS-based anatomy of the anastomotic site is important in order to accurately take a biopsy. On a sagittal view in the midline the anastomotic site is clearly identifiable as the area where the low echogenicity of the membranous urethra suddenly changes to a more echogenic tubularized segment of the bladder neck (Fig. 16) [14]. Local recurrence is commonly located proximal to this area and on the side or posterior aspect of the tabularized segment of bladder neck (Fig. 17) [15]. Identifying the membranous urethra, as described in the normal transrectal prostate biopsy section, also helps orient the true midline of the patient.

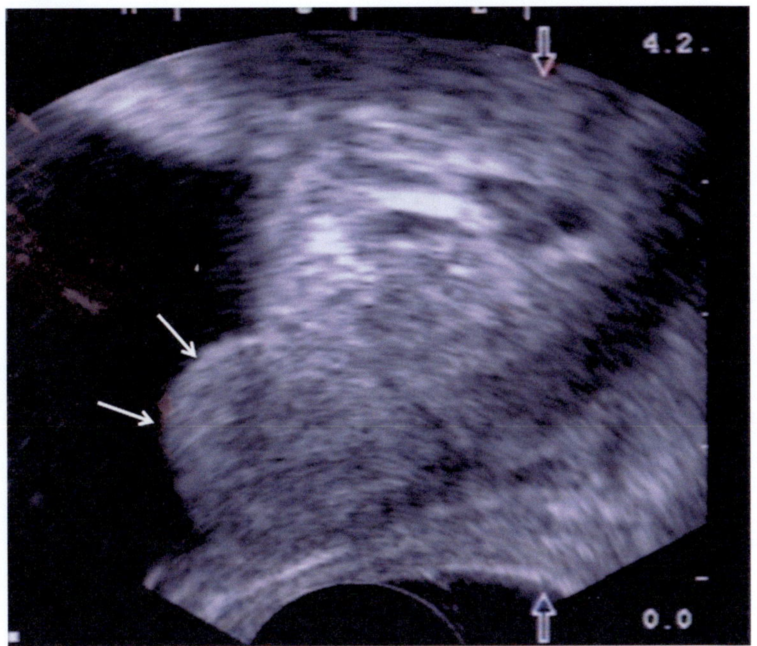

Fig. 18 A 62-year-old man status post radical prostatectomy with detectable PSA of 0.43 ng/ml. TRUS revealed tissue resembling residual median lobe of the prostate (*arrows*). Biopsy of the tissue showed benign prostatic tissue

Biopsy Technique

On the TRUS image, the bladder neck tissue can be seen as a tubularized segment. A local recurrence is frequently seen on the side or posterior aspect of this tubularized segment of the bladder neck as hypoechoic tissue. When the probe is slightly tilted to obtain an off midline image, hypoechoic tissue can be seen isolated from the bladder neck. This finding is very suspicious for local recurrence. Some lesions can be seen as an asymmetrical thickening of the tissue around the anastomotic site or behind the bladder on a transverse image. Occasionally, benign prostatic tissue that persists after radical prostatectomy can be seen as isoechoic tissue (Fig. 18). Local anesthesia is usually not necessary, since only a few samples are taken. However, similar to the apex biopsy, a needle can stimulate the proctocanal when this area is biopsied. The needle tip can easily penetrate through the bladder wall in this population. Observation of the bladder wall by TRUS as described before to confirm the degree of hematuria after biopsy is always necessary for this procedure, since bladder wall bleeding is quite common.

Biopsy of Prostate for Patient Without Anus or With Severe Anal Stricture

Patients that have undergone abdominoperineal resection of the rectum (APR) have no access to the rectum. Digital rectal examination or transrectal ultrasonography cannot be performed, and often prostate cancer diagnosis can be delayed. PSA is the only tool for screening prostate cancer in this population. Transperineal ultrasound-guided prostate biopsy can be performed [16]. Generally, the procedure is performed with the patient in the left lateral decubitus position as in a regular TRUS procedure. In order to visualize the urethra and bladder clearly, placement of Foley catheter in advance is recommended. Intra-prostatic information is very difficult to obtain by transperineal ultrasound. The more important task of ultrasound in this procedure is localization and delineation of the prostate itself. For this purpose, an end-fire probe with a lower frequency setting, 5–6 MHz, is ideal for scanning, since better penetration and visualization of deeper tissue is required. After

Fig. 19 A 64-year-old man status post abdomino-perineal resection of rectum from ulcerative colitis was found to have an elevated PSA of 5.6 ng/ml. Transperineal ultrasound revealed clear image of the prostate gland in transverse view

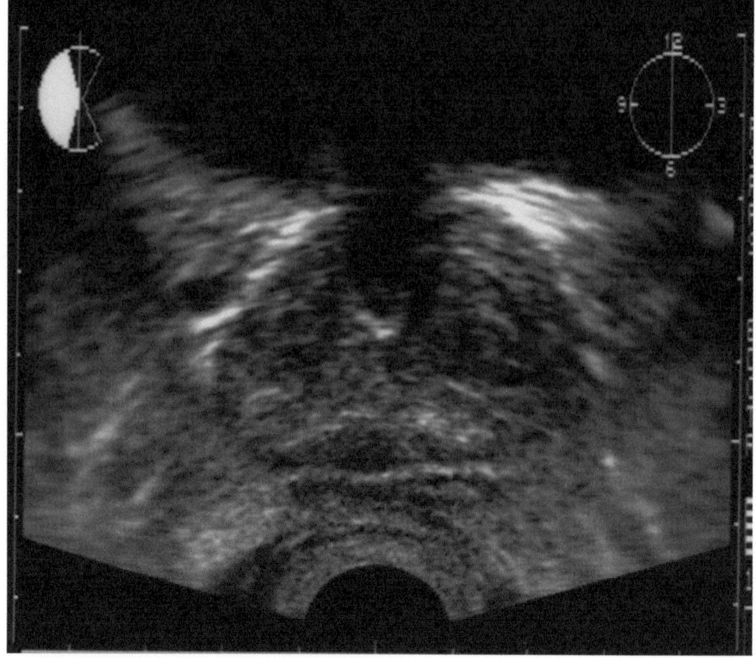

Fig. 20 Same patient in sagittal view in midline. A Foley catheter and a balloon were identifiable

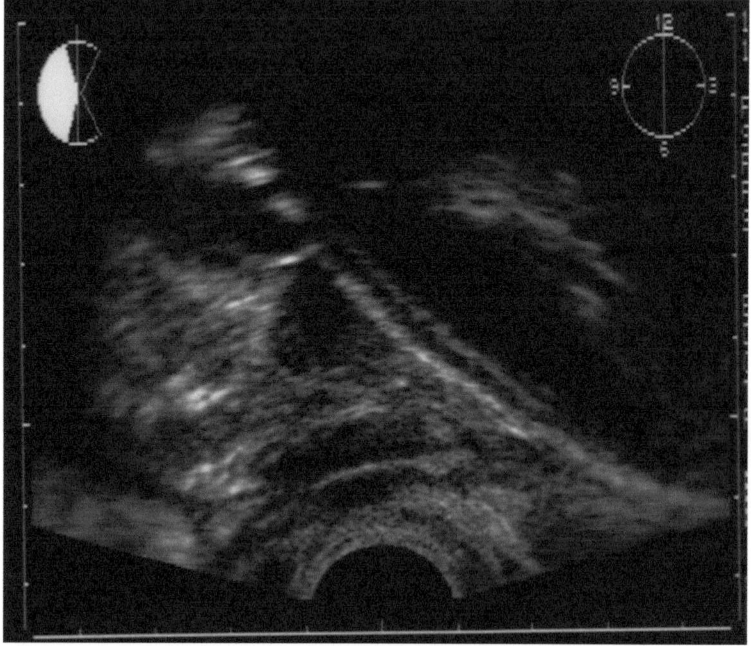

preparation of the skin with antiseptic solution, a probe is applied on the previous anus location that is frequently identifiable by a small skin dimple. Once the Foley catheter is identified, follow the catheter to identify the balloon. At this point, the prostate is seen next to the balloon. The prostate can be visualized either in a longitudinal or cross-sectional image (Figs. 19 and 20). Local anesthesia is given to the perineal skin, pelvic floor, and all the way to the prostate gland by ultrasound guidance. Care must be paid not to inject air during anesthesia, since this will significantly disturb the visual-

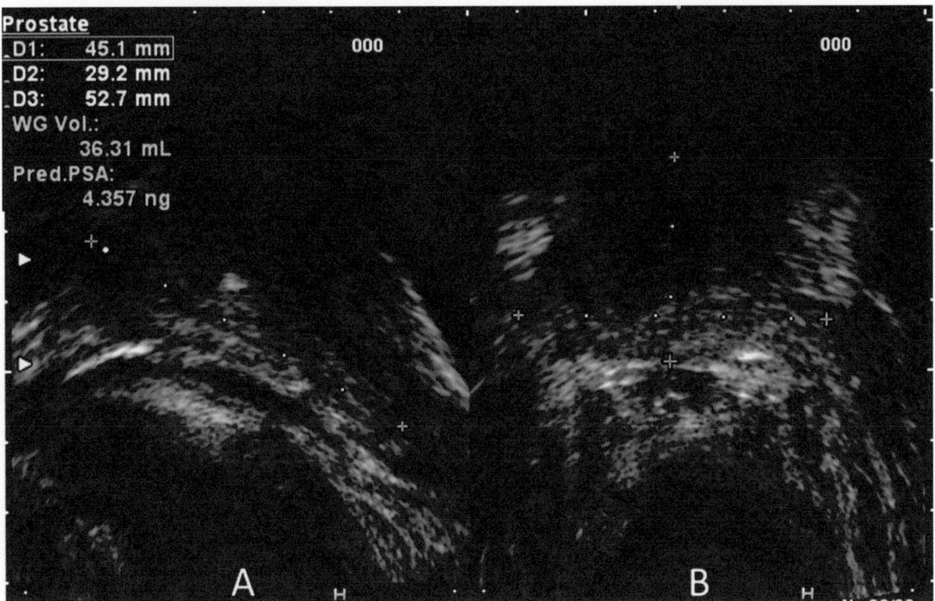

Fig. 21 A 69-year-old man status post low anterior resection of rectum resulted in severe stricture of the proctocanal. TRUS probe was applied over the anus and prostate was clearly visualized in sagittal view (**A**) and transverse view (**B**) for biopsy

ization of the prostate gland. Prostate biopsy can be done either with a sagittal or coronal view. The needle is advanced until it reaches the prostate capsule, as confirmed by ultrasound and a tactile sensation. After the needle tip reaches the prostatic capsule, the biopsy specimen is taken. Extended sextant biopsy of 12 samples can be obtained. Seminal vesicles are frequently biopsied as a staging purpose whenever it is visible, since the local staging cannot be performed by either digital rectal examination or transrectal ultrasonography. For a patient with severe anal stricture due to previous surgery or sphincter spasm, the TRUS probe can be applied over the anus and local anesthesia applied to the perianal tissue anterior to the anus. The prostate gland can be visible in this position and biopsy can be done as in the post-APR patient (Fig. 21).

TRUS Staging

More accurate pretreatment staging of prostate cancer permits the appropriate selection of therapy and increases the likelihood of a favorable treatment outcome. Although there are many imaging techniques available to help assess stage, there is no clear standard modality that is uniformly accurate, sensitive, and specific yet minimally invasive and cost-effective. Although conventional gray-scale ultrasound imaging of the prostate can be performed in a variety of ways, TRUS provides the clearest view of the prostate. TRUS is the most common imaging test for prostate cancer because it is almost universally used to assist in obtaining initial systematic and directed biopsies of the prostate. Additionally, many urologists have familiarity with this imaging technique and the potential side effects of TRUS imaging are minor.

Staging Category

Extracapsular Extension (ECE)

It has been reported that TRUS is superior to digital rectal examination in staging prostate cancer; however, subsequent reports have shown discouraging results [17–20]. Although the criteria for differentiating stages T1 and T2 from non-organ confined stages T3 and T4 are somewhat ambiguous, in general the disappearance or disruption of

Table 1 TRUS staging category

Category	Absent	Probably absent	Indeterminate	Probably present	Present
ECE	Smooth outline throughout the gland	Small hypoechoic area with minimal bulging	Large tumor abuts capsule but minimum bulging	Large tumor abuts capsule with significant bulge	Gross tumor extension seen
	No tissue bulging except for BPH nodule	Capsular distortion without hypoechoic area	Large tumor with capsular distortion	Obscured boundary with double shadowing	Abnormal layer of tissue seen outside of the gland
SVI	Symmetrical clear boundary and separation of ampullae and seminal vesicles	Small abnormal tissue behind the ampullae	Obvious tissue bulge at the base but separated from the seminal vesicles	Obscured boundary posterior to the ampullae	Thick solid looking base of the seminal vesicle
				No clear separation of ampullae and seminal vesicles	Posterior bulging of the seminal vesicle base

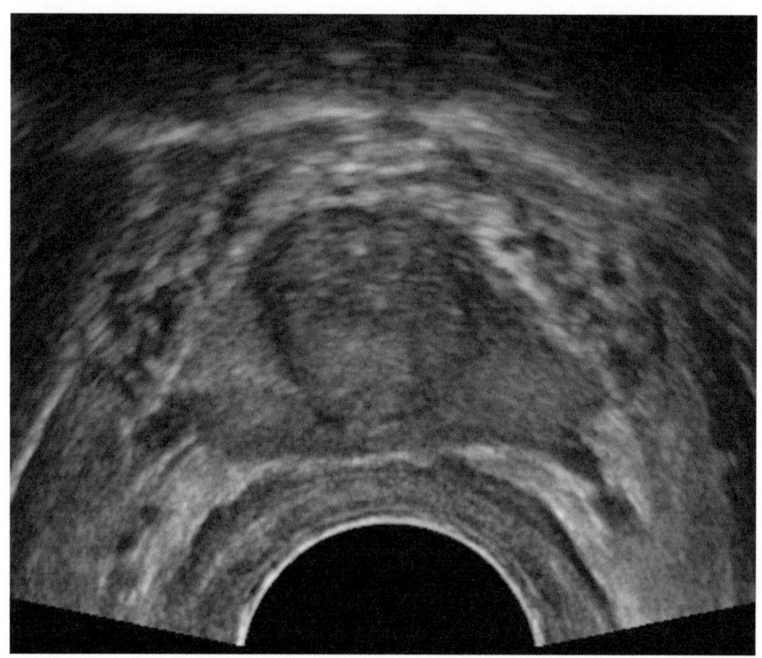

Fig. 22 ECE absent. Prostate gland has smooth outline without capsular bulge or irregularity

the prostate capsule, capsule irregularity, and asymmetry of the prostate or seminal vesicle are all used [21]. Based on these criteria, microscopic tumor extension cannot be diagnosed, although gross tumor extension can be identified. Rosen et al. have reported that a significant number of clinically localized tumors will be shown to be unconfined on surgical pathology. They found elements of non-organ confined disease including extracapsular extension and seminal vesicle invasion in up to 85 and 35 % of stage T2c tumors, respectively; importantly, on pathologic exam a positive surgical margin was found in 40 % of these patients [22]. Furthermore, Ohori et al. have shown that, even if the prostate capsule appears intact, focal tumor extension should be suspected; if the hypoechoic area bulges out from the boundary, the boundary is irregularly serrated, or the prostate contour loses its roundness [23]. At UCSF this author divides the ultrasound-based staging system into five grades with respect to extracapsular extension: absent, probably absent, indeterminate, probably present, and present. The appearance of each is summarized in Table 1 and representative images for each category are shown in Figs. 22, 23, 24, 25, 26, 27, 28, and 29.

Fig. 23 ECE absent. A hypoechoic area is seen in the *left* lobe (*arrow*) without any evidence of ECE

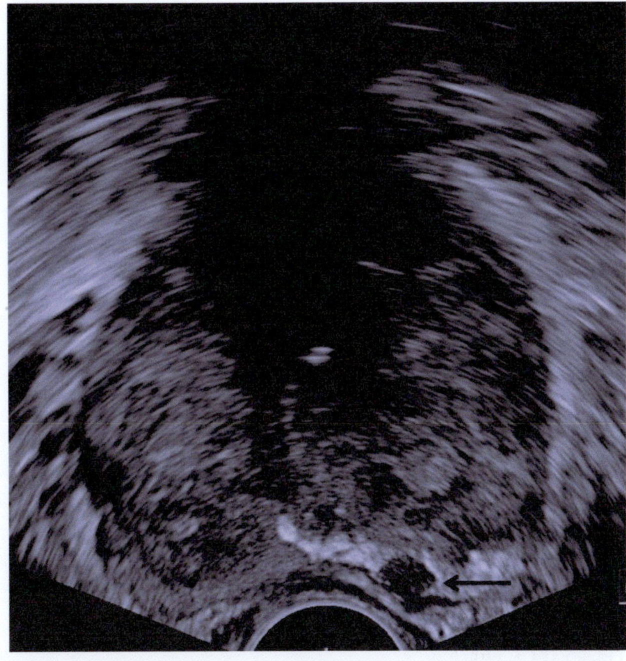

Fig. 24 ECE probably absent. A small hypoechoic area is seen in the *left* lobe with slight bulge of capsule (*arrow*)

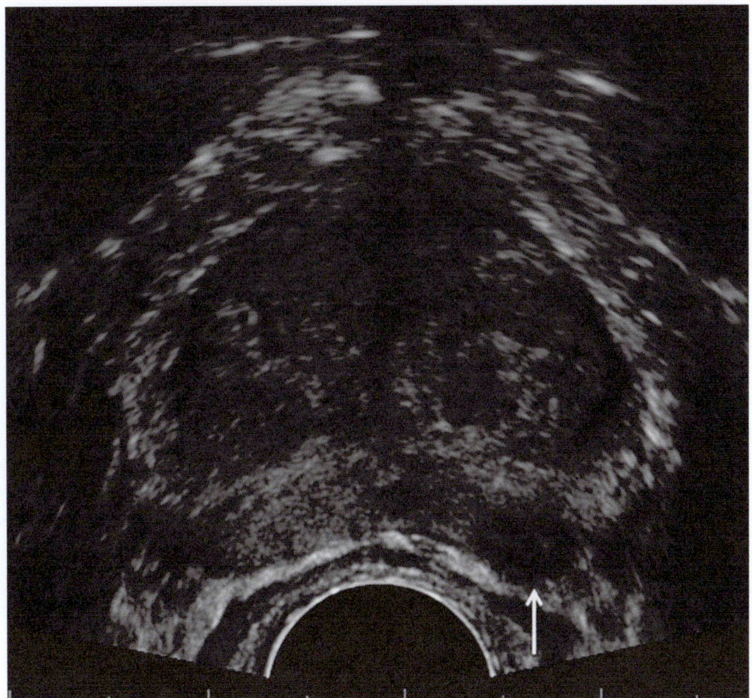

Seminal Vesicle Invasion

Asymmetry of the seminal vesicles is thought to be a sign of seminal vesicle invasion [24, 25]. However, in early invasion, the shape does not change dramatically. In addition, asymmetrical seminal vesicles are not rare in the normal population. Salo et al. and Pontes et al. have reported the specificity of TRUS in seminal vesicle invasion to be very high, but the sensitivity to be only 25–29 % because of overlooked early

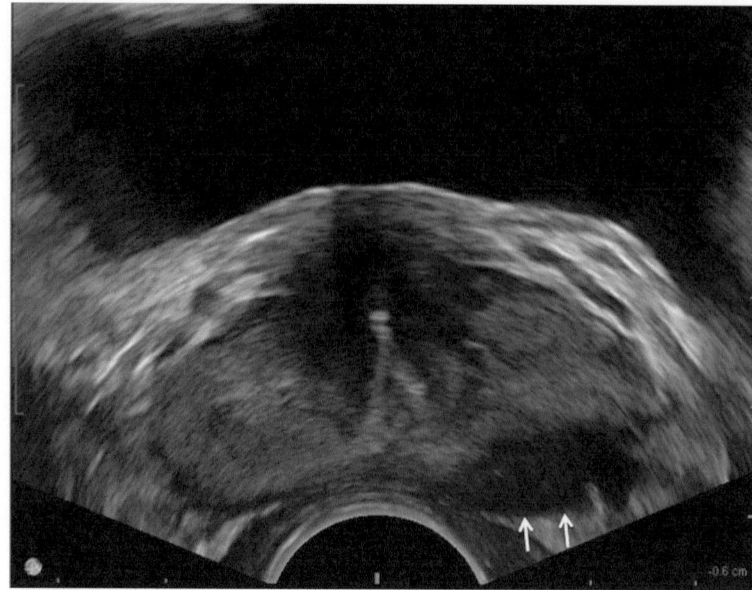

Fig. 25 ECE indeterminate. A large hypoechoic area abuts the capsule in a wide area with minimal capsular bulge

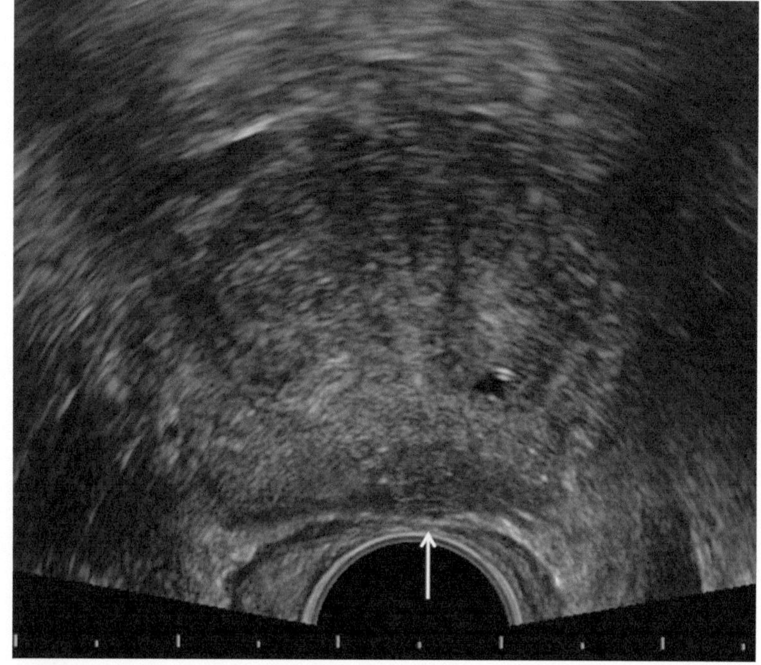

Fig. 26 ECE probably present. A large hypoechoic area abuts the capsule in a wide area with a sharp point of capsular bulge (*arrow*). Of note, microcalcification in the hypoechoic area suggests high-grade disease

invasion [26, 27]. Three routes of seminal vesicle invasion are known: (1) along the ejaculatory ducts with medial invasion into ampulla and seminal vesicles; (2) lateral invasion via the vascular pedicle of the prostate with external entry into the seminal vesicle; (3) metastasis without communication between the prostate and seminal vesicle lesion [28]. In the first case, the seminal vesicle may retain symmetry, but the base of the seminal vesicle thickens and shows convexity towards the rectum (Figs. 30, 31, and 32). In the second case, cancer is located in the lateral aspect

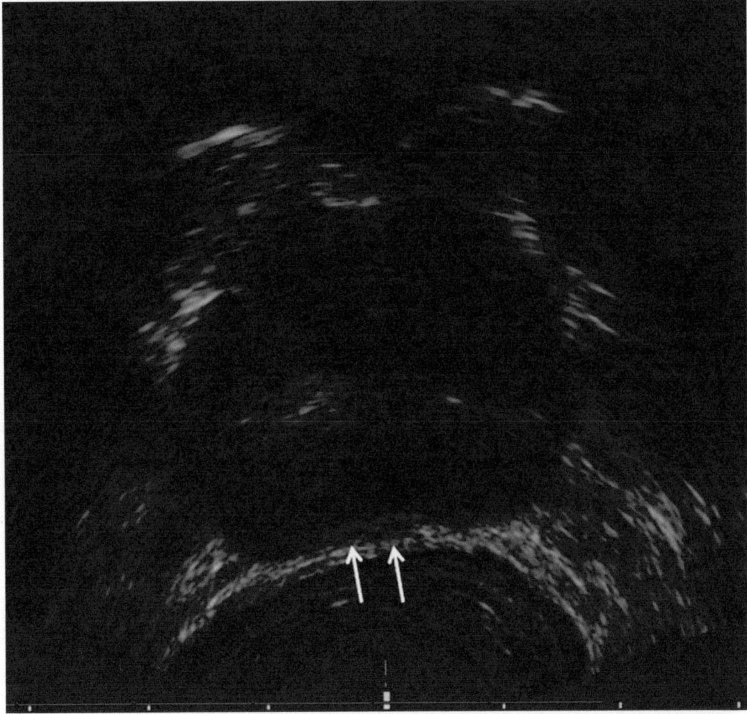

Fig. 27 ECE probably present. Posterior aspect of the prostate gland is obscured. Abnormal fuzzy tissue is seen behind the prostate capsule (*arrows*)

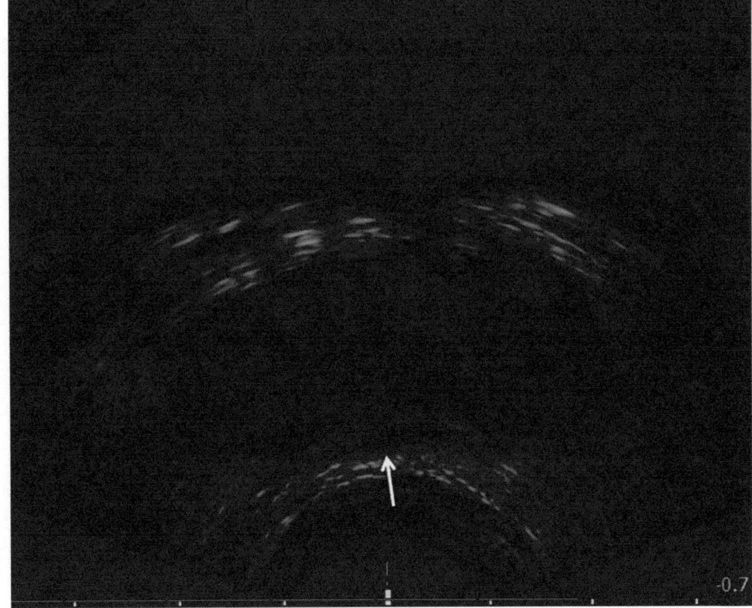

Fig. 28 ECE present. At the base of the prostate, a large amount of abnormal tissue extending behind the prostate creating double boundaries is seen (*arrow*)

of the prostate. Widening of the angle between the prostate and seminal vesicle, a bridge of hypoechoic tissue between, and disappearance of the intervening fat plane are the characteristic signs [29]. Careful observation of the junction of the seminal vesicle and the prostate—not the body of the seminal vesicle—is important in diagnosing early invasion.

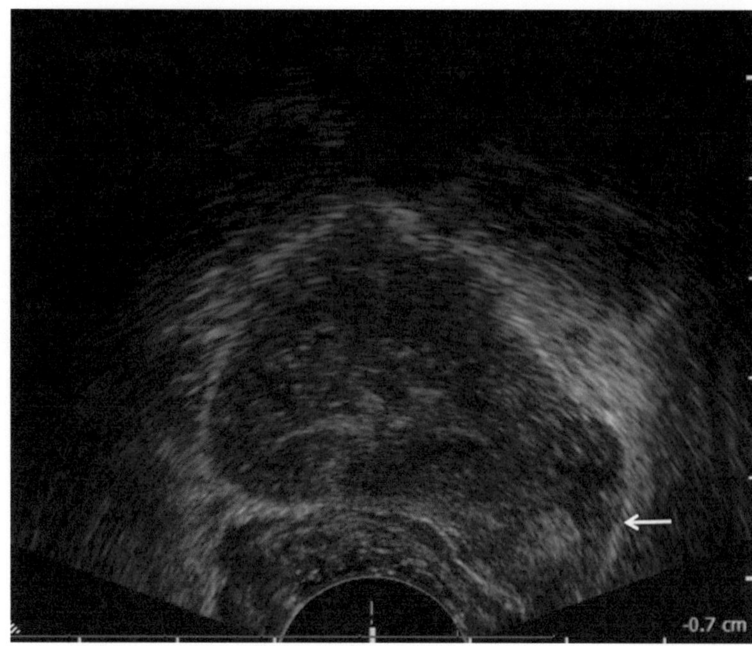

Fig. 29 ECE present. Obvious gross tumor extension is seen (*arrow*)

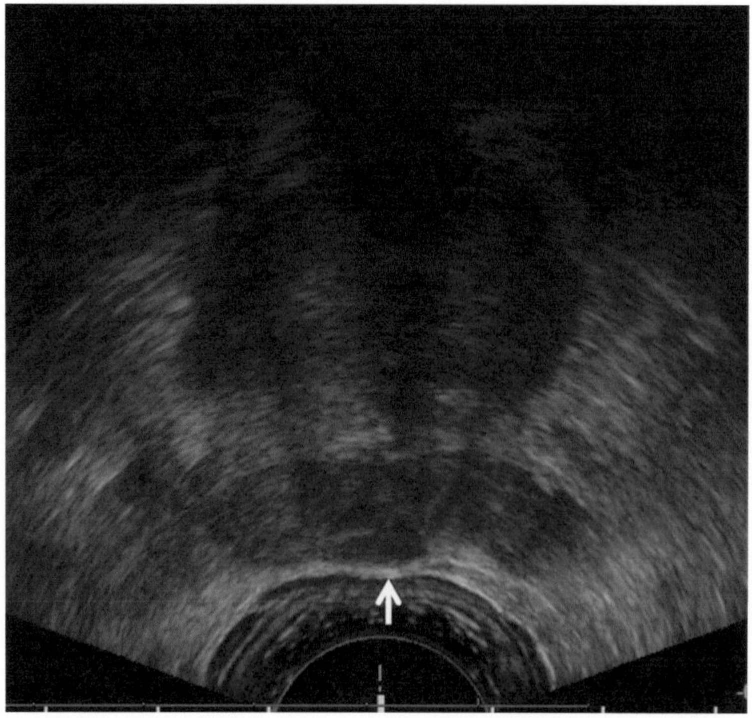

Fig. 30 A hypoechoic tissue is seen behind the ampullae of the vas deferens. SVI is probably present

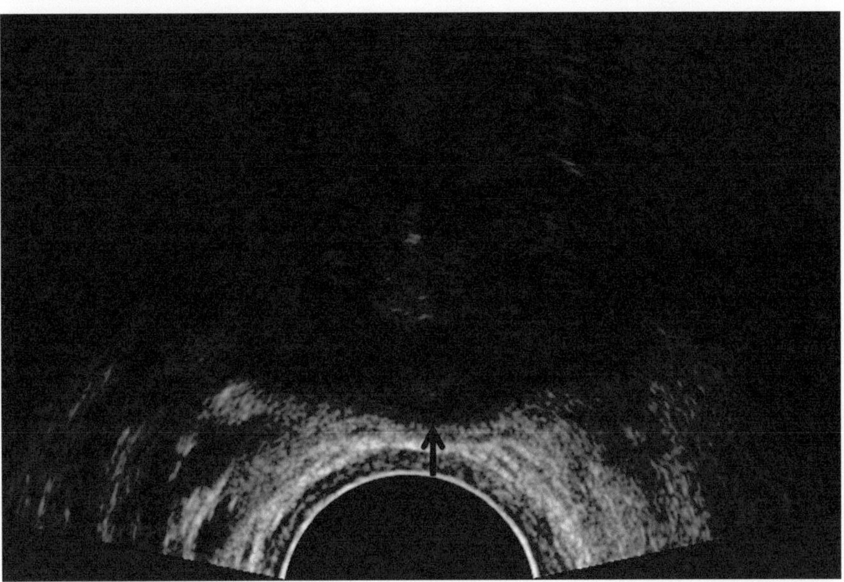

Fig. 31 Smaller hypoechoic tissue bulging posteriorly in the midline and extending behind the ampullae is seen (*arrow*). Obviously, tumor extends beyond the prostatic capsule. However, SVI is indeterminate

Fig. 32 SVI present. Abnormal fuzzy appearing tissue is seen surrounding the posterior aspect of the ampullae and *left* seminal vesicle (*arrows*)

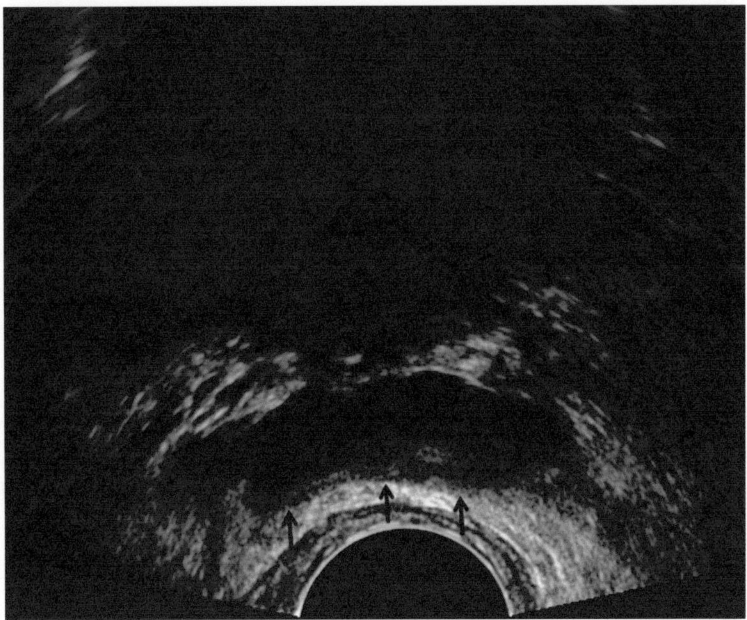

Results of TRUS Staging

A comparison of reported results for staging accuracy by TRUS and radical prostatectomy specimen is shown in Table 2 [20, 30–34]. These reports, however, used different equipment, criteria, and histological methods and were based on the highly selected group of patients who were candidates for radical prostatectomy. Wolf et al. and

Table 2 TRUS staging in the literature

Author	Year		Sensitivity	Specificity	PPV	NPV	Accuracy
Eisenberg et al. [36]	2011	ECE	31	92	58	80	77
		SVI	4	99.8	67	93	93
Bates et al. [39]	1997	ECE	23	86			
		SVI	33	100			
Presti et al. [40]	1996	ECE	48	71	50	69	
		SVI	75	98	75	98	
Rifkin et al. [32]	1990	ECE	66	46	63	49	58
		SVI	22	88			
Hardeman et al. [41]	1989	ECE	54	58	62	50	56
		SVI	60	89	67	86	82
Salo et al. [26]	1987	ECE	86	94	92	89	90
		SVI	29	100	100	75	77

Figures in %

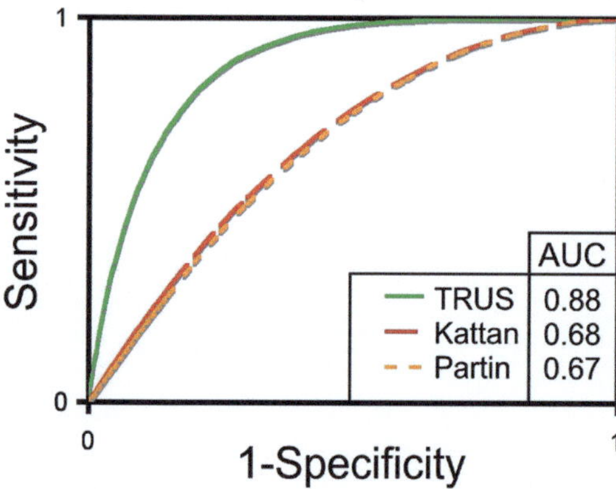

Fig. 33 ROC curve for TRUS, Kattan nomogram, Partin table for detecting ECE or SVI. TRUS alone is clearly superior to the nomogram or table. (Figure cited from [36] with permission)

Gerber et al. reported enhanced TRUS staging results by including PSA value, tumor volume measurement, and Gleason grade [34, 35]. Since 2002, we have established standardized forms to report the extent of the disease on TRUS. Eisenberg analyzed the first 620 patients from 2002 to 2007 by comparing the clinical stage with radical prostatectomy pathological results [36]. This study showed that evidence of ECE by TRUS was associated with pathological stage as well as biochemical failure. TRUS showed an overall sensitivity of 31 %, specificity of 92 %, PPV of 58 %, and NPV of 80 %, with an area under receiver operating characteristic (ROC) curve of 0.77 for detecting ECE (Fig. 33).

TRUS alone was significantly more accurate in predicting ECE than commonly used nomograms or tables. It is important to remember that TRUS also carries the benefit of site specificity when compared to mathematical models, the former being of utmost importance to the surgeon trying to maintain specimen confined disease.

Ekici et al. compared the staging accuracy between TRUS and endorectal coil MRI in 25 patients undergoing radical prostatectomy [37]. MRI was more sensitive in detecting ECE and SVI, while TRUS was more accurate in detecting the site of the seminal vesicles. Overall, MRI was not significantly better than TRUS. Thus, they recommended TRUS for local staging for now. Jung et al. compared T2 weighted MRI to TRUS for staging accuracy by referencing radical prostatectomy results in 101 patients [38]. Both studies used the same criteria for ECE and SVI as described in this chapter. Area under ROC curve was 0.69–0.7 with MRI while it was 0.81 with TRUS, although no statistical significance was noted between the two methods (Fig. 34).

In summary, careful examination along with knowledge and experience in reading TRUS images for early signs of tumor spread should increase the accuracy of TRUS in staging.

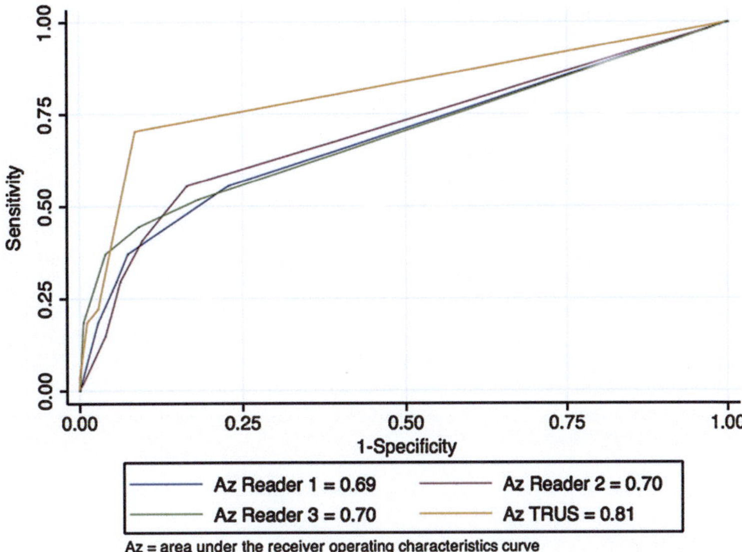

Fig. 34 ROC curve for MRI and TRUS for predicting ECE or SVI. TRUS has a larger area under the curve compared with MRI read by three different radiologists. (Figure cited from [38] with permission)

References

1. Cancer Facts & Figures. 2014; http://www.cancer.org/acs/groups/content/@research/documents/webcontent/acspc-042151.pdf. Accessed 4 July 2014.

2. SEER Stat Fact Sheets: Prostate cancer. 2014; http://seer.cancer.gov/statfacts/html/prost.html. Accessed 5 July 2014.

3. Hodge KK, McNeal JE, Terris MK, et al. Random systematic versus directed ultrasound guided transrectal core biopsies of the prostate. J Urol. 1989;142(1):71–4. discussion 74–5.

4. Stamey TA. Making the most out of six systematic sextant biopsies. Urology. 1995;45(1):2–12.

5. Freedland SJ, Amling CL, Terris MK, et al. Is there a difference in outcome after radical prostatectomy between patients with biopsy Gleason sums 4, 5, and 6? Results from the SEARCH database. Prostate Cancer Prostatic Dis. 2003;6(3):261–5.

6. Chang JJ, Shinohara K, Bhargava V, et al. Prospective evaluation of lateral biopsies of the peripheral zone for prostate cancer detection. J Urol. 1998;160(6 Pt 1):2111–4.

7. Freiha FS, McNeal JE, Stamey TA. Selection criteria for radical prostatectomy based on morphometric studies in prostate carcinoma. NCI Monogr. 1988;7:107–8.

8. Takashima R, Egawa S, Kuwao S, et al. Anterior distribution of Stage T1c nonpalpable tumors in radical prostatectomy specimens. Urology. 2002;59(5):692–7.

9. Meng MV, Franks JH, Presti Jr JC, et al. The utility of apical anterior horn biopsies in prostate cancer detection. Urol Oncol. 2003;21(5):361–5.

10. Franiel T, Stephan C, Erbersdobler A, et al. Areas suspicious for prostate cancer: MR-guided biopsy in patients with at least one transrectal US-guided biopsy with a negative finding–multiparametric MR imaging for detection and biopsy planning. Radiology. 2011;259(1):162–72.

11. Abd-Alazeez M, Ahmed HU, Arya M, et al. The accuracy of multiparametric MRI in men with negative biopsy and elevated PSA level-Can it rule out clinically significant prostate cancer? Urol Oncol. 2014;32(1):17–22.

12. Hambrock T, Somford DM, Hoeks C, et al. Magnetic resonance imaging guided prostate biopsy in men with repeat negative biopsies and increased prostate specific antigen. J Urol. 2010;183(2):520–7.

13. Chade DC, Shariat SF, Cronin AM, et al. Salvage radical prostatectomy for radiation-recurrent prostate cancer: a multi-institutional collaboration. Eur Urol. 2011;60(2):205–10.

14. Foster LS, Jajodia P, Fournier Jr G, et al. The value of prostate specific antigen and transrectal ultrasound guided biopsy in detecting prostatic fossa recurrences following radical prostatectomy. J Urol. 1993;149(5):1024–8.

15. Connolly JA, Shinohara K, Presti Jr JC, et al. Local recurrence after radical prostatectomy: characteristics in size, location, and relationship to prostate-specific antigen and surgical margins. Urology. 1996;47(2):225–31.

16. Shinohara K, Gulati M, Koppie TM, et al. Transperineal prostate biopsy after abdominoperineal resection. J Urol. 2003;169(1):141–4.

17. Rorvik J, Halvorsen OJ, Servoll E, et al. Transrectal ultrasonography to assess local extent of prostatic cancer before radical prostatectomy. Br J Urol. 1994;73(1):65–9.

18. Lorentzen T, Nerstrom H, Iversen P, et al. Local staging of prostate cancer with transrectal ultrasound: a literature review. Prostate Suppl. 1992;4:11–6.

19. Ebert T, Schmitz-Drager BJ, Burrig KF, et al. Accuracy of imaging modalities in staging the local extent of prostate cancer. Urol Clin North Am. 1991;18(3):453–7.
20. McSherry SA, Levy F, Schiebler ML, et al. Preoperative prediction of pathological tumor volume and stage in clinically localized prostate cancer: comparison of digital rectal examination, transrectal ultrasonography and magnetic resonance imaging. J Urol. 1991;146(1):85–9.
21. Scardino PT, Shinohara K, Wheeler TM, et al. Staging of prostate cancer. Value of ultrasonography. Urol Clin North Am. 1989;16(4):713–34.
22. Rosen MA, Goldstone L, Lapin S, et al. Frequency and location of extracapsular extension and positive surgical margins in radical prostatectomy specimens. J Urol. 1992;148(2 Pt 1):331–7.
23. Ohori M, Egawa S, Shinohara K, et al. Detection of microscopic extracapsular extension prior to radical prostatectomy for clinically localized prostate cancer. Br J Urol. 1994;74(1):72–9.
24. Spirnak JP, Resnick MI. Clinical staging of prostatic cancer: new modalities. Urol Clin North Am. 1984;11(2):221–35.
25. Griffiths GJ, Clements R, Jones DR, et al. The ultrasound appearances of prostatic cancer with histological correlation. Clin Radiol. 1987;38(3):219–27.
26. Salo JO, Kivisaari L, Rannikko S, et al. Computerized tomography and transrectal ultrasound in the assessment of local extension of prostatic cancer before radical retropubic prostatectomy. J Urol. 1987;137(3):435–8.
27. Pontes JE, Eisenkraft S, Watanabe H, et al. Preoperative evaluation of localized prostatic carcinoma by transrectal ultrasonography. J Urol. 1985;134(2):289–91.
28. Ohori M, Scardino PT, Lapin SL, et al. The mechanisms and prognostic significance of seminal vesicle involvement by prostate cancer. Am J Surg Pathol. 1993;17(12):1252–61.
29. Ohori M, Shinohara K, Wheeler TM, et al. Ultrasonic detection of non-palpable seminal vesicle invasion: a clinicopathological study. Br J Urol. 1993;72(5 Pt 2):799–808.
30. Perrapato SD, Carothers GG, Maatman TJ, et al. Comparing clinical staging plus transrectal ultrasound with surgical-pathologic staging of prostate cancer. Urology. 1989;33(2):103–5.
31. Andriole GL, Coplen DE, Mikkelsen DJ, et al. Sonographic and pathological staging of patients with clinically localized prostate cancer. J Urol. 1989;142(5):1259–61.
32. Rifkin MD, Zerhouni EA, Gatsonis CA, et al. Comparison of magnetic resonance imaging and ultrasonography in staging early prostate cancer. Results of a multi-institutional cooperative trial. N Engl J Med. 1990;323(10):621–6.
33. Hamper UM, Sheth S, Walsh PC, et al. Capsular transgression of prostatic carcinoma: evaluation with transrectal US with pathologic correlation. Radiology. 1991;178(3):791–5.
34. Wolf Jr JS, Shinohara K, Narayan P. Staging of prostate cancer. Accuracy of transrectal ultrasound enhanced by prostate-specific antigen. Br J Urol. 1992;70(5):534–41.
35. Gerber GS, Goldberg R, Chodak GW. Local staging of prostate cancer by tumor volume, prostate-specific antigen, and transrectal ultrasound. Urology. 1992;40(4):311–6.
36. Eisenberg ML, Cowan JE, Davies BJ, et al. The importance of tumor palpability and transrectal ultrasonographic appearance in the contemporary clinical staging of prostate cancer. Urol Oncol. 2011;29(2):171–6.
37. Ekici S, Ozen H, Agildere M, et al. A comparison of transrectal ultrasonography and endorectal magnetic resonance imaging in the local staging of prostatic carcinoma. BJU Int. 1999;83(7):796–800.
38. Jung AJ, Coakley FV, Shinohara K, et al. Local staging of prostate cancer: comparative accuracy of T2-weighted endorectal MR imaging and transrectal ultrasound. Clin Imaging. 2012;36(5):547–52.
39. Bates TS, Gillatt DA, Cavanagh PM, et al. A comparison of endorectal magnetic resonance imaging and transrectal ultrasonography in the local staging of prostate cancer with histopathological correlation. Br J Urol. 1997;79(6):927–32.
40. Presti Jr JC, Hricak H, Narayan PA, et al. Local staging of prostatic carcinoma: comparison of transrectal sonography and endorectal MR imaging. Am J Roentgenol. 1996;166(1):103–8.
41. Hardeman SW, Causey JQ, Hickey DP, et al. Transrectal ultrasound for staging prior to radical prostatectomy. Urology. 1989;34(4):175–80.

Index

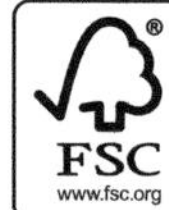